Behavioural Science in Medical Practice

Behavioural Sciences in Medical Practice

Second Edition

Manju Mehta MA DM & SP PhD
Professor of Clinical Psychology
Department of Psychiatry
All India Institute of Medical Sciences (AIIMS)
New Delhi, India

JAYPEE BROTHERS MEDICAL PUBLISHERS (P) LTD

New Delhi • Ahmedabad • Bengaluru • Chennai • Hyderabad • Kochi
Kolkata • Lucknow • Mumbai • Nagpur • St Louis (USA)

Published by
Jitendar P Vij
Jaypee Brothers Medical Publishers (P) Ltd

Corporate Office
4838/24 Ansari Road, Daryaganj, **New Delhi** - 110 002, India, +91-11-43574357 (30 lines)

Registered Office
B-3 EMCA House, 23/23B Ansari Road, Daryaganj, **New Delhi** 110 002, India
Phones: +91-11-23272143, +91-11-23272703, +91-11-23282021, +91-11-23245672,
Rel: +91-11-32558559 Fax: +91-11-23276490, +91-11-23245683
e-mail: jaypee@jaypeebrothers.com, Website: www.jaypeebrothers.com

Branches

- 2/B, Akruti Society, Jodhpur Gam Road Satellite
  Ahmedabad 380 015 Phones: +91-79-26926233, Rel: +91-79-32988717
  Fax: +91-79-26927094 e-mail: ahmedabad@jaypeebrothers.com
- 202 Batavia Chambers, 8 Kumara Krupa Road, Kumara Park East
  Bengaluru 560 001 Phones: +91-80-22285971, +91-80-22382956, +91-80-22372664
  Rel: +91-80-32714073, Fax: +91-80-22281761 e-mail: bangalore@jaypeebrothers.com
- 282 IIIrd Floor, Khaleel Shirazi Estate, Fountain Plaza, Pantheon Road
  Chennai 600 008 Phones: +91-44-28193265, +91-44-28194897,
  Rel: +91-44-32972089 Fax: +91-44-28193231 e-mail: chennai@jaypeebrothers.com
- 4-2-1067/1-3, 1st Floor, Balaji Building, Ramkote Cross Road
  Hyderabad 500 095 Phones: +91-40-66610020, +91-40-24758498, Rel:+91-40-32940929
  Fax:+91-40-24758499 e-mail: hyderabad@jaypeebrothers.com
- No. 41/3098, B & B1, Kuruvi Building, St. Vincent Road
  Kochi 682 018, Kerala Phones: +91-484-4036109, +91-484-2395739, +91-484-2395740
  e-mail: kochi@jaypeebrothers.com
- 1-A Indian Mirror Street, Wellington Square
  Kolkata 700 013 Phones: +91-33-22651926, +91-33-22276404, +91-33-22276415
  Rel: +91-33-32901926, Fax: +91-33-22656075, e-mail: kolkata@jaypeebrothers.com
- Lekhraj Market III, B-2, Sector-4, Faizabad Road, Indira Nagar
  Lucknow 226 016 Phones: +91-522-3040553, +91-522-3040554 e-mail: lucknow@jaypeebrothers.com
- 106 Amit Industrial Estate, 61 Dr SS Rao Road, Near MGM Hospital, Parel
  Mumbai 400012 Phones: +91-22-24124863, +91-22-24104532, Rel: +91-22-32926896
  Fax: +91-22-24160828 e-mail: mumbai@jaypeebrothers.com
- "KAMALPUSHPA" 38, Reshimbag, Opp. Mohota Science College, Umred Road
  Nagpur 440 009 (MS) Phone: Rel: +91-712-3245220, Fax: +91-712-2704275 e-mail: nagpur@jaypeebrothers.com

USA Office
1745, Pheasant Run Drive, Maryland Heights (Missouri), MO 63043, USA, Ph: 001-636-6279734
e-mail: jaypee@jaypeebrothers.com, anjulav@jaypeebrothers.com

Behavioural Sciences in Medical Practice

© 2009, Jaypee Brothers Medical Publishers

All rights reserved. No part of this publication should be reproduced, stored in a retrieval system, or transmitted in any form or by any means: electronic, mechanical, photocopying, recording, or otherwise, without the prior written permission of the author and the publisher.

This book has been published in good faith that the material provided by author is original. Every effort is made to ensure accuracy of material, but the publisher, printer and author will not be held responsible for any inadvertent error(s). In case of any dispute, all legal matters to be settled under Delhi jurisdiction only.

First Edition: **1998**
Second Edition: **2009**

ISBN 978-81-8448-629-2

Typeset at JPBMP typesetting unit
Printed at Sanat Printers, Kundli

To
My parents

To
My parents

Preface

Medical practice and medical education, at the end of twenty first century, are being driven by several factors. Behavioural Sciences can be considered as one of the most influential of these factors. There was a time when medicine was equated with the study of pathophysiology, diagnosis and treatment of diseases. We are now beginning to understand that the diseased individual is a part of the complex human ecosystem, with several levels of organisation ranging from the molecular to psychosocial and culture. Our recognition of the limitations of curative biomedicine has also opened up alternative strategies such as behavioural and cognitive therapies, which have enriched the field of medicine.

There has been a paradigm shift in the disease pattern of the society. While the age-old infectious diseases and poverty-related illnesses are still haunting us, there has been sudden upsurge in the lifestyle-related illnesses such as cardiovascular diseases, cancers, trauma and chronic degenerative disorders, which cannot be tackled by biomedical sciences alone. The trauma of a terminally-ill patient, the tale of an ill-fated HIV/AIDS positive individual or even a victim of stress in a fast moving society have their genesis in the behavioural aspects of medicine.

The need for introducing behavioural science components in the curriculum of undergraduate medical students has been keenly felt but hardly implemented. Many of the committees on medical education and other forums have strongly expressed the need for introducing behavioural sciences. A study conducted by the consortium of medical institutions, adopting inquiry-driven strategies for innovation in medical education has clearly revealed that the young graduates are deficient in communication and interpersonal skills, and humanistic aspects of medicine. Though the need for incorporating behavioural sciences has been keenly felt, the attempts to formulate a well-structured programme have been few and sporadic. This is mainly because of dearth of good textbooks and resource materials. The present book is an attempt to bridge this void.

The contents of this book have been divided in six parts. *The first part* is an introduction to the subject. The *second part* deals with basis of behaviour, which are core psychological processes that determine human behaviour. These processes like learning, memory, stress are not only relevant to medical practice, but an understanding of these processes can be of great importance to the students themselves. Many psychosocial problems are related to the developmental process; thus, the *third part* of the book is on development of behaviour from birth to death. A special emphasis is given to adolescence and oldage as these periods are concerned with new emerging specialities: adolescent psychiatry, medicine and geriatrics. A chapter has been devoted to enhance the skills of medical students to deal with difficult situations like dying patients, breaking news of death to the family members and to understand the bereavement process. *The fourth part* is primarily related to social issues important in patient care, these being the attitudes, family and compliance behaviour. Qualitative as well as quantitative research in any medical speciality often borrows methods and tools from behavioural sciences; hence *fifth part* deals with assessment methods and various psychological methods of management; the most important of these being counselling. A chapter on behavioural medicine has been included, as behavioural methods have been integrated in management of certain disorders. The *sixth part* deals with special applications of behavioural skills like communication skills, understanding illness behaviour and psychology of pain.

The overwhelming response to the first edition of this book has encouraged me to work for the second edition, which brings additions in some chapters. I hope these additions would be helpful for the students. Behavioural Sciences need human dimensions, thus an attempt has been made to explain the concepts and theories in simple manner. Real case studies with fictitious names have been given in the beginning of each chapter, and clinical applications are discussed to make the students comprehend, relate and use this information in their practical work. It was not feasible to include some other important aspects of health care like economics, ethics, etc. simply to keep the volume of information at a readable level. Again, not much emphasis has been given on latest research finding as the objective of this book is to help the students understand the relevance of behavioural sciences to medicine.

It is impossible to acknowledge all the sources of inspiration and information that I used while writing this book. But first of all, I must thank my patients, whom I have met over the last three decades; the experiences I have gained from them have helped me understand the clinical applications of behavioural sciences. I am also grateful to Professor NN Wig, former Regional Director, WHO, for stimulating my achievement motivation. I am greatly indebted to Mrs Roxana Samuel, Ms Renuka Dutta, Ms Anubha Dhal and my students for the help provided to me, with their valuable suggestions and the editing of this book.

Mrs Nani Gangadharan has painstakingly typed and retyped manuscript of this book, and she deserves my whole-hearted gratitude. I also appreciate the enthusiasm of Sameer and Aditi in making graphic illustrations on computer.

Last but not the least, this work would not have been possible without the patience, support and encouragement that I received from my husband, Dr Anil Mehta and other members of my family.

Manju Mehta

Contents

PART 1: Introduction
1. Behavioural Sciences 1

PART 2: Basis of Behaviour
2. Sensory Processes and Perception 7
3. Attention 19
4. Memory 24
5. Learning and Studying 35
6. Intelligence 48
7. Thinking 58
8. Motivation 67
9. Emotion 77
10. Stress and Coping 88
11. Personality 100

PART 3: Development of Behaviour
12. Development—Infancy to Adolescence 111
13. Adulthood to Ageing 124
14. Dealing with Death and Bereavement 132

PART 4: Social Behaviour
15. Attitudes 138
16. Family 146
17. Compliance with Health Care 155

PART 5: Assessment and Management

18. Assessment in Behavioural Sciences 161
19. Counselling 177
20. Behaviour Therapy 185
21. Cognitive Behaviour Therapy 196
22. Behaviour Medicine 206

PART 6: Applications of Behavioural Sciences to Health

23. Communication Skills 212
24. Illness Behaviour 222
25. Psychology of Pain 229

Bibliography *243*

Index *253*

PART 1: Introduction

Behavioural Sciences

While taking ward rounds you examine Mr R aged fifty-five years on bed no. 5, and Mr S aged forty-eight years on bed no. 6, both the patients have similar symptoms and have been diagnosed as carcinoma of lungs. From physical point of view you have knowledge of human anatomy, physiology, and learning of pharmacology helps you to prescribe medicines. Yet you find that both the patients are reacting to illness and responding to the medical treatment differently. How do you explain these differences? Mr S is restless, gets irritated easily, is always complaining of other staff working in the ward. On the other hand Mr R is accommodating and is grateful for whatsoever care is given to him. They are not only patients of bed no. 5 and bed no. 6, but are two human beings with their unique personalities, abilities to cope with stress and varied family responsibilities. These differences in behaviour are due to one's own personality and reactions to illness. It is not sufficient to have knowledge about the biological and organic aspects of the disease only, it is important to understand the person having the disease and his psychosocial background.

Definition

The branch of science, which can help you in understanding your patients as unique individuals, is known as Behavioural Sciences. This term has been used to denote the study of human behaviour both of the individual and of groups of people, small or large. It emphasises on individual behaviour and on the application of such basic knowledge to medical and allied disciplines.

Thus behavioural sciences have become part of the undergraduate medical education all over the world. Though this course is fairly well-established in many developed countries, it is included in some medical schools in India also. The Indian Medical Council has recommended its inclusion in all the undergraduate medical schools. Behavioural Sciences draws upon various disciplines and sciences related to the study of human behaviour like: psychology, sociology, anthropology, economics and statistics (Fig. 1.1). Psychology is the study of human individual behaviour. Sociology is more about social and group behaviours. Anthropology deals with culture and natural history of mankind of different races and their development. Economics has to do with the distribution of scarce resources within a society. The statistics helps in testing hypotheses and measurement. The treatment to all these branches cannot be given at par in this book more concentration is given on the understanding of the individual patient.

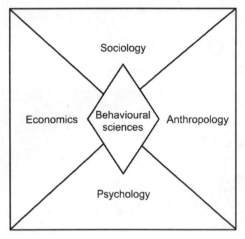

Fig. 1.1: Subject content in behavioural sciences

Need for Behavioural Sciences

The aim of this book is to help the students to develop an understanding of human behaviour, and its relationship with medical practice. The understanding of conceptual and methodological basis is required for subsequent clinical instructions. An understanding of human behaviour is desirable in most branches of clinical practice; it is especially important in medicine, psychiatry, community medicine, pediatrics and geriatrics. There are ample examples to illustrate the need for the disciplines of behavioural sciences (which mainly consists of psychology and sociology) to provide a systematic academic foundation in the preclinical period for these clinical subjects.

Developments in medical education have come about mainly as a response to scientific and technological advances made in the field of medicine. There is a growing danger that the student may become so preoccupied with the minutiae of the specialities and with the technologies of the laboratory that he loses sight of the patient as a "whole person", functioning in a social context. Moreover little attention is paid to changes in community patterns of disease or to changes in the social functions of medicine.

This has led some medical educators to search for a counter-balancing element to build into the medical curriculum. It seems that behavioural sciences can provide this element. They can have a significant effect on the outlook and attitudes of medical students, both through their subject matter (human behaviour and social processes) and through their central premise that the problems they deal with are susceptible to scientific investigation and explanation.

Behavioural Sciences can be of more direct medical relevance also. In medical practice the doctor's main concern is individual patient. Often one encounters differences in response to pain, illness, hospitalisation, and other stresses; the influence of personality and social class on illness. Patient's personalities and relationships may be important factors in the disease process and in medical care. A doctor also needs to communicate effectively with patients, their relatives, with colleagues-doctors, and nurses. He faces resistance to attitude and behaviour change in the context of preventive medicine—these are a few examples of everyday problems of medical care, which require the doctor to form judgement and make decisions based on an understanding of human behaviour and institutions. Biological training alone does not prepare a doctor to deal with such situations.

Furthermore, psychological knowledge can be valuable in developing the effectiveness of the student's and doctor's own cognitive processes. Clinical practice involves complex routines of observations, discrimination, and interpretation, acquiring and retaining factual information, of problem-solving and decision-making. There is an extensive body of psychological knowledge concerning these processes and the variables which influence them (e.g. the effects of fatigue, attitudes, and expectancy on accuracy of perception and recall); and it is believed that students can profit from awareness of these problems and of the principles underlying them.

Culture as Determinant of Health

Culture is shared learned behaviour that is transmitted from one generation to another for purposes of human adjustment, adaptation, and growth. Culture has both external and internal referents. External referents include roles and institutions. Internal referents include attitudes, values, beliefs, expectations, and consciousness.

Culture is something that mediates and shapes virtually all aspects of human behaviour. It is the way in which human beings define and experience reality. It includes their sense of morality and personhood. These dimensions of human behaviour are not inborn but rather are shaped by the socialisation process. An ethno cultural group's language and its religion, economic, political, and social systems are institutional reflections of culture and help to shape the internal referents as part of a reciprocal or interdependent system.

As children are reared, they are conditioned directly and indirectly to think, feel, and act in certain ways. These ways constitute their reality. Their language helps to shape reality and is also in turn shaped by it. Culture is a critical determinant of human behaviour, to the extent that culture varies, human behaviour must also vary. Compare the two adolescent males grown up in two different places like one in North India and the second in down South, you would find that their differences in the appearance, food, dress, and rituals also produce differences in the way they think and define reality. The individual is the representative product of biological, psychological, social and cultural determinants. Figure 1.2 presents this conceptualisation of human behaviour.

The illness behaviour is also influenced by the cultural determinants, e.g. in many cultures males are not likely to cry or express pain or suffering, during an illness. If you are not aware of these determinants, then probably your assessment of that patient's pain and suffering will be biased.

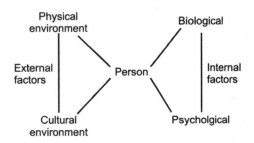

Fig. 1.2: Determinants of behaviour

Scope of Behavioural Sciences

Training in the behavioural sciences is essential for the appropriate education of physicians as major health problems of today can lead to premature death or disability. Cardiovascular disease, substance abuse, AIDS, cancer, and adolescent pregnancy are directly caused by risk-taking behaviour and can be prevented by people only by modifying their lifestyle and behaviour. Many diseases require major modifications of lifestyle to ensure benefits of therapy. The primary purpose of teaching behavioural science in medical schools is to prepare physicians to understand the role of social and psychological factors in the aetiology and course of disease. The knowledge can be applied to reduce the burden of disease by changing the patient's behaviour. Some other causes of illness stem from sociocultural forces, such as poverty, low socioeconomic status, and industrialisation. These factors are very common in developing countries, though they lie beyond the realm of the individual doctor-patient relationship; yet understanding these factors can help physicians plan appropriate medical services and preventive efforts.

The scope of behavioural sciences is envisaged in the following areas of medicine.

The Doctor-Patient Relationship

The clinical knowledge base now includes a large amount of research on doctor-patient relationships which has been demonstrated to be important to patient care outcomes. It includes information about the understanding of intimacy-relations of trust and power between doctors and patients, and how interpersonal influence works in doctor-patient transactions.

Effective interviewing techniques are among the most essential skills that all physicians need to learn. Many studies have demonstrated that physicians who fail to obtain accurate information may misdiagnoses or recommend inappropriate therapies. Examples of successful outcomes due to skillful inquiry provide useful stimulus for students to learn behavioural sciences.

Social Class and Health Behaviour

Social class is broadly associated with almost every indicator of morbidity, disability and mortality. Factors associated with lower social class increase susceptibility to illness and injury. Understanding specific risks and vulnerabilities associated with social status provides physicians opportunities for more effective communication and therapy, and for preventive initiatives.

Several investigators have demonstrated that disadvantaged social environments increase the risk of serious health problems especially in children and adolescents. One of the examples is the low birth weight child when reared in disadvantaged environment, has an increased prevalence of acute and chronic illness for as long as eleven years after birth.

Physicians often underestimate the extent to which the patients of lower socioeconomic status desire information. Such patients are often less expressive and less questioning than the better educated patients and physicians commonly give them less treatment relevant information.

Human Development: Life Cycle, Health and Illness

Physicians need to understand how life experiences at one stage of development influence later behaviour, susceptibility to illness, and use of medical services. Previous life experiences also modify physiologic and immunologic responses. Longitudinal studies of life span in humans have illuminated the cause-and effect relationships of early nutrition to later heart disease and the effect of early life stress on later immunologic response.

Psychophysical Relations

This is one of the most rapidly advancing fields is in the mind-body relationship. Parents with a child who is dying from leukaemia have markedly different cortisol and T-lymphocyte responses, depending on whether they can grieve openly or not. Those who cannot grieve have greater elevation of cortisol and more illness in the year after the death of a child than those who can.

Data from primate laboratories have demonstrated that about twenty per cent of monkeys are shy and withdrawn from birth, and if left on their own, grow up to have low status in the group. These studies not only demonstrate the biological basis of such behaviour but the possibilities of modification by early experience.

Children who are taught self-imaging (i.e. self-hypnosis) respond with greater secretory IgA in their pharynges than those who are not, and self-imaging has been shown to be as effective in treatment of migraine headaches in children as standard pharmacologic treatments.

There are marked individual differences in cortisol and neuroimmunologic response to stress from early life. Physicians need to recognise the mind-body relationship, which has been extensively documented. Physical disease cause behavioural changes. Psychological stresses cause physical changes.

Health and Illness Behaviour

Differences in behaviour account for much of the variation in the health of different populations. These include not only personal health behaviours such as smoking, diet, substance abuse and exercise but also exposure to environmental risks and interpersonal, work-related and community-related stresses. Risks to health are often inadvertent consequences of personal choices and routine activities. Understanding these risks and developing strategic approaches for intervention enhance physician's opportunities to assist their patients in leading healthier lives controlling many extremely serious risks to health and to life itself such as HIV infection depends exclusively on successful modification behaviour and exposure to risk.

The Impact of Social Support

Many studies show that the presence of social support, the quality of social networks, and the degree of participation in them have substantial effects on coping health status, and longevity.

The Importance of Self Efficacy

A large literature now attests to the importance of self efficacy in supporting social adaptation and health. The deterioration of frail elderly persons who move to new environments is often linked to their sense of loss of control. Haggerty et al (1993) have quoted experiments carried out in nursing homes, which show that increasing the elderly person's sense of control results in enhancement of health. Similar finding have been reported on patients with chronic pain, that experience of pain is less in patients who think controlling power is with the person himself (see Chapter 25). While there is still much to be learned, several areas of research converge in demonstrating the importance of a person's sense of control over his or her immediate environment.

The Hole of Self-Attention on Symptom Amplification

Numerous lines of investigation show how focussed attention on physical states amplify the intensity of experience and concern about health status (see Chapter 3). Understanding of this work has relevance for pain management and for understanding symptom prevention and response.

The Illness-Disability Perception

Disability caused by the illness depends on a range of factors that intervene between the occurrence of illness and disability. These factors include personal variables such as attitudes and motivation; aspects of the social context, such as opportunities for participation, stigma, and physical accessibility; and the health workers' management of the initial condition over its longitudinal course. The understanding of these factors is crucial in the appropriate care of persons with physical impairments, the elderly, and individuals with chronic disease.

Adult Sexuality, Loss, Grief, Mourning, Aging, and Death These issues are concerned primarily with the interaction of psychologic and sociologic aspects of individual behaviour and need few specific examples to demonstrate their importance. Behavioural science seeks to understand the social organisation of the communities in which patients live, the institutions involved in the provision of medical care, and their influence on health.

Selye described the general adaptation syndrome and developed the general concept of stress and the neuroendocrine mechanisms involved, particularly the role of catecholamines and the steroids. Since that time, steady progress has been made toward working out step-by-step the biological mechanisms involved, whereby stress can lead to cardiovascular changes that cause heart attacks and stroke or have profound effects on the immune system for example, we still have a long way to go in learning the details of these mechanisms, but we know enough already to begin to see how behaviours such as smoking and high fat/high calorie diets, for example, affect these same mechanisms and exacerbate them and how exercise can ameliorate them. We also know that behavioural change leading to prenatal care, good nutrition, and immunisation will make the difference in improving our infant mortality rates. Furthermore, violence, teenage high-risk behaviours, and suicide are major cause of mortality and morbidity. Finally, we know that adherence to medication, especially in the adult and the elderly, remains a major problem in managing chronic diseases.

With chronic diseases such a major portion of modern medicine and so dependent on lifestyles, behaviour modification and coping strategies, health-promoting and disease-preventing behaviours become of great importance in the practice of medicine not only for their value in cost containment but also for the general welfare of our society.

SUMMARY

Behavioural sciences is the branch of science which can help you in understanding your patients as unique individuals. This term has been used to denote the study of human behaviour both of the individual and of groups of people, small or large. It emphasises on individual behaviour and on the application of such basic knowledge to medical and allied disciplines. Behavioural sciences draws upon various disciplines and sciences related to the study of human behaviour like psychology, sociology, anthropology, economics, and statistics.

An understanding of human behaviour is desirable in most branches of clinical practice, especially in medicine, psychiatry, community medicine, paediatrics and geriatrics. Behavioural sciences are of direct medical relevance, as in medical practice the doctor's main concern is individual patient. To understand variations in response to pain, illness, hospitalisation, and other stresses; the influence of personality and social class on illness, knowledge of normal range of behaviour should be known. Patients personalities and relationships may be important factors in the disease process and in medical care. A doctor also needs to develop communication skills to deal effectively with patients, their relatives, with colleagues-doctors, and nurses.

Psychological knowledge can be valuable in developing the effectiveness of the one's own cognitive processes. Clinical practice involves complex routines of observations, discrimination, and interpretation, acquiring and retaining factual information, of problem-solving and decision-making.

Culture shapes not only the normal behaviour but it also influences illness behaviour. Thus the patient's behaviour and his symptoms should be understood in their cultural context.

Thus the scope of behavioural sciences ranges from doctor-patient relationship to various aspects of health care such as, social class and health behaviour, developmental life cycle, psychophysical relations, social support, self efficacy, aging and bereavement.

PART 2: Basis of Behaviour

Sensory Processes and Perception

Ranjeet, a young man comes to you with severe anxiety, Ranjeet is a music teacher in a private school, he is blind due to congenital defect, and he is married but does not have children. His wife has normal vision, but she is not educated. The anxiety was precipitated after a neighbour suddenly passed away following cardiac arrest. The incident has caused concern and fear in Ranjeet's mind that being blind, how can he handle such a situation if the need be. Any sensory defect can have negative psychological impact on the individual's personality and adjustment.

We live in a world of objects and peoples—a world that constantly bombards our senses with stimuli, bringing us information and presenting us with decisions, first on how we'll perceive these stimuli and then on how we'll behave in response. The sensory organs—vision, hearing, smell, touch and taste are highly complex systems and they do not make a straightforward response to each stimulus encountered. The knowledge comes to each one of us through our senses. We know about the world around us from what we learn directly about it, using our bodily sensations. We can understand the external world only from what our senses can detect of it. Therefore, sensation becomes the primary source of all human knowledge. In human being unlike simple organism, sensation is only a small part of much more complicated information processing systems.

Let us define some terms here. A stimulus is any form of energy to which we can respond (light waves, sound waves, and pressure on the skin). A sense is a particular physiological pathway for responding to a specific kind of energy. Sensation is the feeling we have in response to information that comes in through our sensory organs. Perception is the way our brain organises these feelings to make sense out of them. This involves recognition of objects that comes from a combination of sensations and the memory of previous sensory experiences.

SENSATION

Sensations contain both a 'quantity' element (size, hardness, coldness), and a 'quality' element (attractive, bad or dangerous). For example if you get burnt from a hot pressure cooker, you may think of all pressure cookers as being dangerous equipment. The physical property of heat may therefore, take on the psychological property of dangerousness. Thus the physical and physiological events are collectively called 'sensation'. That is the way in which the body responds to energy impinging upon it from the environment.

PERCEPTION

Sensation refers to the process of receiving information, whereas to perceive means to interpret and understand. Perceiving is not seeing, believing. Perception refers to what is immediately experienced by a person. Sensory events are translated into patterns of activity in the sensory channels and the central nervous system. Some of what we perceive is very closely linked to these activity patterns. Perception is the process of knowing the world outside you, by forming some mental representation. Perception is a complex process, extending far beyond the mere registering of light, sound, and other impulses from the external world. This external information must be internally coded and transformed before anyone can know what is really out there. Often your beliefs and expectations about some external stimulus prove to be more important in determining your behaviour than the physical characteristics of that external object. Perception is like solving a complicated puzzle. You must take bits and pieces of information that are present in the external world and fit them together somehow to form a comprehensive internal picture.

It may at first appear that every object in the external world makes direct contact with the brain via the sense organs: the eyes, ears, skin, and so on. But this view of perception is much too simple. There is no direct one-to-one relationship between the image formed by your eye and your perception of that image. The situation is indeed even more complex, since many physical arrangements in the external world can produce exactly the same image upon the eye. For example, it follows from elementary principles of geometry that a small triangle near you will produce the same image in the eye as that of a large triangle further away. Since any single external cue is likely to prove insufficient to narrow down the possibilities about the external world, we are forced to rely upon various combinations of cues. Although each cue by itself may be unreliable, if we consider enough cues together, we can often come up with an accurate mental picture of the external situation.

However, for much of what we perceive, the sensory patterns merely provide the 'raw data' for experience. The sensory information is transformed elaborated and combined with memories to create what we actually experience or perceive.

Perceptual Processes

We do not perceive world as loud sounds, bright lights or patches of colours. We perceive the world around us as objects like, book, glass, and plants. We hear doorbell, footsteps and songs. That means the sensory inputs at the focus of our attention have form and meaning. Perceptual processes which provide meaning to what we see or hear are classified as—form, visual depth, constancy, movement perception, plasticity and individual differences. We shall very briefly examine these processes.

Form Perception

The sensory inputs we receive come into our awareness as shapes, pattern and form. The basic element needed for visual form perception is the presence of contour. A contour is an area within the visual array where there is an abrupt change in luminance. The normal optic array is filled with contour information and an area completely enclosed by a contour is usually seen as distinct and separate form.

Another fundamental process in form perception is the recognition of a figure on a ground. We see objects as standing against a background. The words on this book are figures against the background of the page. We must be able to differentiate between the figure and these backgrounds, from which they are emerging. But in a reversible figure ground stimulus; perception of figures is a psychological act of interpretations and not necessarily, directly predictable from the stimulus array. Reversible figure ground relationship illustrates the multistability of perceptual organisation, i.e. some stimulus inputs can be organised differently in perception.

Organisation in perception partially explains our perception of complex patterns as unitary forms or objects. We see objects as objects only because grouping process operate in perception. Some laws of organisation are:
1. *Law of proximity*—items close together in space or time tend to be perceived as belonging together.
2. *Similarity*—similar objects tend to be grouped together.
3. *Symmetry*—there is a tendency to organise things to make a balanced or symmetrical figure that includes all the parts.
4. *Continuation*—there is a tendency to perceive a time that starts in one way as continuing in the same way.
5. *Common fate*—elements, which are perceived as moving together from an organised group.
6. *Law of closure*—refers to perceptual process sees, which organize the perceived world by filling gaps in stimulation.

Depth Perception

Artists, philosophers, and psychologists have long been challenged by the everyday fact of 3D seeing. The problem is set by the very structure of eye, which forms an optical image on a 2-dimensional surface, the retina. We make use of information, or cues in the sensory input to generate the 3D perception. The depth cues, were first studied by artist Leonardo da Vinci (1452-1519) to keep artists portray depth and distance on a flat canvas. We use monocular and binocular cues to create such effect.

Monocular cues: These operate when only one eye is looking. The artist to give us depth experience from a flat painting generally uses these. The depth perception is created by-Linear perspective (the distances operating the images), clearness, interposition (one object obstructs view of another), shadows, gradients of texture (change without abrupt transition) and movement.

Binocular cues: Many of the cues for depth perception require only one eye. Individuals with vision in one eye have adequate depth perception in most conditions. When we observe with two-eye vision, at the world we add binocular cues to the depth perception to the monocular cues. As the two eyes receive slightly different view of the world thereby producing binocular cues.

Nonvisual cues of depth and distance: There are two possible cues to the perception of depth namely convergence and accommodation. The conception was that subject adjusted this accommodation and convergence until he had a sharp and single image of the object.

Visual Pattern Perception

When we consider all the processes that underlie the recognition of complex, everyday pattern, we find they can be classified in two ways:
1. Data-driven processing—begins with the arrival of sensory information reaching the receptors (data). This input is said to drive a series of analyses, beginning with registration of luminance differences in image, colours, lines, angles, etc. This analysis proceeds from retina up through various levels of visual pathways, until it reaches higher centres of brain.
2. The other type is called "conceptually-driven processing—it uses higher level conceptual processes including memories of past experiences; general organisational strategies; knowledge of world and expectations based upon surrounding context or situation. Both

type of analyses can be occurring simultaneously, or they may occur one after the others.

Constancy of perception: Our perceptual experiences are not isolated; they build a world of identifiable things. This world as we perceive is a stable world. An object that has been constituted perceptually as a permanent and stable thing is perceived as such regardless of the illumination on it; the position from which it is viewed; or the distance at which it appears. This stability of environment as we experience is termed as 'perceptual constancy'.

Size constancy refers to the fact that as an object is moved further away we, tend to correct it for distance and still see it as more or less normal in size, when we, see an object at a distance, we might judge its size in one of the 3 ways:
1. *Perspective size:* According to the geometry of perspective, i.e. size inversely proportional to distance. This size would correspond to size of image on retina.
2. *Object size:* If object constancy is perfect we might judge an object by its known size.
3. *Compromise between perspective size and object size:* It might compromise and see the objects smaller at a distance, but not as much smaller as geometry of perspective indicates.

Size constancy develops largely as the result of experience. Similarly, the tendency to see an object, as of standard shape regardless of the viewing angle is shape constancy. The tendency to see an object as of normal colour regardless of light and shadow is called 'colour constancy' and brightness respectively, finally, the fact that objects retain their same positions, even as we move about is known as 'location constancy'. Although the word constancy is an exaggeration, but it dramatises our relatively stable perception of objects.

Movement Perception

When we perceive movement, we sense action in space taking place over time. We usually explain the perception of movement according to the stimulation of successive parts of sensory surface. Adaptive behaviour requires that we perceive movement accurately; otherwise one would land up in the hospital following an accident. Perceived motion also occurs without any energy movement across the receptor surface or without a successive pattern of stimulation, and is called apparent motion. In contrast to this there is real motion, the perception of the actual physical movement of the objects.

Apparent motion It is movement perceived in the absence of physical movement of an image across the retina. This is caused by the following factors:
a. *Autokinetic effect*—if we stare at a single spot of light in a completely dark room, after a few seconds light will appear to move in an erratic manner. This apparent movement of stationary light is called Autokinetic effect.
b. *Stroboscopic motion*—This illusion of motion is created, when separated stimuli, not in motion are presented in succession. This motion is used in making of cartoon films. Each frame of a film is slightly different from the preceding one, but when frames are presented rapidly enough, the picture blends into a smooth motion. A simple form of stroboscopic motion is called "Phi-Phenomenon", according to this, in a dark room if these are four lights and one of these four lights blinks on and off, followed shortly by another, there is an illusion of a single light moving from first position to the second. When all four lights flash on and off in a rapid sequence, it appears that single light is travelling in a circle, but the perceived size of the circle is smaller; than would be the case if lights were actually rotating.

Real motion: The perception of real motion depends upon relations between objects within the visual field. Whenever there is movement, the brain has to decide what is moving and what is stationary with respect to some frame of reference. We generally tend to assume that large objects are stationary and, smaller objects are moving. "Induced movement" is experienced when we look at the moon through a thin cover of moving clouds. In a clear sky, the moon appears to be stationary. When framed by moving clouds the moon will appear to race across the sky, while clouds appear stationary.

Plasticity: Visual deprivation or plasticity is restriction of the visual output. This is generally caused during the development stage in early infancy. Individuals born with congenital cataract face this type of problem.

Individual differences: Individuals differ in the ways they process sensory inputs to give rise to what they experience. Two individuals watching sunset in the western coast beach may have very different perceptions of the sunset. One may report it was breath taking or pure magic, whereas the other may report a red circle gradually descending. These differences in the perception are the result of the following factors.

Perceptual learning: Eleanor Gibson (1969) has defined perceptual learning as "increase in the ability to extract information from the environment as a result of experience or practice with the stimulation coming from it". This learning influences behaviours and experiences; and also determines the focus of attention. There are many examples to show that learning can mould perception. The one common example that we commonly encounter is the competence of individuals trained in various professions, as compared to untrained individuals. Skills in any variety are result of perceptual learning, which is achieved only through practice. Another very relevant example of perceptual learning is that blind persons learn to extract information from the environment, which generally the sighted people can not do, e.g. very sensitive discrimination of auditory sounds.

Related with learning one often wonders whether the perception is inborn or is influenced by the environmental factor. Those who advocate nature's role, say that brain organisation is determined by genetic codes and is so innate. The perception that depends upon this organisation is thus also innate. They say that sensory deprivation or special sensory experience during critical period results in a loss of brain connections that were genetically determined, because they needed environmental input, or nurture, for their maintenance. On the other hand, supporters of environment, argue that while genetic codes may provide a rough blueprint nurture interacts with the genetic outline during critical periods to direct growth and cause the proper brain connections to be made, so according to them alterations in the environment during critical period actually change the way the brain grows and the connections are made.

Perceptual set: We frequently perceive an event or object because we were mentally prepared for a particular object or event to arise. Set refers to the idea that we are ready to receive certain kinds of sensory input. Such set or expectancies vary from individual-to-individual. Imagine the time when you were expecting your result for admission to a medical college, you will be able to recollect that you were able to spot the result in the newspaper in no time whereas your friends who were not expecting did not even look at this news. Perceptual sets are related to the actual physical environment of the stimulus itself or to the internal factors, such as emotion or motivation.

Motives and needs: Several experiments have been conducted to study the effect of need and motive on perception. We attend to and organise sensory inputs in ways that match our needs. When you are hungry or thirsty, you are likely to pay more attention to places that would satisfy your need.

Illusions: Visual illusions are a dramatic example of how perceptual cues can be assembled incorrectly. Many illusions do not support the traditional view of perception that we infer from what we see. An illusion is any figure that gives rise to a bizarre interpretation of reality. The illusions demonstrate that what we perceive often depends on processes that go far beyond the 'raw data' of sensory input. Illusions show that perception results from transformation, elaboration and combination of sensory inputs. Specific instances in which the apparent curvature or length of a perceived line are not predictable from the curvature or length of its stimulus pattern, have been called the "Geometrical illusions". But this does not mean that they occur only with regular lines and patterns; they can also be demonstrated with quite irregular drawings and with real objects in normal environment. The illusions are important because they may provide clues for our understanding of processes of shape perception.

We shall examine some illusions that have a direct basis in our perception of ordinary objects and scenes. In these cases it may be that our senses have become so used to interpreting a particular stimulus in a given way that they cannot readily be dispensed with the 'stereo type'. The famous Muller-Lyer illusion (Fig. 2.1) shows that people usually perceive the vertical lines of different lengths. In reality both the vertical lines

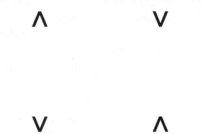

Fig. 2.2: Measure the space between the two sets of arrowheads at their point

are equal in length. This illusion arises because of the architectural perspective implied in these two arrangements of lines.

However, Figure 2.2 shows, even when the vertical lines are removed from the figure the illusion still persists; the inward pointing arrowheads still seem to be further separated at the point than are those in the outward pointing version. The reason for this illusion is that even in normal circumstances we do not utilise all the available information when we perceive objects.

Same illusion is evoked even when arrows are replaced by circles (Fig. 2.3). In this presence of the circles now generate the illusion of one line being longer than the other.

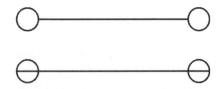

Fig. 2.3: Which of the straight lines is longer

Lines that converge suggest an appearance of distance. The common example of this is a stretch of long road or railroad tracks that remain parallel and equally wide as they disappear into the distance (Fig. 2.4). The Ponzo illusion also occurs due to the converging lines suggest depth (Fig. 2.5).

Illusions make clear that the context in which a given stimulus appears will determine how it

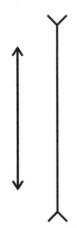

Fig. 2.1: Which of the lines is longer? The Muller-Lyer illusion

Sensory Processes and Perception

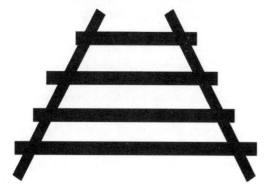

Fig. 2.4: Converging railroad

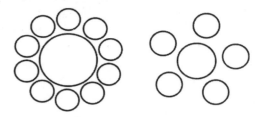

Fig. 2.6: Perceive these circles. The context of the circles that surround the centre circles influences our perception

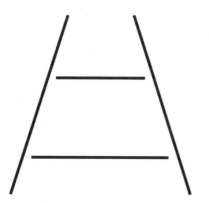

Fig. 2.5: Ponzo illusion

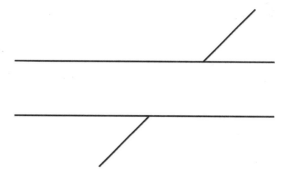

Fig. 2.7: The Poggendorf illusion

is perceived. Figure 2.6 demonstrates the importance of context in determining perception that we cannot ignore. In spite of our knowing that we do not perceive accurately, still we are unable to prevent the false interpretation arising out of these figures. These illusions show that our perception is independent of our conscious will. Information reaching us in normal circumstances may frequently contain inaccuracies imposed by these unconscious processes even though we are unaware of it happening.

At times the illusions can have serious effects. The Poggendorf Illusion can cause serious tragedy like, crashing aeroplanes, or misguiding the surgeons while operating. This is the simple illusion, which occurs when there are two parallel lines and a third line intersects them (Fig. 2.7). As you can see that the diagonal lines do not appear to intersect, though in reality they are extensions of the same line. The Poggendorf illusion can be explained by a combination of physical and cognitive factors. These factors are called structural effects and processing strategies. The structural effect depends upon the biological and optical construction of the eye. The processing strategy depends upon the cognitive decisions that are shaped by learning, experience and motivation.

Perception as Developmental Process

Is perception a developmental process? Like any other psychological processes, perception is also different in children as compared to the adults.

Moreover, throughout the life span of an individual some changes occur in the perceptual processes. Basic perceptual functions in children may continue to mature during first year due to the actual normal functioning of the visual system. At behavioural level, we can find some responses in newborns to the direction, distance or movement of stimuli. Infants are capable of directing their age movements toward targets. Neonates tend to make convergent and divergent eye movements. Even repetitive eye movement sequence in the presence of a moving pattern called optikinetic nystagmus, is seen. But visual acuity of neonates is quite poor. Infants can discriminate between patterns. Fontz (1963) found that infants younger than one month, reported a looking preference for stimuli containing facial features; but could not differentiate between normal and a scrambled face. This suggests they are discriminating patterns on basis of simple elements rather than on the basis of total stimulus organisation. However, by 4 months, there is definite preference for unscrambled face; indicating they can identify human face. Process of habituation can be seen from the very first days of life. So, the newborn child does have a reasonable set of perceptual capacities, quite soon after the birth.

One of the most informative ways to monitor changes in perceptual discrimination, recognition and information processing is to observe the way in which child selects information from external stimuli. By monitoring eye movement patterns in children we can determine the manner in which they are viewing and hence constructing. As child becomes older there is gradual movement toward a consideration of more global aspects of a pattern and its elements. Older children are more efficient at extracting details. But there is one form of pattern discrimination error, which is characteristic of young children. This involves mirror reversals (common around 3 year and gradually decrease, until child is about 10 or 11 years). Letter reversals, in children suggest that a child is relatively insensitive to orientation of a stimulus.

Perceptual change in adults involve basic sensory function especially like dark adaptation which tend to diminish with age, response to more complex visual problems becomes better, or more accurate with age.

As we grow older, there seems to be gradual decrease in efficiency of sensory structures. This is, however accompanied by gradual improvement in our abilities to perform complex, perceptual integrations and discriminations.

Extrasensory Perception (ESP)

You would have heard that some persons have reported correctly about their previous birth, or can predict about some event which is about to occur in very near future, like some accident is to take place or such a person sitting 500 kms would be doing a particular task. These extraordinary types of perceptions require no sense organ stimulation whatsoever. Though, ESP is a controversial issue, yet some research has been carried out even in India. ESP stimulates also called as parapsychological phenomenon is of two main kinds—
1. ESP
   a. Telepathy or thought transference from one person to another.
   b. Clairvoyance or, perception of objects or events not influencing the senses (e.g. telling the details of the contents sealed in an envelope.
2. Psychokinesis (PK) or mentally manipulating objects without touching them.

There is skepticism about ESP, one of the chief reasons being that no method has been formed for reliably demonstrating the phenomena. Also, the results do not vary systematically with the introduction of different experimental manipulation. But still, it is desirable to keep an open mind about issues that permit empirical demonstration, as some ESP phenomena do.

Social Perception

We meet someone for the first time and talk with or observe him or her for a few minutes. Even in this short space of time we make judgements about a number of characteristics. Social perception is concerned with our interpretation of behaviour in social settings and generally refers to how we perceive others, favourably or unfavourably. Social perception is of great relevance to medical profession. How the patient perceives the physician determines his trust for physician's healing power. Similarly physician's perception of the patient, his illness, agony and pain influences physician's involvement and efficacy of treatment. In the present era of consumer protection social perception of both the physician and the patient has gained even more importance. We form opinion of other persons by means of initial impression formed, the reasons for prejudice and discrimination, and also the development of liking and relationships with specific individuals through interpersonal attraction.

Attribution

As we do not have access to the personal thoughts, motives, or feelings of others, we make inferences about the traits based on the behaviour we observe. If we infer that something about the person is primarily responsible for the behaviour our inference is called "dispositional attribution." But if we include that some external force is, primarily responsible for the behaviour, it is called "situational attribution".

Basic tendency to ascribe causes to events is believed to be an inherent part of how people process information in both their social and physical world. A particular behaviour is considered to be caused by environmental forces plus personal forces, which is further divided into motivation and ability. Motivation involves both an intention to do something and an exertion of efforts to accomplish it. There is also relation between personal force of ability and environmental forces such as task difficulty. Together, these qualities form the perception of 'can' if the personal force of ability outweighs environmental force, then individual can do action.

Behaviour is seen as involving choices and intended effects on the part of the individual. A perceiver is said to take into account not only what other person does but also what the person might have done. What a person does is a chosen action. Some of the effects of chosen and unchosen actions are same, but other effects are uncommon to both chosen or unchosen actions. It is these uncommon effects, which yield clues regarding the intentions of another person. A perceiver gains most of the information about personal characteristics of another person, from a small number of uncommon effects, which have low valance.

According to Kelley (1967) the observers evaluate the motives for the behaviour of others using a number of criteria. Observers use this information to form a casual schema with which they make sense of things happening around them.

Attribution theory and social cognition has been applied in a number of different settings. Of our relevance is cognitive theory of depression by Beck (see Chapter 21). This theory describes the faulty inferences people make when in a depressed state. These depressed persons blame themselves when something goes wrong, think others have interfered and nothing can be good for them even in the future.

Self-perception: We use, much the same processes for self-attribution, as that for other attribution. When we want to make attributions about our own behaviour, we become observers of that behaviour and make attributions much as if we were observing someone else. Therefore, with our behaviour we would first determine whether the environment, has caused the behaviour through some strong external force. If this does not seem likely, we then, assume, the behaviour occurred because of some internal motives or personality traits. Internal states are inferred by ruling out external forces.

Errors in attribution: We underestimate the situational causes of behaviour, jumping to conclusions about dispositions of person. This bias toward disposition rather than situational attributions is called fundamental attribution error. Due to the expectation people tend to see, what they want to see and hear what they want to, our motives and emotions may also lead us to expect to perceive certain things. Projective tests, capitalise on these influences of motivation and emotion on perception. Perhaps, the greatest influence of motivation on perception is to be found in perception of such complex events as social and interpersonal relationships. This is so, because social situations are often indefinite and ambiguous. Our perception of them are less, definite and stable than our perceptions of physical objects. Expectancy or set, refers to the idea that we may be 'ready' and 'prepared for' certain kind of sensory input. Expectancy has much to do with selection of what we perceive or attend to. It also has a large role to play in the way, we perceive ambiguous situations.

Clinical Applications

Sensory Defects

When sensory apparatus is damaged or partially destroyed the impairment of perception may not be an accurate reflection of sensory damage. In Hemianopia, for example destruction in visual cortex of brain can render one half of visual receptor apparatus inactive, so that patient's visual field is cut in half vertically. Surprisingly patient may not report this as a handicap to his everyday activities, as he has been able to readjust or compensate for it. Gestalt psychologists investigated such patients to demonstrate their principle of closure in perception. A circle presented to such a patient, so that it overlapped the functioning and blind areas was reported as a complete circle. As in other situation where, closure operates hemianopic perceived the whole figure when the amount presented was sufficient to determine the nature of whole. Similar closure effects have been seen in patients suffering from deafness; affecting only certain sound frequencies, and in patients with disorder of tactile sensations.

A more elaborate instance of this tendency to closure after defect occurs in phenomenon known as "phantom limbs". Following amputation the patient may continue to experience realistic sensations in missing limb for sometime even for years. This odd phenomenon is related to the "perception of bodily self" or bodily image derived from sensations in muscles, tendons, joints and balancing mechanism, as well as from vision, hearing, taste, touch and smell.

Perceptual Function

Perceptual functions have been tested which basically are based on Gestalt principles. The Ishihara test for colour blindness is one of the examples, the subject is shown the series of cards, and each contains a mosaic made up of hundreds of little dots of different colours. Embedded in mosaic might be a numeral, which can be presented on the basis of the principle of similarity. A normal person will use colour, as basis of similarity but colour blind, will use brightness as basis of similarity.

Pain Perception

Melzack and Wall (1965) have proposed a "Gate control" theory of pain, which takes into account psychological variables as well as sensory inputs (see Chapter 25). Perception of intensity of pain, tolerance and its impact on the global functioning of the individual is dependent on perception of pain.

Hallucinations

Hallucinations are defined as percepts, which occur without an external stimulus. They can occur, in any of the senses and have all characters of normal perception, yet there is nothing in environment, which stimulate the sense receptors to produce experience. It is different from illusion, as in an illusion some of the sensory features of stimulus are identified but recognition of whole is incorrect. Hallucinations occur in patients with psychotic disorders especially chronic schizophrenics and in patients having organic psychosis. They can be classified in terms of particular sense through which they are apparently experienced, visual, auditory or tactile.

Sensory Deprivation

Sensory deprivation can lead to considerable psychological disturbance. Such disturbances are also known to occur in patients admitted for a very long duration in the hospital especially those patients confined for long periods or indefinitely in respirators, those restricted by attachment to various pieces of recording equipment and life-support systems in intensive care units, and those deprived of sight for a period after eye surgery. Even more generally, we may note that the manifestations of impairment of consciousness in delirious states are commonly at night, which may in part be due to the lower level of sensory and perceptual stimulation at that time. The active modification of the sensory input is required in certain clinical situations.

SUMMARY

The sensory organs—vision, hearing, smell, touch and taste are highly complex systems and they do not make a straightforward response to each stimulus encountered. The knowledge comes to each one of us through our senses. Sensation is the primary source of all human knowledge. In human being unlike simple organism, sensation is only a small part of much more complicated information processing systems.

A stimulus is any form of energy to which we can respond (pressure on the skin), a sense is a particular physiological pathway for responding to a specific kind of energy. Sensation is the feeling we have in response to information that comes in through our sensory organs. Perception is the way our brain organises these feelings to make sense out of them. This involves recognition of objects that comes from a combination of sensations and the memory of previous sensory experiences. Sensation contains both qualitative as well as quantitative element, and both physical and physiological events are collectively called 'sensation'. Sensation refers to the process of receiving information, whereas to perceive means to interpret and understand. Perception is the process of knowing the world outside you, by forming some mental representation. Perception is a complex process, extending far beyond the mere registering of light, sound, and other impulses from the external world. This external information must be internally coded and transformed before anyone can know what is really out there.

Since any single external cue is likely to prove insufficient to narrow down the possibilities about the external world, we are forced to rely upon various combinations of cues. Much of what we perceive, the sensory patterns merely provide the 'raw data' for experience. The sensory information is transformed elaborated and combined with memories to create what we actually experience or perceive.

Perceptual processes, which provide meaning to what we see or hear, are classified as—form, visual depth, constancy, movement perception, plasticity and individual differences.

Visual illusions are a dramatic example of how perceptual cues can be assembled incorrectly. An illusion is any figure that gives rise to a bizarre interpretation of reality. The illusions demonstrate that what we perceive often depends on processes that go far beyond the 'raw data' of sensory input. Specific instances in which the apparent curvature or length of a perceived line are not predictable from the curvature or length of its stimulus pattern, have been called the "Geometrical illusions". But this does not mean that they occur only with regular lines and patterns; they can also be demonstrated with quite irregular drawings and with real objects in normal environment. The illusions are important because they may provide clues for our understanding of processes of shape perception. Throughout the life span of an individual some changes occur in the perceptual processes.

Extrasensory perception or ESP, stimulates also called as parapsychological phenomenon is of two main kinds:

1. ESP
   a. Telepathy or thought transference from one person to another.
   b. Clairvoyance or, perception of objects or events not influencing the senses.
2. Psychokinesis or mentally manipulating objects without touching them.

Social perception is concerned with our interpretation of behaviour in social settings and generally refers to how we perceive others, favourably or unfavourably. Social perception is of great relevance to medical profession. How the patient perceives the physician determines his trust for physician's healing power. Attribution is making inferrences of others behaviour. Basic tendency to ascribe causes to events is believed to be an inherent part of how people process information in both their social and physical world. Sensory deprivation, phantom limb, hallucinations, perception of pain and perceptual disorders are some of the examples of clinical application of understanding of perceptions. Social perception and attribution are important for physicians as these are related to their interpersonal relationship with the patients.

Attention

Vimal, a college going student complains of decline in his academic performance for the last two months, he wants to get a college degree but whenever he sits to study, his mind wanders he is not able to comprehend, and is lagging behind. Similarly you would encounter number of patients: children, adolescents, adults and old aged, complaining of poor attention and difficulty in concentration.

Definition

Attention is the perceptual processing of selected inputs for inclusion in our conscious experience, or awareness, at any given time. We do not react equally to all stimuli that impinge upon us; we focus upon only a few. In other words, this perceptual focussing is called attention. Concentration is the ability to sustain attention for a specific period, on a particular object or subject.

The processes of attention divide our field of attention. Consider being in the sports stadium watching a cricket match. While your focus of attention is on the batting of the player, yet you are also aware of the scoreboard, you would also be trying to focus on the commentary and you also would be dimly aware of other observers sitting next to you, or occupying front rows. Here though your focus was on the player, the marginal inputs (awareness of other events) illustrate characteristic of attention that it is constantly shifting. What is at the focus one moment may be in the margin the next moment and the objects being in the margins may become the focus.

Attention is needed for the efficient assimilation of information and generation of coordinated behaviour. It is like a computer system that gets stuck if it tries to process at each level a large number of simultaneous events. The attentional limitation is not necessarily one of response in compatibility though this might sometimes be a factor. You can understand this by an example that in an experiment on conditional salivation reflects to a sound new light can suppress processing of the sound as indexed by inhibition of salivation. This is a competition for a limited processing capacity rather than motor output (Rizzolatti, 1983).

A basic process in attention is considered to be a kind of filtering of the sensory information we receive. We cannot process all the information in our sensory channels, so we filter out, or block irrelevant information (Broadbent 1958). There is evidence, that stimuli to which we are not actively attending still register in some form in our perceptual system, even though we may not recognised them at that time. There are two types of processing, known as parallel processing and serial processing. The parallel processing is when we are able to pick up information from two different conversations or sources simultaneously. On the other hand serial processing is when we pick up information in a serial order from different sources.

Factors Facilitating Attention

There are certain factors, which are either external or internal factors, which direct and facilitate our filtering of inputs.

External Factors

There are many external factors, which attract our attention more easily than other stimuli. The features that call for selection of focus of attention are stimuli, which are of higher intensity, like loud music, or lecture delivered with microphone. Stimuli of larger size generally arouse attention, thus you would experience that in seminars or conferences emphasis is placed on bold and large lettering for audiovisual presentation. Contrast and novelty are other characteristics of the stimuli, which easily catch attention. These principles are often used in making of commercial advertisement, designing fashion clothes, architecture of a building. You also use these methods in your academic presentations. Repetition and movement of stimuli are also used by the media to facilitate attention, as moving objects are more attended to, as when compared to static objects.

Internal Factors

The internal factors are those present within the individuals that cause them to attend to one event instead of other. One of them is 'motive' or need, if you want to buy a car, your attention would go more easily on advertisements related to selling of cars, similarly if you are hungry, you attend more to the eating places. Preparating set, i.e. a person's readiness to respond to one kind of sensory input, but not to other kinds, is another factor, which determines attention and was dicussed in Chapter 2 (Sensation and Perception). Interest, also influences the selectivity of attention. These internal factors may be the temporary or permanent state of our mind at a given time, e.g. motives keep changing interest may be more or less permanent as interest in sports. These factors provide us with a certain amount of consistency in the events to which we pay attention. So they give our experience, or perception of the world some direction and stability.

Types of Attention

Attention can be subdivided into different subsystems. These are based on somewhat different brain regions. Perry and Hodges classify attention as follows:

Selective Attention

Imagine you are in the library preparing for your seminar. While you are going through the latest research in the journal, you also hear some of your fellow students talking to each other, the attendant helping someone to find a book, the telephone ringing, noise of hammers coming from one corner of the library where the carpenters are at work. Despite all these potential distractions you are probably still able to focus your thoughts on the article that you were reading. Our ability to attend one main event whilst being remotely conscious of others provides us with the paradox of how attention can be both a selective and a divided process simultaneously. The restriction of mental processing to one event at a time is called 'selective attention'.

This type of attention provides the means by which we reduce the workload on our mental systems. Schizophrenic patients have been found consistently deficit in their ability to focus on a particular task. They show marked impairment inability to avoid distracting stimuli.

Broadbent (1958) has explained how attention is controlled by a filter. According to him, the information that becomes filtered out of the system (consciously unattended) will receive only a low level of analysis. How we select what to select, and on what criterion, is decided very early in the processing of information.

Selection is based upon the physical properties of the stimulus and is also referred to as sensory selection. Broadbent's filter theory of attention has been used in number of experiments with normal individuals as well as with schizophrenic patients and this still holds a popular place in theories of attention.

Generally most of the individuals cannot perform more than one task without taking their mind off the other. However, there is some evidence that people may be able to be trained to perform two difficult tasks at the same time.

Divided Attention

It is our every day experience that we are able to divide our attention between two or more events or tasks, such as listening to music while studying, knitting while watching television, or engaging in conversation while driving. Psychologists studying the selective aspects of attention have always emphasised how limited our ability is for diverse attention. In the typical experiment of dichotic listening it was always found that subjects were unable to attend more than one thing at a time. However, in these experiments generally the tasks given were very intellectually demanding, hence subjects had very little mental power left for attending to another task.

It is fairly recently that more attention is being focussed on the divided attention. Kahneman (1973) proposed the 'resource allocation' theory of attention.' Resources' refer to a reservoir of mental energy from which is drawn the appropriate amount when dealing with specific tasks. The more difficult the task, the greater will be the demands of the mental resources required to complete it. The less energy one particular task demands then the more of that energy will be available for allocation to other things being done simultaneously. It is not the task themselves that determine the allocation of the resources but the person who performs them. For instance, even though a particular task may require a lot of resources we may perform poorly on the task simply by not putting enough effort into it. This allocation of cognitive resources to the task, is under conscious control and we are free at any time to switch our attention to other events.

Our capacity for dividing attention between tasks increases with practice on them. It has been suggested that our mental resources do not have limited capacity but may actually expand with practice. It may, therefore, be possible to develop our cognitive resources in more efficient ways, once the principles are more clearly understood.

Sustained Attention

Sustained attention or vigilance is required to process stimuli of long duration. Sustained attention underlies the capacity to detect a signal over long periods (Perry and Hodges 1999), for example to inspect a screen and report when a signal appears. Sustained attention can be assessed on continuous performance test. The test consists of rapidly presented set of task with varied spacing and timing of target and nontarget stimuli.

Automatic and Conscious Processing

Compare a person who has been driving for long to that of a novice. One notices that after acquiring the skill a person can drive and converse or listen to the music at the same time, whereas the novice will have to put in all his mental resources in driving, e.g. his concentration on the road, on the steering wheel, accelerator, brakes, etc. This fundamental difference between our ability to perform a complex task as a beginner and later as a skilled person is that of degree of mental effort involved. The way that a skilled person applies a little effort in order to perform a task fluently is a source of constant frustration to the struggling novice. Skilled performance seems to require few cognitive resources such as that involving attention to detail. Shiffrin and Schneider (1977) proposed that attention occurred in two domains, which they named 'dom A' and 'dom B'. Dom A processing describes general, undivided attention, the features of which are that it is passive, automatic, has a relatively large capacity and makes a multilevel analysis of the attended information. Conversely, dom B processing is consciously controlled and is an active system having limited capacity and having no control over the processing that occurs in dom A. The dom A system continuously receives input about the environment that it processes unconsciously. Tasks that are well learnt have their elements stored in long-term memory, so they are available during the automatic processing of events when such tasks are subsequently performed.

Clinical Applications

Attention and concentration are the psychological processes, which are the first to get affected in illness and especially in psychiatric disorders. The patients with schizophrenia exhibit deficits in attention, which is evident even from the casual clinical contact with these patients. Some schizophrenics lack the capacity to perceive and respond to situations objectively, due to their inability to achieve a major 'set'. The schizophrenic is characterised by segmental set, in which response preparation is compromised due to an inappropriate focus on minor or irrelevant aspects of the stimulus array. The attentional deficits in schizophrenic have been assessed on immediate serial recall tasks, span of apprehension, reaction time, dictomic listening, backward masking and continuous performance tests. Assessment of attention and concentration has been discussed in Chapter 18, on assessment.

Undue preoccupation with memories of recent and/or past events associated, for example, with bereavement, an anxiety state or a depressive disorder, results in diminished attention to the external world, so that information is not registered and the individual becomes forgetful and unable to pursue a task requiring sustained attention such as reading.

In some patients who complain of physical symptoms for which no organic cause can be discovered, it is probable that their complaints are, at least in part, due to an excessive focussing of attention on the site of the symptom and that what they are experiencing is a bodily sensation which does not normally reach the level of awareness. Just as in some patients input may be selectively enhanced, so in others it may be blocked for psychological reasons. There are patients who, though free from organic disease, present with a loss of skin sensation in part of the body, or of a special sense such as vision or hearing. Such complaints usually do not correspond with those produced by organic disease and they are commonly described as hysterical. It has for long been suggested that the mechanism by which they occur is a process of involuntary dissociation between a limited part of consciousness (e.g. that concerned with skin sensation from a particular area or with visual or auditory perception) and the rest of consciousness. Thus these parts are dissociated or shut off from the rest of awareness and the individual no longer experiences the appropriate sensations or perceptions.

Some of the phenomena produced by hypnosis may be related to alterations of attention, and indeed the fundamental basis for the process may be a highly selective focussing of attention by the subject on the hypnotist with a corresponding lowering of attention to all other stimuli. Thus in a suitable subject the hypnotist is able to suggest a selective inattention to particular stimuli, resulting in, for example, an area of skin anaesthesia or a loss of a special sense such as vision or hearing.

Diseases affecting the brainstem (i.e. including the reticular formation), such as inflammation (e.g. encephalitis lethargic or sleeping sickness) or pressure from a tumour, can cause drowsiness, sleep or complete loss of consciousness. Conditions affecting the functioning of the brain more generally (e.g. through lack of oxygen or blood supply) may cause a state of delirium, with impairment or 'clouding' of consciousness; the patient may become confused, or disoriented—not knowing the present time or place and hallucinated, may have difficulty in concentration and subsequently have little or no memory for events at the time. Finally, episodes of unconsciousness occur in some forms of epileptic seizure, a condition associated with an electrical discharge in the brain which, in some individuals, 'epileptics', arises spontaneously from time-to-time, but can be provoked in anyone by chemical or electrical means (e.g. electroconvulsive therapy or ECT). Attention deficit hyperactive disorder is a common clinical condition in children. This disorder has onset before seven years of age, is four to five times more common in boys than girls. Attention disturbances are manifested as failing to finish the tasks that were started, easy distractibility, and difficulty in tasks requiring sustained attention. Children with poor attention may have average intelligence yet their school performance is very poor. These children often have comorbid problem of conduct disorder or specific learning disability.

SUMMARY

Attention refers to the perceptual focussing on certain stimuli with the aim of including them in the conscious awareness. Ability to sustain attention for some time is called concentration. Attention is influenced by external and internal factors. The former includes intensity and size of the stimulus, novelty, contrast and movement. The internal factors include motivation and interest. Attention is of three types, namely, selective attention, sustained attention and divided attention. Selective attention refers to the ability to focus the thoughts on a particular stimulus, despite the presence of other factors. Sustained attention refers to the ability to hold attention over considerable period of time (vigilance). Divided attention implies focussing attention on two or more tasks simultaneously. Attention also involves automatic and conscious processing. Study of attention is important since attentional deficits are commonly seen in patients, especially those having anxiety, schizophrenia, somatic complaints and certain neurological conditions. Poor attention and difficulty in sustaining concentration is the primary complaint in children diagnosed as attention deficit hyperactivity disorder.

Memory

Fifty-eight years old, male, senior executive in a good company comes to you with the complaints of not being able to remember his appointments. At times he has difficulty in recalling names of his colleagues, but remembers all the details of his past life. Otherwise he is able to carry on his work quite effectively.

Just before the exams, many students complain about forgetting everything that they have learnt. You would have wondered why one forgets in these situations. Though you would have read about the neurophysiology of memory, here we shall examine the psychological and clinical aspects of memory.

You would have realised learning emphasises that one must also remember the information or skill learned. Imagine, if you were unable to retain or remember all that you 'have earlier learned. Even animals have some system by which they remember. Memory plays a very important role in our learning and psychological growth. Through memory of our past experiences, we handle new situation, it helps us in our relearning, problem solving and thinking.

Memory Process

Memory is the storage of learned behavioural potentials over time. It brings a persistent change in the central nervous system brought about by environmental input and by the activities of the organism. Memory process can be divided into stages for the purpose of understanding (Fig. 4.1). Memory starts with the sensory input or stimulus from the environment. The input is through sensory channels, like vision, hearing or touch and is held briefly (seconds) in a sensory register. Information is passed through sensory register to short-term memory (STM) store where it is held for 20-30 seconds. Some part of the information from STM is further processed in

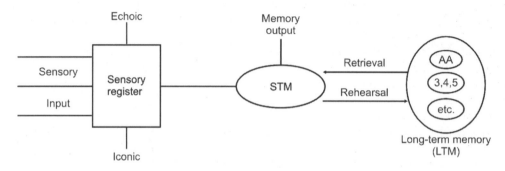

Fig. 4.1: Memory process

rehearsal buffer that is information is repeated, and in some way linked with other information already stored in memory. From the rehearsal buffer processed information is passed on to long-term memory store (LTM) where it is organised in categories and stored for years. Information not so processed is forgotten. This process can be compared with your day-to-day experiences. To learn new technical words, or names, you have to rehearse several times.

Memory is viewed by cognitive theorist as an attempt to isolate some of the processes that act between the input of the stimulus and the response output. Memory is divided into three stages, encoding, storage, and retrieval. Encoding means transforming the sensory input into a form that can be processed by the memory system. The encoded information is transferred to storage. Retrieval involves locating memorised information when needed. Figure 4.2 summarises this model.

Input→Encoding→Storage→Retrieval→Output

Fig. 4.2: Information processing model of memory

This could be compared with your experience of attending a particular class. You hear lecture and make notes that is you encode the lecture, then the notes are stored in some file using date or topic name. When later this information is required you retrieve by searching that particular file by it's topic name. Thus any memory system must perform three functions—
a. Input—allow information to be fed into the system
b. Storage—to maintain information
c. Retrieval—to access information when required.

There is another way of looking at the way the memory works. Craik and Lockhart (1972) disagree with the concept of memory as a division into three completely separate memory structures—sensory, short-term, and long-term memory. They identify only one kind of memory and maintain that the ability to remember is dependent on how deeply we process information. We process material along a continuum of ever-increasing depth, running it through on levels that range from quite shallow to very deep. The deeper we process it, the longer it lasts.

This concept of memory sees it as more of an active than a reactive process with memory performance a direct result of the learner's mental activity. The shallowest level of processing, according to this model, involves your awareness of a sensory feature-what a word or number looks like or sounds like, what a food smells or tastes like, and so forth. As you recognise some kind of pattern in your sensory impression, you will process it more deeply. And when you make an association, that is give a meaning, to your impression, you will be at the deepest level of processing of all, the kind that will form the strongest and most enduring memory trace (Fig. 4.3).

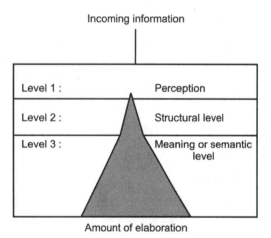

Fig. 4.3: Levels of processing memory

Memory Systems

Recall of information is most often required in daily activities and especially in educational performances. We also recognise the material, or persons or places by acknowledging it.

Familiar material can be learned more rapidly than the unfamiliar material. There are at least three distinct ways of classifying memory. These are based on (1) neurological structure of the brain, (2) experimental model of psychology and (3) clinical practices of mental examination. On the basis of neurological, theory, memory is divided into verbal and non-verbal. On the basis of experimental model, memory is divided into sensory memory, short-term memory and long-term memory. On the basis of clinical practice, memory can be divided into remote, recent and immediate. Their levels of processing also differentiate short-term and long-term memory. Some detail of these memories is as follows:

Sensory Memory

Sensory memory is the first stop of an incoming stimulus. All sensory modalities (visual and auditory, tactile, olfactory and kinesthetic) are involved in receiving these first impressions. These impressions are either lost with time or processed further for later remembering. The duration of sensory memory is very short and it varies in time for different sensory modalities. Iconic memory or visual sensory memory may last from 250 msec to 500 msec, echoic or auditory sensory memory from 2 to 10 sec tactual memory about 4 sec and motor memory (kinesthetic) as long as 80 sec.

Short-term Memory

You have just seen that information from sensory register is passed on to short-term memory (STM). This is also known as primary memory and can be called as immediate memory. While you have no voluntary control over what happens to information in sensory storage, you can control what is stored in STM by rehearsal. Information is held; in STM store upto about 30 seconds, but the length can vary depending upon many factors. Short-term memory has very limited storage capacity; six to seven items can be stored at one time. With new stimulus input, the original items get erased or fade away. The storage capacity ran be increased by chunking, i.e. combining several items. Unfamiliar items fade out faster than familiar items. Items can be recalled at will while the information is in short-term store.

Coding for short-term memory involves speech sounds, visual images and words. Generally visual stimuli is translated into sounds, for example, if a card of unfamiliar letters is flashed for half a second after 15 seconds and you are asked to repeat it, chances are that you would reproduce the sound resembling that letter.

Some experiments have also demonstrated that the material presented in the beginning of the next and at the end are recalled relatively well than those appearing in the middle. This is called serial position effect. When recall is better in the beginning of the text then it is known as primacy effect while if the recall is better for the last part of the text then it is called recency effect.

Working Memory

Working memory is at times used as an alternative term to STM. The concept of working memory is similar to STM with the only difference on its processing as well as its. storage functions. Working memory occurs between the short time of sensory memory and the long-term memory. A number of characteristics distinguished this memory processing phase.
- Working memory has very limited capacity.
- Retains material for a very short duration of time, for 18 to 20 seconds unless one tries to hold consciously.
- Material is consciously processed and retention last as long as it is held in attention.

This system is called working memory because the material transferred either in sensory memory or long-term memory has to be worked on, thought about and mentally organised. Working memory provides a mental working space to help in sorting and processing new information (Shiffrin, 1993). You can understand process of working memory by recalling that you tend to remember the telephone numbers till you have to dial it, after using the number it is discarded and it is no longer in the memory.

Rehearsal

Rehearsal means repeating items of information, silently or aloud and it helps to keep these items of information in the centre of attention. Experiments have shown that rehearsal could be maintenance rehearsal where in information is just repeated as it is. This is not very helpful in remembering for a longer duration. Elaborative rehearsal organises the material and gives meaning while rehearsing. This is an active process of transferring material from short-term memory to long-term memory. The amount of rehearsal given to items is important in the transfer of information from short-term to long-term memory, the more an item is rehearsed, and the more likely it is to become part of long-term memory. In elaborative rehearsal, people use strategies that give meaning and organisation to the material so that it can be fitted in with existing organised long-term memories.

Long-term Memory

Long-term memory also known as secondary memory seems to be very complex as it stores many different aspects of our experiences. The storage capacity has no known limits and one can remember information for days, months, and years. It records the salient features of sensory inputs and files these according to various memory categories. It also creates an auditory representation of the input and it also records how to reproduce the information when required.

Long-term memory is of two types—procedural and declarative. Each one holds different kind of information. Procedural memory stores memory for how things are done. It is used to acquire retain and use perceptual cognitive and motor skills. Procedural memory is related to action sequence, you recall skill memories like swimming, driving, giving an injection. The interesting characteristic of this memory is that you remember the initial phase of learning. Once you have acquired the skill, you may perform without consciously thinking about the task. Declarative memory is for remembering explicit information. It is also known as 'fact memory'. Declarative memory contains two different categories of information.

Semantic Memory

Conains meaning of words and concepts, rules of using these in language. Semantic memory is not easily forgotten, as the information is stored in highly organised way in logical hierarchies, from general to specific ones. Such organisation makes it possible for us to make logical inferences from the information stored in semantic memory.

Episodic Memory

Contains personal experiences of long-term memories. It is a record of what has happened to us, or remembrances of past things. Episodic memory seems to be organised with respect to certain events that happened in our lives. The episodes do not have to have a logical organisation. It is less organised, episodic memory seems more susceptible to being forgotten than semantic memory.

Long-term memory is highly organised. Information is categorised in number of ways. One of the evidence of organisation is seen in 'tip of the tongue phenomenon'. You all would have experienced while trying to retrieve a person's name you cannot quite remember it but the name is at your tongue. If we look at this tip-of-the-tongue (TOT) phenomenon in greater detail, we find evidence for the organisation of long-term memory. The search through the memory store in the TOT state is not random. If the name we are looking for is Shalu, we may come up with Shalini or Shobha, but not Meena. If you try to experiment within this phenomenon, you would observe that when the subjects are in the TOT state, on hearing the definition but not able to hit the "target" word, they would tend to retrieve words from their long-term memories that (1) sounded like the target word, (2) started with the same letter as the target word, (3) contain the same number of syllables as the target word, and/or (4) have a meaning similar to that of the target word. The TOT phenomenon indicates that information is organised in long-term memory. Types of memory are summarised in Figure 4.4.

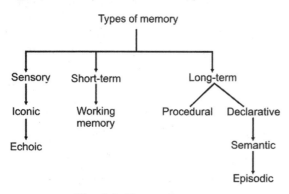

Fig. 4.4: Types of memory

FORGETTING

Forgetting is failure to retrieve information from long-term memory store. Much of the information is lost but enough remains, so that we have sketchy record of our lives. Sometimes what we think is forgotten in real sense is not forgotten because it was never encoded and stored in the first place. Many students complain that they do not remember the contents after attending the class or forget after reading the text. This happens due to lack of attention. Some information does not reach short-term memory from the sensory register or due to inadequate encoding and rehearsal; the information may not have been transferred from short-term to long-term memory. Information was not stored in long term memory because rehearsal was not sufficiently elaborate.

Many times we forget, as memory does not match events, which had occurred. This happens due to the constructive processes, i.e. during encoding, the to-be-remembered information, especially if it is a complex life event or something you have read, is modified. Certain details are accentuated, the material may be simplified, or it may be changed in many other ways so that what is encoded and stored is far from a literal copy of the input. Constructive processes of encoding distort what is stored in the memory and distortions are remembered. We remember the gist, or meaning of what we have read or heard but not the actual words themselves; inferences constructed at the time the information was encoded for storage is remembered, or portions of the to-be-remembered informations is encoded. Besides the faulty memory processes, some of the other common factors of forgetting are as following.

Interference

According to this explanation, what we do in the interval between learning and recall, determines the course of forgetting. Experimental studies have shown that learning new things interferes with memory of what is learned earlier and prior learning interferes with memory of things learned later.

Retroactive inhibition: This is a technical name for new learning that may interfere with material previously learned. This has been demonstrated in experiments as following.

	Activity		
Group	I	II	III
Experimental	Learn A	Learn B	Recall A
Control	Learn A	Unrelated activity	Recall A

As an example you may learn one chapter of physiology in activity I, then learn one topic of Anatomy in activity II, then try to recall what you had learned in physiology. The amount of information you forget would be due to interference caused by learning anatomy. Compared to this, if you learn a topic from Physiology, rest for sometime, then recall physiology you would find that your recall is better than that of the previous chapter.

Proactive inhibition: When prior learning interferes with the learning and recall of new material, it is called proactive inhibition. To demonstrate this type of interference experiment is designed as following.

	Activity		
Group	I	II	III
Experimental	Learn A	Learn B	Recall A
Control	Rest or unrelated activity	Learn B	Recall A

Supposing you learn English, then learn French and recall French, you would find that study of English interferes with your recall of French. Here what you have learned earlier, interferes with the subsequent memory.

Even though lots of experiments have been conducted, yet the process of interference is not very clear. One idea is that the interferences disrupts the various kinds of associations between stimuli and responses formed during learning. Another idea is that interference has its greatest effect on the memory of retrieval cues. You have seen in the earlier section that memory depends on retrieval cues, so if interference results in problems with these cues, forgetting will result.

In both types of interference it has been found that the effect of interference is less with meaningful material and after attaining some mastery in the subject. In initial period of your course you should try to allot different study times to similar subjects.

Encoding, Organisation and Retrieval Problems If the stored information is not encoded well or organized at the time it was learned, it is forgotten. Retrieval cues are also important in memory, as we may not be able to recall some information in one situation but may spontaneously remember in the other situation. Retrieval is facilitated by organisation of the stored material and the presence of retrieval cues that can guide our search through long-term memory for stored informations. In the absence of proper retrieval cues, the sought for items stored in long-term memory are not found. Many times you would have experienced that you cannot recall something while actively searching for it, but after giving up that search while doing something else, you recall that object. The new activity in which you engaged, or the new context gives another set of reminders, which helps to retrieve that information. It is a good idea to give up and do something else in order to generate new retrieval cues.

Motivated Forgetting

Emotional factors also play an important role in forgetting. If we encode information while in one emotional state and try to recall it while in another, recall suffers. Many lapses of memory in daily life illustrate motivated forgetting. We may forget the names of people we do not like. Repression theory holds that we forget because the retrieval of memories would be painful or unacceptable in some way to the person. Freud, in his book "The Psychopathology of Everyday Life" had illustrated many examples of repression in forgetting. Repression includes retrieval failure for the association of the threatening, anxiety-provoking information.

Anxiety or guilt producing material is more often forgotten than pleasant experiences. Supposing in a particular class you were scolded by the teacher, chances of forgetting what happened in that class would be higher. Psychologist have also found that some persons cannot forget unpleasant experiences easily, they have related this phenomenon with personality. Some stored information is so threatening and anxiety arousing that it's retrieval is possible only under special circumstances like hypnosis, free associations.

Zeigarnik Effect

A Russian psychologist demonstrated through experiments that incomplete tasks are remembered better than the completed tasks. This is sometimes called "Zeigarnik effect", "Ego-oriented" persons remember more of completed tasks as incomplete tasks generate more anxiety. On the other hand task-oriented persons remember more of incomplete tasks, as for them the incomplete task is more painful while completed tasks are not so.

Amnesia—Forgetting during Sickness

Amnesia refers to loss of memory due to disease. Amnesia is a general "disorder of memory". The person may forget his past experiences or may have impaired ability to encode, store and to retrieve, thus forming of new memory is difficult. Amnesia is a profound memory deficit due to either the loss of what has been stored or to the inability to form new memories. Amnesias are classified under two categories: (i) biological and (ii) psychological.

Biological amnesias: Forgetting could be due to any of following reasons—diseases of the brain like senile dementia, Korsakoff syndrome, concession from blows on head, brain damage, brain infections, tumour, stroke, temporary disturbances in the blood supply or effect of high dose of alcohol and drug abuse.

Senile dementia: It is characterised by deficits in many intellectual abilities like memory, attention, judgement, and abstract thought, that could occur in aged people. The person has trouble remembering events that happened after the onset of the disease. Thus the person with this disorder has trouble learning and cannot recall well what happened last month, yesterday, or even a few hours ago. Senile dementia is usually the result of a reduction in blood flow to the brain.

Transient global amnesia: These are profound memory problem with no loss of consciousness. It comes on suddenly without any obvious cause, and it typically lasts for only a few hours or days before memory becomes normal again. Fortunately, most people who experience such amnesia have it only once. This type of amnesia is called global because much of what has already been stored in memory is forgotten and because even though the person is conscious and can go about the routine business of daily life, no new memories are formed while the attack is in progress.

Alcohol and drug abuse: These also cause amnesia, a person may have amnesia for the events occurring while under the influence of alcohol because encoding and storage processes have been disrupted by the effects of the alcohol on the brain. Heavy drinking over a period of years however, can result through vitamin-B deficits and other chemical imbalances, in irreversible brain damage and a pattern of symptoms known as the Korsakoff syndrome. Interograde amnesia the inability to form new memories is one of the prominent symptoms of this syndrome.

Psychological amnesia: These types of amnesias occur due to psychiatric diseases where the person forgets his identity also. There may not be a permanent loss.

Childhood amnesia: is due to the differences in the ways young children and older people encode and store information. As adults, much of our memory is encoded verbally and tied into networks, or schemata, that are based on language. But the young child without language encodes memories in a nonverbal form, perhaps storing information as images or feelings. Early childhood memories are thus said to be stored in forms no longer available to us as adults. Our language-dominated memories, do not have retrieval cues appropriate for gaining access to the image and feeling memories of early childhood. Perhaps the memory machine is just not able to store long-term memories until its maturation is essentially finished. Language ability and memory develop together because both depend on brain maturation. You all experience that dreams are forgotten on waking up. Dream amnesia may actually have a biological basis. The dreaming brain seems to be in a special state different from that of the waking brain.

Defensive amnesia: People with defensive amnesia may forget their names, where they have come from, who their spouses are, and many other important details of their past lives.

It is called defensive because this type of amnesia is usually considered to be a way of protecting oneself from the guilt or anxiety that can result from intense, intolerable life situations and conflicts. Defensive amnesia is thus an extreme form of repression.

Normal aging: has its problems too, but the typical forgetfulness of old age is hardly severe enough to be called amnesia. In normal aging, the memory problem, centres largely on the storage of relatively recent events; it is anterograde in nature. But, in marked contrast to senile dementia patients, normal old people are able to compensate for their mild memory problems. They try to do less and thus put a smaller burden on their information-processing systems, they provide themselves with reminder cues, perhaps by writing down what is to be remembered, and they organise their lives into routines so that fewer new things need to be remembered. In other words, normal old people adopt adaptive memory strategies.

Methods to Improve Memory

With training, practice and motivation memory can be improved. Some well-practiced methods, verbal as well as visual mediators to improve memory are listed in this section.

Mnemonics

You can recall when a list of difficult technical words in pharmacology or unfamiliar words in foreign language is to be remembered. Mnemonics are devices that facilitate the learning and recall of many such forms of difficult material. One of the method is to associate whatever you want to recall with something already established in your memory bank, e.g. colours of rainbow are associated with name "Roy G. BIV", i.e. Red. Orange, Yellow, Green, Blue, Indigo and Violet.

Method of Loci

You visualise a scene and fit the items to be remembered in that scene. The scene can be a street, a building with rooms, the layout of a college campus, a kitchen, or just about anything that can be visualised clearly and contains a number of discrete items in specific locations to serve as memory pegs. Supposing you want to remember for examination classical conditioning, then start by imagining a dog, experimental room, food, bell and any person as an experimenter. Rehearse this image over and over until it is well-established in your mind. After you have formed your image, associate the events, the stimulus substitution, and extinction with this. The trick is to make associations with as many concepts as needed.

Pegword Method

Pegword method is another technique through which a list of items and their relative positions can be learned effectively. To establish the main idea in your long-term memory, a well-organized set of images to which the to-be-remembered items could be linked. For letter systems you can establish mnemonic pegs by forming strong distinctive images of words that start with the sounds of the letter of the alphabet.

In number systems, you form an image with each number.

Rhyming

Rhyming can be used for learning of long list involving numbers like the numbers 1 through 10. You can organize or arrange the first letters of words in such a way that it rhymes. In Anatomy many students use rhyming to remember names of the different bones.

Making a Story

Making a story in this you can fit the facts in the story like you read in elaborative rehearsal.

Chunking

This technique illustrates systematic ways of encoding information. If you want to remember a long list of digits, e.g. 1989609065 you can break the numbers into chunks, the first four digits could be remembered as the year you passed your school or associated with any significant thing that happened in that year. Next three digits could also be taken as date, e.g. for someone's birthday. The last 3 digits can be an address code. Like this chunks can be associated with some important thing for lasting memory.

Remembering Names and Faces

As first steps in establishing a good memory for names and faces, we should: (i) be sure we hear the name clearly when introduced, (ii) repeat the name when acknowledging the introduction, and (iii) if the name is unusual, politely ask the new acquaintance to spell it. While we are making sure we have heard and rehearsed the name, we should be paying close attention to the individual's face.

The important thing for good memory is your motivation and ability to organise the material. One strategy in remembering things well is to organise, or arrange the input so that it fits into existing long-term memory categories, is grouped in some logical manner, or is arranged in some other way that makes sense. The organisational encoding may be inherent in the input itself or it may be supplied by individuals as they learn and remember new things.

Here are some tips to help you to improve your memory.

1. Plan your study content and make a time schedule to cover that content. Stick to this schedule firmly.
2. For academic and nonacademic activities. One can make use of methods that help us to study better for the exams and do well. These methods are listed in the section below.
3. As you have seen rehearsal is important to transfer information into long-term memory, and elaborative rehearsal is more effective than maintenance rehearsal. So make notes of important points as all the details of information cannot be remembered. Revise these notes.
4. You can use imagery to visualise the material you are learning and give auditory stimulation by reading aloud. For example while studying nervous system, visualise the structure of nervous system with minutest details and also read loudly. Multi-channel stimulation would improve your memory.
5. Try to organise your material with retrieval cues or reminders. Make a map of contents in your mind.
6. Give a feedback to yourself by testing your memory. Revise areas where you could not remember.
7. Review before examination. Try to learn but do not get anxious as you have seen high anxiety level would interfere with your remembering.
8. Give some short rest pauses between your study times. It would help to consolidate the material you are learning.

Clinical Assessment of Memory

Measurement of memory is a complex task because a number of variables interact in recall. All these variables can be divided in three groups: (i) nature of the material, (ii) the methods used for testing the recall, and (iii) characteristics of the individual. A combination of these three factors is necessary for testing the memory. Methods to assess memory are given in Chapter 18.

The method employed for testing the memory includes, immediate recall, delayed recall, sequential recall, associative recall, reconstruction, recognition both filled and unfilled interval between presentation of material and their recall. Recall is also affected by individual's characteristics. A person who is more attentive and receptive can recall better. The physical state of the individual taking test, his motivation, age, sex, education, do play role in the recall; irrespective of the material and methods used for testing the memory.

We are much more concerned about memory disturbances and its quantification. There are two types of memory disturbances—period specific memory disturbances and generalised slowing in memory. The former includes retrograde amnesia and anterograde amnesia. Retrograde is a defect of recall whereas anterograde amnesia is a defect of registration/retention, from the point of occurrence of a significant life event.

Longer the time duration of washout of previous traces in case of retrograde and the difficulty in forming the images for subsequent recall in case of anterograde amnesia forms the degree of severity of memory disturbances. Conventional techniques of memory testing do not quantify these period specific memory disturbances.

The generalised slowing in the formation and retrieval of the traces however, can be quantified from the available psychological tests of memory.

Clinical Applications

Memory is the most recognised cognitive function. It is markedly sensitive and easily influenced by emotionality, problems of daily life, psychiatric disturbances, sleep deprivation, over work, fatigue, consumption of intoxicants, electroconvulsive therapy (ECT), exposure to anaesthetic gases, head injury, etc.

In your clinical practice you shall come across many patients having minor memory disturbances, but you may also come across patients with very severe memory disturbance, where the patient may even forget his name, to which place he belongs. He may go from one place to another and have total loss of memory for the incident. In memory loss due to normal aging sometimes the individual may remember everything of the past, but is unable to form new memories. Memory problems are very common amongst students. Children with below average intelligence also have memory problems. Similarly poor memory is reported in children with attention deficit disorders. High anxiety state in students during examination impairs retention.

Psychological strategies for enhancing memory or aids to rehabilitation especially for patients with neurological problems have been developed. These are of special importance in rehabilitation of patients with head injury, and amnesias of all types. As any memory process includes three functions namely—encoding, storage and retrieval thus the strategies to enhance these processes are given in brief in the following section.

Encoding

To improve encoding of the information advise patients/family members to:
  i. Simplify information
  ii. Reduce the amount
  iii. Make sure he has understood

iv. Repeat the information
v. Make associations
vi. Encourage to organise and group the information
vii. Process at deeper levels—think about makes it meaningful.

Storage

To improve storage process first of all rate of forgetting should be objectively assessed. Then attempts should be made to rehearse, then test and retest the memory. Use method of expanded or reconstruction rehearsal method as this is more effective than repetition.

Retrieval

As retrieval is better in context where the patient is learning, so advise patients to go to the situation in which retrieval is required. Retrieval can be done by:
  i. First letter prompts
  ii. Alphabetical searching
  iii. Mental retracing of events.

In addition to this certain other strategies can be used for rehabilitation of patients with memory impairment. Environmental adaptations for patients having very impaired memory can be made by using labels, sign post, or colour coding. External aids can be used. These are of two types: (1) those aids that we use to store information externally, e.g. lists, plans, diaries, and (2) cueing devices. Also some of the methods listed above to improve memory can be used, like mnemonics. While helping such patients it is also important to advise family members not to make fun or laugh at these patients. An encouraging attitude towards the patient should be adopted.

SUMMARY

Memory is an ability to remember, this is a very important cognitive process for our learning. The memory process is divided into three main stages—encoding, storage and retrieval. There are three distinct ways of classifying memory: (i) neurological structure of the brain, which divides memory into verbal and nonverbal, (ii) on the basis of experimental model, memory is divided into sensory memory, short-term memory and long-term memory, and (iii) on the basis of clinical practice, memory can be divided into remote, recent and immediate. Their levels of processing also differentiate short-term and long-term memory. The two primary and secondary types of memory are, short-term memory wherein information is stored for maximum 30 seconds and has limited capacity. In long-term memory store, information is organised in semantic memory or in episodic memory.

There are four main causes of forgetting: (i) interference due to similar material, (ii) faulty encoding, storage and retrieval. If the sensory registration or input of information is faulty then memory will not be established. Similarly each of these stages are important for good memory, (iii) motivated forgetting, and (iv) amnesias which could be biological, due to diseases of the brain or psychological.

Memory could be improved with good planning, organisation, review and feedback. The other methods to improve memory are mnemonics, method of loci, pegword method, rhyming, making a story, and chunking. Some strategies have been developed to help and rehabilitate patients with severe memory defects such as head injury, dementias, normal aging. These strategies provide steps to enhance memory at different stages of processing.

There are several methods to assess memory, which have been given in Chapter 18.

Clinical applications of memory extend from various psychiatric; child psychiatric disorders to neurological disorders especially head injury and dementia. Methods to improve memory are of relevance to the students themselves.

Learning and Studying

Try to remember the first time you tried to solve problem on Rubrik's Cube or played badminton. Probably now you will laugh at that behaviour, as at that time you found that difficult to perform or play because of the errors made one after another. But you can also recall that with gradual practice, you got better and better at each time. This illustrates an important principle of 'Learning,' the capacity to 'profit' from experience and practice. Learning is an important process as it has applications not only to learn new things, but also to modify maladaptive behaviours. For a student, learning also has relevance as it can help in understanding one learning process, and methods to improve learning styles.

Definition

Learning is the central process to all our behaviour, as we learn to do various activities like speak, write, think, or play. Our attitudes and emotional expressions are also learned behaviours. All our adaptive as well as unadaptive, cognitive as well as affective behaviour are formed by learning processes. These are of vital importance in helping the person to adapt to his changing environment.

Learning is the acquisition through insight of cognitive structure. It is an internal process, not necessarily observable, in which information is integrated into the structure of what student already knows and understands. Learning is a process resulting in some modification, relatively permanent, of the way of thinking, feeling, and doing of the learner. The characteristics of learning is producing a behavioural change in the learner, leading to a relatively permanent change, that is also gradual, adaptable and selective resulting from practice, repetitions and experience, and not directly observable. There are three important factors in learning:

1. Learning brings change in behaviour.
2. Change takes place through practice or experience. It emphasises that all changes due to growth or maturation or by drugs, brain injury, are not learning.
3. The change in behaviour should be permanent, to be called as learning.

Learning is not only acquisition of a body of knowledge, but it governs our total behaviour from simple to complex. There are a variety of ways by which we learn, which are detailed in the following section:

How do we Learn?

There are a number of theoretical explanations about the process of learning. Some theories emphasise on stimulus response (S-R) relationships, and interpret learning as an associative process. Classical conditioning and operant conditioning are based on associative learning. Other psychologists argue that all types of learning cannot be explained on simple forms of S-R relationships. They give importance to perception and understanding for learning complex forms of learning. Cognitive theories are an offshoot of this explanation. However, we are social beings and we learn number of tasks in social context, so another group of theorists have given the social learning model. In the following section, all these methods of learning shall be examined in detail.

Classical Conditioning

Classical conditioning is the simplest form of learning based on experiments of Pavlov, a Russian physiologist. Conditioning is a term used to describe the process by which the previously neutral stimulus (CS) gains the power to elicit the conditioned response (CR). Pavlov had noticed during the experiments that his experimental dogs salivated not only to the sight of food, but also to the sound of experimenter's footsteps. To study this phenomenon systematically, he associated the presentation of food to the dog with another stimulus, such as the sound of bell. After giving some trials in which the bell preceded the presentation of food, the dog started salivating at the sound of the bell. To explain this phenomenon, some technical terms are used; food is called unconditioned stimulus (US), and salivation elicited for food is called unconditioned response (UR). The sound of bell in the experiment was conditioned stimulus (CS). It was initially a neutral stimulus because except for an alerting or attentional response during the first few times it is presented; it does not evoke a specific response. The response of salivation to bell is called conditioned response, as it was originally a neutral conditioned stimulus; it evoked a specific response due to learning (Fig. 5.1) the conditioning procedure.

Innate stimulus   Response connection
    (US)   (UR)
Food ———————————————— Salivation

Learned stimulus   Reponse connection
    (CS)   (CR)
Bell ———————————————— Salivation

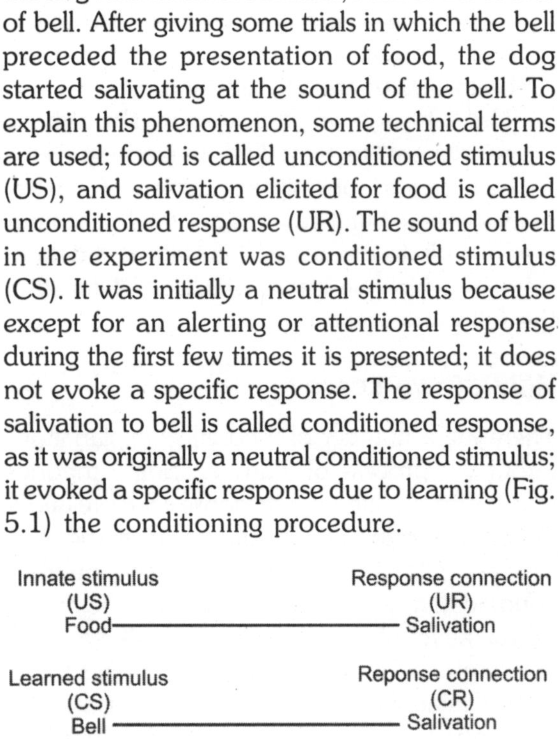

Fig. 5.1: Classical conditioning procedure

The acquisition of a conditioned response is gradual and becomes stronger with repeated trials. There are certain acts of classical conditioning which require consideration.

Acquisition: Each paired presentation of the CS and the US should be presented a number of times, and the interval between CS and US should be short. In simultaneous conditioning, the CS begins a little earlier than the onset of US and continues along with it until the response occurs. In delayed conditioning, the CS begins much before the onset of US. In trace conditioning, the CS is presented and then removed before the US starts.

Stimulus substitution: An association or pairing of CS with US acquires the capacity to substitute for the US in evoking a response. With conditioning, a link or bond is formed between the CS and US, and as a result of this CS becomes equivalent to US in eliciting a response. Stimulus substitution occurs if CS is similar to US. But the recent theorists do not agree with this simple process of stimulus substitution. According to their viewpoint, CS becomes a signal for the US; when CS is presented, the US is expected and the learner responds due to expectation.

Stimulus generalisation and discrimination: When the conditioned response to a stimulus has been acquired, other similar stimuli can also evoke the same response. This is known as stimulus generalisation. In Pavlov's experiments, the dog gave CR to slightly different bell also. It has also been demonstrated that the closer the similarity to US with other stimuli, the greater is the CR.

Discrimination is to make one response to one stimulus and a different response, or no response to another. This process is complementary to generalisation. In experiments it is demonstrated by using two different tones CS1 and CS2. On some trials CS1 is paired with US and on other trials CS2 is given alone without US. The subject learns to respond only to CS1, after learning takes place (Fig. 5.2).

Generalisation	Discrimination
Tone 1 Response	Tone 1 NO Response
Tone 2 Response	Tone 2 No Response
Tone 3 Response	Tone 3 Response

Fig. 5.2: Generalisation and discrimination learning

Behaviour	Positive Consequences.	Recurrence of behaviour (positive reinforcement)
Behaviour	No reward or punishment	Behaviour disappears (extinction)

Fig. 5.3: Operant conditioning process

Extinction and spontaneous recovery: If the unconditioned stimulus (US) does not follow the conditioned stimulus CS repeatedly, the conditioned response gradually diminishes. Repetition of the conditioned stimulus without unconditioned stimulus is called extinction; this is not forgetting, as a specific procedure is involved in this.

Extinction is used for modification of problem behaviours in clinical practice. A response that has been extinguished, does recur later on its own, this is called spontaneous recovery. If there is a period of rest after extinction, the CR tends to re-emerge. This tendency is more marked after continuous than distributed practice of the response during extinction. At this stage, if reinforcement or US is not presented with CS, the response extinguishes permanently.

Operant Conditioning

Operant conditioning, a term coined by BF Skinner, means that the likelihood of a behaviour depends on the significance of the event immediately following it to person showing the behaviour. If the event following the behaviour is positively reinforcing or rewarding, then it will recur. If it is not reinforced or is punished, then it is less likely to recur and eventually stops completely, a process known as 'extinction'. An alternative related approach is 'stimulus control'—changing the preceding event. When a response operates on the environment, it may have consequences that can affect the likelihood of the response occurring again. This form of learning is also known as instrumental conditioning, because some action or behaviour of the learner is instrumental in bringing about a change in the environment, that makes the action more or less likely to occur again in the future. For example, putting food in your mouth (an operant) is likely to be repeated because of its pleasant consequences (Fig. 5.3).

This is an effective method for teaching new behaviour patterns and for modifying undesirable behaviours. A number of treatment strategies used in behavioural therapy and behavioural medicine are derived from this method (see Chapters 20, 22). The basics of operant conditioning are reinforcement and punishment. Thus, use of reinforcement and punishment shall be examined in detail.

Reinforcement: The basic principles of operant conditioning are that when a behaviour occurs and is followed by reinforcement, it is more likely to occur again in the future. A great deal of our behaviour has been learned because it has been rewarded. For example, you study because you may find it reinforcing in terms of marks attained or praise from your colleagues. Many responses can be made to occur more frequently by following it with reinforcement. The behaviour can be shaped and moulded by appropriate arrangements of responses and reinforcers.

Nature of reinforcers: Whether something is positively reinforcing or punishing, depends on the effect it has on behaviour. What may be positively reinforcing to one child may not be so for another. For example, usually food will be positively reinforcing, but to an anorexic girl, who hates the sight of food, it may be punishing. Pain is usually punishing, but to a child preoccupied with guilt with masochistic tendencies, it will be positively reinforcing or rewarding. Further, the strength and direction of reinforcement will depend to some degree on the child's relationship with the person administering or involved in it. A game of football is likely to be more positively reinforcing for a boy if it involves his father than his mother. A star chart for bed-wetting worked out in cooperation with a mother with whom a 6 years old has a good relationship, is likely to be more effective than if the mother and child are in serious conflict.

Reinforcements are divided into two types: (i) primary or material rewards, such as snacks, sweets, food, etc. and (ii) secondary or social rewards, such as praise, smile. Events or consequences, which strengthen behaviour when they are presented, are called positive reinforcers. In negative reinforcement, the response causes the termination of a painful event. Removal of painful or unpleasant consequences can also strengthen or reinforce behaviour. For instance, offering a screaming child an ice cream may result in a child stopping screaming. The adult is likely to continue to give ice cream (operant) to stop the child from screaming (negative reinforcement for the adult).

In children, the most common form of positive reinforcement is praise and attention. Children are likely to repeat behaviour, which gives pleasure to those whom they are fond of. Usually their parents and teachers are the most important people to give positive reinforcement; as they get older, other children/peers increasingly take on this role. If a teacher plays gratifying attention to bad behaviour (even if the attention takes form of shouting at the child), then bad behaviour will recur. Material rewards such as money, sweets, chocolates, other favourite foods, and watching television are also used as reinforcers.

Schedule of reinforcement: According to Skinner, at the beginning of training you should reward each and every move the child makes toward the goal. However, once the child has mastered a given response in the chain, you may begin slowly fading out the reward by reinforcing the response intermittently. Continuous reinforcement is necessary at first, both to keep the individual to perform and to let him know that he is doing something right. However, once the child learns what that "something" is, you may begin reinforcing the response every second time, then every third or fourth time, then perhaps every tenth time. If you fade out the reward very gradually, you can get a child to make a simple response several times, for each reinforcement.

During the fading process, the exact scheduling of the reward is crucial. If you reinforce exactly every tenth response, the child will soon learn to anticipate which response will gain him reward. Skinner calls this fixed ratio reinforcement, because the ratio between the number of responses required and the rewards given is fixed and never varies. Instead of reinforcing exactly the tenth response, we can vary the schedule, so that sometimes the third response yields reward, sometimes the twentieth or any response in between. A hundred responses will yield about 10 rewards, but the child will never know when the next reward is coming. When trained on variable ratio schedules, individuals respond at a fairly constant pace.

Extinction generally occurs most rapidly following withdrawal of things that are positive reinforcers. Thus the withdrawal of love from people of whom the child is fond is often the most effective way of achieving extinction of the undesirable behaviour. In other children, the withdrawal of material goods, such pocket money, special food or drink, and opportunity to watch television are more important.

Shaping: Refers to the gradual forming of the behaviour. Desirable new behaviour can be built up through successive reinforcement of a sequence of components parts of that behaviour.

It is commonly used in teaching skills to mentally subnormal.

Punishment: When we wish to eliminate an unadaptive behaviour, punishment tends to decrease the likelihood of occurrence of the responses. Any unpleasant consequence of behaviour, which makes that behaviour less likely to occur, can be seen as punishing. Physical punishment by parents is the most frequently used, but many children do not respond to it by a reduction in their undesirable behaviour. Probably, the attention they get when they are punished has a positive reinforcing rewarding effect, and this result overrides negative experiences of physical pain. The experience of negative emotional states like anxiety, depression and a sense of failure, are like strong punishment. In other words, punishment decreases the frequency of a response and stops the behaviours leading to it. Some of the common methods based on principle of punishment are time out from reinforcement, overcorrection and response cost. These methods, if used consistently and systematically, have been found to be very effective in modifying problem behaviour in children (Mehta, 1989).

Comparison between Classical Conditioning and Operant Conditioning

Both classical and operant conditioning are the important methods of learning, but you would have observed that these two types of conditioning are different in their process of learning from each other. These differences have been highlighted in the following Table 5.1.

Cognitive Learning

In learning more complex tasks, perception and knowledge or cognitive processes play an important role. Cognitive theorists state that learning cannot be satisfactorily explained in terms of stimulus response association. They propose, that a learner forms a cognitive structure in memory, which organizes information into relationships and meaning. Without any known reinforcement, new associations are formed and new relationships are perceived among events,

Table 5.1: Comparison between classical conditioning and operant conditioning

Classical conditioning	Operant conditioning
1. Stimulus oriented	Response oriented
2. UCS is given irrespective of the organism's behaviour	Organism's own behaviour determines whether or not the UCS will be presented
3. Time interval between the CS and the UCS is rigidly behaviour	Time interval depends on the organism's own fixed
4. CR is reflexively forced by UCS	Response is more voluntary and spontaneous
5. CR and UCR are similar but not identical	Similarity is the exception rather than rule
6. Responses involuntarily medicated by autonomic nervous system like eye blink	Responses under voluntary control, mediated by the central nervous system
7. The unconditioned stimulus (UCS) occurs without regard to the subject behaviour	The reward is contingent upon the occurrence of response
8. Association between stimulus response (S-R) is on the basis of law of contiguity (things occurring closer time and space get associated)	Association between stimulus response (S-R) is on the basis of law of in effect (effect of reward and punishm'
9. Reinforcement comes first, as food is presented first to elicit the response	Reinforcement is provided after the response is mac' by the organism
10. Stress is laid on time control	Place of motivation and reward is stressed
11. The essence of learning is stimulus substitution	The essence of learning is response modificatio'

simply as a result of having experienced these events. Links are made among stimuli, so that stimulus-stimulus (S-S) associations are learned. These theories take account of concept formation, in which the learner actively tests his ideas, rules and principles, in order to make sense of incoming information. Bruner et al (1966) hypothesised that the learner interprets and transforms any incoming stimulus in the light of previous experience. Gagne suggested that learning is an eight stage hierarchical process, involving events both internal and external to the learner and which incorporate many different types of learning (see Box 5.1).

> **Box 5.1: STAGES OF LEARNING**
> - Motivation (desire to learn new things)
> - Apprehending or attending (perceiving the relevant information)
> - Acquisition (the learner codes the information)
> - Retention (the information is stored in memory)
> - Recall (the information is retrieved from memory)
> - Generalisation (the information is applied to novel situations)
> - Performance (or practice of what has been learned)
> - Feedback (The learner receives knowledge of their performance)

Cognitive learning includes some of the following methods of learning.

Insight learning: Kohler, a German psychologist, on the basis of this experiments on chimpanzees, emphasised that while working on a problem, one grasps three inner relationships through insight, not through mere trial and error, but by perceiving the relationships essential to solution. In his typical experiment, a chimpanzee in the bars was given two unequal sizes of sticks and the fruit was kept outside the bars, which could not be reached by one stick alone. After several trials, the animal all of a sudden joined the two sticks together to make it a single long stick, and with that he could reach the fruit.

Insight is often used in problem solving, puzzles and riddles. To emphasise the suddenness of the solution, it is also called by some as "Aha experience" (see Chapter 7).

Sign learning: It is an acquired expectation that one stimulus will be followed by another in a particular context. What we learn is a set of expectations or a cognitive map of the environment, rather than specific responses.

Toleman believed that some learning is sign learning. We develop a sort of cognitive map or structure, instead of learning a sequence of the task. On the basis of understanding, we tend to make spatial relationships.

Social Learning

There are many forms of learning, which cannot be explained through conditioning or through cognitive learning. We also learn through observation. Social learning theorists stress upon observational learning or modeling, in which a person acquires a response to a specific situation, by watching others make a response (Bandura, 1969).

Imitation is one of the important methods based on this theory, which could be applied in learning of many skills. For example, many of your skills like giving an injection, measuring blood pressure, dressing of a wound or surgical skills, are learned by simply observing seniors performing those skills. Even maladaptive behaviours, like aggression are learnt through imitation. The learner acquires and stores internal (representations) response through images and verbal coding, which may be expressed later. Social learning methods are also applied in behaviour therapy (see Chapter 20).

Observational Learning

Imagine the following events:
1. A student watches a consultant surgeon operating on an infant for diaphragmatic

hernia. In this way, he begins to acquire the complex skills needed for this type of surgery.
2. A group of young men and women listen to a detailed account of an unusual, but highly successful bank robbery on the evening news. Later, they plan and carry out a similar robbery themselves.

These two situations are different, yet they share one important feature of learning through observation. In each case, new forms of behaviour were acquired simply by observing others' actions.

There has been rising recognition of the key role played by observational learning in the behaviour of young children. Many experiments suggest that youngsters acquire a wide range of responses, including attitudes, values, and self-control, through exposure to their parents or other persons that is, through exposure to social models (Rushton, 1976; Bandura, 1977). In several early studies, Albert Bandura and his colleagues exposed children to brief films, in which an adult model acted aggressively toward an inflated plastic doll. Observational learning is increased when we pay close attention to the actions of others, but is reduced when such attention is absent. It is also increased when we attempt to first summarise or code others' behaviour in some manner, and then rehearse it (Bandura, 1977; Berger et al 1979).

Latent Learning

This type of learning refers to any changes that are not evidenced by behaviour at the time of the learning. It occurs without any reinforcement for particular responses, and seems to involve changes in the way in which information is processed. You can get ample examples of latent learning from your own experiences. This is different from observational learning, as you have not consciously put an effort to learning, but later you can perform that particular skill or responses.

Biological Learning

You would have seen that in spite of using similar methods of learning, devoting similar time, yet all persons are not able to learn in a same way. Some people take more time to learn as compared to others. Thus, important process of learning cannot be fully understood without some grasp of the biological functioning of different people. We possess different capacities to receive and process different abilities to learn. The study of learning has acquired a new perspective, one in which the impact of biological factors is given increased emphasis. The most important concept that emerged out of this perspective is concept of preparedness, proposed by Seligman (1970). According to this concept, persons are prepared by their biological structure and function, to accomplish certain kinds of learning but not others. Learned behaviour can be divided into distinct categories.

Prepared: These actions are closely related to the survival of the persons and very little training is required.

Unprepared: The tasks are learned slowly as and when required by the person. These are not related to the survival.

Contraprepared: These are responses, which are contrary to the persons' natural tendencies, for example, fears.

These findings seem to suggest that as human beings, we are prepared to acquire fears of some stimuli, e.g. snakes, lizards, etc. but not others, e.g. houses, flowers. This possibility is also seen in clinical practice. While individuals come for help in over-coming fears of some animals, objects and situations, but not on others.

Principles of Learning

Learning is primarily controlled by the learner. It is unique and individual. It is affected by the total state of the learner. It can be cooperative and collaborative, it is an evolutionary process. It is a consequence of experience and is not directly observable. There are four principles of learning:

Individuality of the Learner

Each learner is a unique individual in terms of the style of learning and rate of learning. However, given adequate time and flexibility in approach all individuals can attain required level of competence.

All Learning is Contextual

Learning takes place when a person 'interacts' with a problem/situation, and 'processes' information in the light of his/her own previous learning and experience. By providing real life experience or using simulated situation, learning can be made more meaningful. Participatory training techniques, in which the trainee actively participates in the learning process, should be used, such as group discussions, case studies, demonstration, role play, games, exercises, projects, field work, etc. New learning should be built on the previous experience of the trainees. Asking questions about previous learning, not only activates the learner, but also helps in proper understanding of the subject.

Role of Motivation

Motivation holds the key for all learning. Motivation depends upon the needs felt by the individual, which varies from individual-to-individual, and from one situation to the other. However, one can make following generalisations regarding the factors motivating an adult learner:

- Physiological needs: (self-preservation/existence, hunger, sex)
- Security: job security, living conditions, etc.
- Social status: recognition, fellow feeling
- Esteem: ego fulfillment
- Self-actualisation: working for the sake of excellence.

These are organised in a hierarchical manner. Unless the lower level need is met, the higher ones usually do not operate; e.g. an under-paid nursing orderly is more concerned about his pay, perks and making living. A doctor whose such needs are fulfilled might work for esteem or recognition.

Positive reinforcement of the correct response in course of learning greatly facilitates learning. The reinforcement could be in the form of verbal response (e.g. excellent, fantastic, ideal, that is great, etc.); it could be a nonverbal gesture (e.g. a pat, or a smile, etc.). Rewards have a positive effect on motivation and the punishment has negative influence. While promotion, higher pay, perks, awards medals, etc. represent extrinsic form of motivation; self-satisfaction, working for sake of work, pursuit of excellence represent intrinsic motivation. Intrinsic motivation lasts longer than extrinsic motivation.

Motivation is heightened, when a person has clear idea of the 'goals', and when he perceives value of reaching the goal. If the goal is not clear or not achievable at all, a person is not likely to put in efforts. Adult learners always think: is it worth pursuing? What do I get out of it? Does this task help in any way in my present or future job performance? The extent to which the answer is 'yes', the person is likely to put in effort. If the goal is not clear or not achievable at all, a person is not likely to put in efforts.

Motivation calls for a 'nonthreatening' environment in learning. Though learning is a cognitive activity, it is also an emotional experience. People learn when they are happy, cheerful. The training atmosphere must be cordial. The attitude of the trainer to a large extent determines this factor. A democratic and friendly trainer is more effective than an authoritarian, conservative trainer.

Feedback

Learning is very much facilitated, when individuals are helped to set the goals and given continuous feedback on their progress. The knowledge of success or failure includes not only the extent of achievement or failure, but also the logic and the cause of failure. Successful performance of tasks increases confidence, which again breeds success. The failure may either lead to frustration or may enthuse the person to take alternate approach leading to success.

How is Learning Facilitated?

Over the last few years, research studies have been focussed on how students learn. Learning process is influenced by a host of factors such as ability to concentrate, memory, organisation of learning material. Some of the students have difficulties with their studies, arising not just from lack of application or psychosocial problems, but from specific problems with the way they study and learn. There seems little doubt that good study skills contribute to academic success. With the skills, the student should have a positive attitude and motivation to the subject. It is very important to organise the time and resources available to the learner. Here are some tips by which you can learn more effectively.

Definite Goal

In any learning, student should have clear goal in view, as with a goal in mind, one works towards a definite and sure purpose. Students should get specific, immediate and achievable goals, as they enhance your motivation to learn and ensure better learning.

Knowledge of Results or Psychological Feedback

The learner must also have conscious assurance that he is making progress towards his achievement. Frequent and regular review of the amount of progress being made toward the goal, act as a strong motive to promote continuing effort on the part of the learner.

Distribution of Practice Periods

A number of experiments have demonstrated those shorter practice periods are more economical than longer periods, and when distributed over several days; they yield better returns that when they are concentrated into a single sitting.

Whole versus Part Method

Whether the entire topic should be learned all the way through in each trial, or by breaking it into small portions and learning in turns? The former is known as whole method and latter as part method. With easy units, whole method should be adopted. If material is difficult in relation to the learner's ability, smaller units should be learnt; but they still are as large wholes as a learner can manage efficiently. Try to learn in natural units.

Logical Learning

This means that instead of learning by heart, rote memorisation, you should try to grasp meaning and idea of the text. Logical learning calls for an arrangement and assimilation with other ideas in mind.

Rest Pauses

Take brief rest pauses in between your studies as mental fatigue blocks your ability to remember and think.

Avoid undue Anxiety

Worry, apprehension or nervousness interferes with good performance. Forgetting is more in state of anxiety.

Rhyming

To improve memory, rhyming can be helpful, as it is well known that certain kind of material (poems Vs. prose) can be learnt better by rhyming.

Rational use of Media

When information is given through multiple channels (viz. audio and visual), it makes stronger memory traces. Moreover, in medical education, the students need to understand and develop ability to see relationship among various topics. With the use of media (e.g. video films of self-instructional programmes), a learner can go through the material at his own pace.

Overlearning

Continuing repetitions of stimulus response learning, even after 100% reproductions, help retain learned material over a longer period of time.

Reading Aloud

Better learning can be ensured at times with reading aloud than silent reading, especially if one has habit to get into day dreaming. This method of learning can be applied to many clinical situations like treatment of speech disorders.

LEARNING STYLES

Kirti studies day and night, yet barely manages to pass. Ravi can learn better through group discussions, whereas Amit learns better by self-learning. These differences in learning reported by these students as well as by some others, indicate that all students do not have the same method of learning. They have different methods of reading, interpreting and coding the information. There are individual differences in a student's ability to assimilate, retain and reproduce at the required time. Often, their strategies or methods of processing information are useful. However, some students may develop pathological learning strategies.

Different students describe their learning experience differently. Some students describe learning as the retention of knowledge achieved through repetition and recitation, while others describe it as an interpretative process aimed at understanding reality. Several studies have led to elucidation of the concept of learning strategies.

How does Students Learn?

Every student implements a set of procedures for accomplishing learning. These procedures denote that learning strategies are determined by student's perception and personal attributes. Two basic approaches to learning have been identified, namely, the "surface" and the "deep" approach.

The students with surface approach tend to memorise important parts of the text, from which they anticipate questions in assessment. The learning outcome is essentially a reproduction of the words from the textbook. Their focus of attention is limited to the specific facts, or disconnected information, which is rote, learned. Furthermore, the surface approach does not include perception of the holistic structure of information, but instead atomises it into disconnected bits and pieces that are memorised through repetition. This means that students taking a surface approach fail to derive full meaning, including implications and connections from information they have gone through.

On the other hand, students with deep approach try to understand the meaning of the materials and relate it to previous knowledge, concepts and experiences. A deep approach involves perception of the holistic organisation of the material studied, organised in a hierarchical manner. A student using this approach is able to extract the meaning from words, not focussing on words as an end in themselves. The learner is sensitive to relationships among topics and to the structure.

A medical student needs to have a versatile approach. He should be able to use both deep as well as surface approaches as required, for a particular learning task. It is also important that he looks for the meaning and comprehends the learning material. In a study at AIIMS, it has been observed that in the 1st semester, undergraduate students adopt the surface approach. But by the time they reach the 7th, 8th semester, their approach changes towards deep. This change is linked to the demands of the curriculum assessment, teaching style and learning environment (Fig. 5.4).

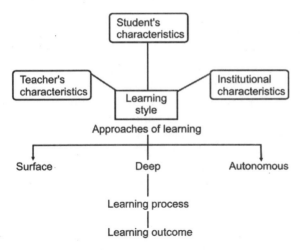

Fig. 5.4: Factors affecting learning outcome

Student Autonomy

Medical students ultimately need to become more effective learners, to enable themselves to respond to the variety of situations faced by them during their medical profession. A medical student learns a great deal on his own pace. Student autonomy refers to student independence and responsibility with regard to his learning. A medical student needs to develop an ability to decide which areas of study require more focus than others, and also which type of approach should be used in learning specific skills or subject matter.

Ability to think independently can be promoted by developing certain skills like choosing, deciding, deliberating, reflecting planning and judging. Cognitive and emotional development of the students also have a bearing on the development, which leads to increasing differentiation of perceptual categories revealing the uniqueness of events. On the emotional side, self-esteem and self-confidence in the student helps in the development of autonomy.

Skills Requisites of an Autonomous Learner

Autonomy in learning does not come naturally to all students; it is a capability, which needs to be developed. If the student is exposed to the autonomous methods of learning without internalising the values of autonomy, then it will not result in the change of his approach. To be an autonomous student, one needs to have an ability and willingness to approach a situation with an open mind, to suspend critical judgement, and to act in accordance with rules and principles which are the product of the autonomous person's own endeavours and experiences.

Certain attributes of an autonomous learner need to be inculcated, in order to be an effective learner in higher education. The most important characteristic is that students should take responsibility for their own learning. Following are some steps to initiate autonomous learning in medical students (Table 5.2).

Table 5.2: Steps in autonomous learning

- Identifying learning needs
- Setting goals and planning learning activities
- Finding resource learning material
- Conjuring up problems to tackle
- Using teachers as guide
- Undertaking additional nonteacher guidance
- Self-assessment and reflection on their learning process

In the setting of medical education, autonomous approaches to learning are of great relevance. One such approach is in the form of problem-based learning. The basic idea here is that the starting point for learning should be a problem, a query or a puzzle that the learner wishes to solve. Organized forms of knowledge and academic disciplines should be introduced, when the demands of the problems require them.

Role of Teachers in Facilitating Learning

The teachers should help the students to be autonomous learners. This can be achieved by guiding them to learn to focus in meanings of the contents. This can also be achieved by using advance organizers. Prior to teaching a new topic, the student goes through the main points of the study and gets a clearer idea of the subject. According to Ramsden, the factors influencing include teaching methods, the degree of enthusiasm/commitment of the teachers, the structure, pace and the level at which information is presented. The teachers need to provide opportunities for students to learn in a way, which suits the students preferred style of learning. Thus, teachers have an important role in helping students to learn successfully, control their cognitive processes, including learning to learn, to remember and to think.

But a student has a major responsibility in learning by developing skills to use learning strategies judiciously according to the topic, and develop motivation to learn and to handle his emotions.

Clinical Applications of Learning

Learning is fundamental to the development and modification of behaviour; knowledge concerning the process may be usefully applied to many clinical situations, not only for the patients but also for the students and professionals. Many of our subjective feelings, emotions and attitudes are probably conditioned responses. Through generalisation, it becomes difficult to identify the origin of our emotional responses. Both our adaptive emotional responses as well as unadaptive responses are learned and can be unlearned through principle of learning.

Behaviour modification or behaviour therapy is a group of techniques commonly used in the treatment of various psychiatric disorders, and in the training of mentally handicapped children. Cognitive learning methods are also applied in clinical settings.

Learning methods have wide applications in educational setting. In programmed learning, the material to be learned is broken up into small easy steps, so that the learner can accomplish without frustrations. Also with programmed learning, learner can master the task at his own pace. With versatile and flexible learning you can improve your learning style. Use of reinforcement principles can often, increase productivity, both in studies as well as in vocation.

The principles of operant conditioning have also been applied to various clinical problems. One example concerns the attempt to improve the social behaviour of long-stay patients in psychiatric hospitals.

Other conditions of clinical interest, where operant conditioning principles may be important—both in causation and treatment—are those disorders of behaviour, for example, excessive gambling, smoking, over eating and addictions. These behaviours are maladaptive in the sense of being harmful to the individual, yet become habitual. Other examples of maladaptive behaviour familiar to general medicine are abnormal illness behaviour, and noncompliance of treatment, can also be modified using behavioural techniques.

Learning theories have not only been applied to clinical problems of patients, but have also been applied in development of techniques to acquire clinical skills by health professionals. Some of these skills are related to interpersonal relationships. These skills are required for *'bedside'* examination of patients, dealing with family members of the patients, and with colleagues, seniors and junior staff. Although personality differences may contribute to variation in this respect, clinical skills have to be developed through the process of learning. Many of such skills are learnt through imitation, modelling and role-playing.

There are certain disorders in which individual's ability to acquire new information is impaired (e.g. clouded consciousness, dementia). There are psychological tests to detect and measure the extent of impairment of learning. These are generally based on speed with which new material can be learned by the patient.

SUMMARY

Learning is defined as any relatively permanent change in behaviour that occurs as a result of practice or experience. Methods of learning are classified as: classical conditioning, operant conditioning, cognitive learning and social learning, observational learning, latent learning and biological learning. In classical conditioning, a neutral stimulus CS is presented before the unconditioned stimulus (US), that evokes an unconditioned response (UR). As a result of association, the previously neutral stimulus begins to elicit a conditioned response (CR). In operant conditioning, an action of the learner is instrumental in bringing about a change in the environment that makes the action more or less likely to occur again in the future. Reinforcement is basic in this form of learning. Cognitive learning refers to changes in the way information is processed as a result of experience a person has had. Insight learning and sign learning are examples of cognitive learning. Social learning emphasises the role of observation, imitation and modelling in learning. Biological learning places emphasis on differences in the capability of individuals. There are four principles of learning, namely, individual differences in the learner, all learning is contextual, motivation and feedback is important for learning to progress. Learning can be facilitated by defining a definite goal, giving feedback, spacing your study time, learning unit size that is easily grasped, understanding the material rather than rote learning and by avoiding anxiety.

There are different learning styles used by the students. These are surface, deep and versatile; these learning styles also influence the learning outcome. In medical education, the students need to adopt their own autonomous approaches to learning. Teachers and education environment play a crucial role in helping students to develop the learning styles.

Clinical applications of learning are related to development of phobias, depression and other maladaptive behaviours. Behaviour therapy, social skills training and cognitive therapy are offshoot of learning theories. Learning pathologies cause failure and learning styles determine the learning outcome. Thus faulty learning styles can be modified.

Intelligence

Ramesh had recently celebrated his fifth birthday. His joyous parents got him admitted in a public school. Ramesh enthusiastically started going to the school. He had made one friend in his class. Gradually, Ramesh's mother got complaints from the teachers that he was NOT able to cope up with the task in the class, which other children were doing quite well. His parents started teaching the child at home, and also arranged an extra tuition class for him after the school hours. Yet Ramesh was either making too many spelling mistakes, or was not able to memorise, his handwriting was also very poor. Ramesh was no longer keen to go to the school. Ramesh's parents were advised to get his intelligence assessed. On standardised intelligence test Ramesh got a score of 70, borderline intelligence. He was advised admission in a special school for slow learners. Ramesh's parents could not judge his intelligence because it cannot be observed like height or weight, it can only be inferred from behaviour.

Intelligence as a concept is used very commonly in our day-to-day life. We often make comments that this person seems to be very intelligent or seems to be dull. But what is this intelligence? Different people would give different meaning to intelligence. Similarly psychologists have attributed a variety of factors to the concept of intelligence.

Definition

Most commonly accepted view is that intelligence is a general capacity for comprehension and reasoning that manifests itself in various ways. The most widely accepted definition is, "Intelligence is the global capacity of an individual to act purposefully, to think rationally and to deal effectively with his environment" (Weschler 1944). It includes the power of adaptation of an individual to his milieu, his ability to learn and for abstract thinking.

Difference between Intelligence and Aptitude

A distinction has to be made between intelligence and aptitude. Intelligence is the capacity or the potentiality that a person has, whereas aptitude is a combination of characteristics indicative of an individual's capacity to acquire some specific knowledge, or skill. Aptitude means an individual's aptitude for a given type of activity, the capacity to acquire proficiency under appropriate conditions.

Nature of Intelligence

Different theories have been proposed to understand the nature of intelligence.

Two Factor Theory

Charles Spearman (1927) proposed that individuals possess general intelligence factor (G) in varying amounts (degree). This determines the individual's overall ability. In addition to G, individuals also possess specific abilities, (S) G is universal inborn ability, and it is general mental energy. The amount of 'G' differs from individual-to-individual. Higher the 'G' in an individual, higher is the success in life. 'S' is learned and acquired in the environment, it varies from activity-to-activity even in the same individual: the individuals themselves differ in the amount of 'S' ability (Fig. 6.1).

Two individuals in a class may be comparable on their G factor, yet one may be very good with numbers while the other possesses higher musical ability.

Multifactor Theories

a. Thurstone (1936) felt that intelligence could be broken down into a number of primary mental abilities. He had derived 7 primary mental abilities on the basis of factor analyses. These abilities, as shown in the Table 6.1 are represented in items in test construction.

b. Guilford has broadened the concept of intelligence. According to him there are two types of thinking: (a) convergent thinking—solving a problem that has a defined correct answer and (b) divergent thinking—arriving

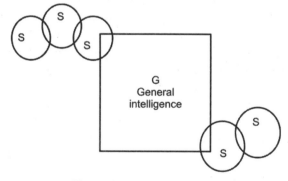

Fig. 6.1: Two factor theory

Table 6.1: Primary mental abilities

Ability	Description
Verbal comprehension	Understanding meaning of words.
Word fluency	Ability to think rapidly
Number	Perform calculations
Space	Visualise space form relationship
Memory	Recall verbal stimuli
Perceptual speed	Grasp of visual details
Reasoning	Ability to find a general rule, logical thinking.

at many possible solutions to a problem. This is predominantly creative thinking. He had proposed a three dimensional theory represented in a cubical model shown in Figure 6.2. Guilford maintained that intelligence test items should distinguish in terms of the operations performed upon the content and the product that results. This model provides for 120 factors of intelligence, which is a combination yield of 4 contents, 5 operations and 6 products. Assume that a subject is asked to rearrange jumble of words, e.g. CEIV, NERTE, to form a familiar words (VICE, ENTER). The content is symbolic; since the test involves a set of letter symbols; the operation is 'cognition' because it requires recognition of information and the product unit is a word.

Process Oriented Theories

These theories have focussed on intellectual processes—the pattern of thinking that people use when they reason and solve problems. These theorists prefer to use the term cognitive processes in place of intelligence. They are often more interested in how people solve problems and how many get the right solution. They have focussed on the development of cognitive abilities. Piaget's work is a significant contribution in this area (see Chapter 12). He viewed intelligence as an adaptive process that involves interplay of biological maturation and interaction with environment.

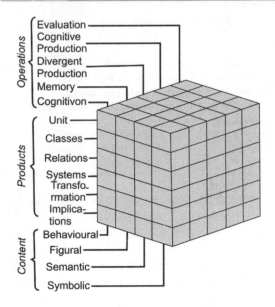

Fig. 6.2: Guilford's model of intelligence

Information Processing Theories

These theories break intelligence down into various basic skills that people employ to take in information, process it, and then use it to reason and solve problems. These basic skills may be simple or complex. Robert Sternberg (1984), distinguishes between information processing "components" and "metacomponents". Components are the steps to solve a problem and metacomponents are the basics of knowledge that one has to know to solve the problem. The information processing theory has often been compared with computers in which attention and memory have been designated as the intellectual hardware whereas the action schemes (Piagetian notion) are similar to specific, repeatable intellectual sequences, and executive schemes, similar to plans and strategies. The neo Piagetians are of the opinion that people's software becomes more sophisticated as they mature, with their schemes expanding in complexity and their amount of available mental energy increasing. Such changes in their view, promote the growth of intelligence. Other approaches focus on the rules involved in intelligent behaviour or the skills required for various tasks.

Hebb (1966) has distinguished two meanings of intelligence on neurological basis. Intelligence A is the innate potential based on the developmental process. This type of intelligence is dependent upon 'the possession of a good brain and a good neural metabolism'. Intelligence B involves the functioning of the brain, and is observable indirectly from the individual's behaviour. Intelligence A is not observable and cannot be measured, whereas intelligence B is measured through tests.

Cattell (1971) on the basis of factor analysis, has divided general factor of intelligence (G) into two parts—fluid intelligence (GF) and crystallised intelligence (GC). The former being innate, biologically or genetically determined and the latter is acquired based on cultural and educational experience. Fluid intelligence is related to ability to solve problems, thus is assessed on intelligence test like block design test on progressive matrices. Crystallised knowledge thus is measured on tests of information, arithmetic and vocabulary.

Eysenck (1973) distinguishes between speed and power components of intelligence. Speed is measured by the time required to complete the task and power is measured through test of reasoning.

Jensen (1980) splits intelligence into two levels. Associative ability being the capacity to learn, remember and recall information. It represents the lower level of continuum. Cognitive ability is concerned with reasoning and is located at the higher level. Cognitive ability depends upon associated ability but not *vice versa*.

Earl Hunt (1983) proposed that individual differences in intelligence are due to the different processes people use in solving problems. Hunt identifies these ways of cognitive processes that makes difference in people. These are: (1) way to internally represent a problem, (2) strategies for manipulating mental representation and (3) abilities necessary to execute basic information processing steps, according to the strategy requirement.

Howard Gardner (1983) has proposed seven types of intelligence, each one of those is important. The seven intelligences identified by Gardner are—
1. Linguistic ability
2. Logical-mathematical ability
3. Spatial ability (navigating in space, using mental images)
4. Musical ability
5. Bodily-kinesthetic ability
6. Interpersonal ability (understanding others)
7. Intrapersonal ability (understanding oneself).

Robert Sternberg (1986) has suggested triarchic (three points of origin) components in intelligence—in this knowledge acquisition, performance and metacognition is for learning new facts, for problem solving strategies and techniques for selecting a strategy and monitoring process towards success. According to Sternberg individuals can improve their experimental, contextual intelligence and componential intelligence by practice and effort.

Emotional Intelligence (EI)

Emotional intelligence refers to the way we handle the each other and ourselves. Peter Salovey and John Mayer (1990) coined the term emotional intelligence. Later Daniel Goleman (1995) did extensive work on the concept of emotional intelligence. Though personal intelligence is important for academic abilities yet emotional intelligence contributes towards a balanced personality. Emotional intelligence helps 'to be angry with a right person, to the right degree, at the right time, for the right purpose and in the right way' (Aristotle). The competencies of the emotional intelligence are crucial for success in work and in interpersonal relationships. It trains people to manage emotions and develop to skills to handle relationships. The five domains of emotional intelligence are—
- Knowing one's emotions
- Managing emotions
- Motivating oneself
- Recognising emotions in others
- Handling relationships.

It is feasible to enhance emotional intelligence through training. Currently attempts are being made to include training in emotional intelligence in the school curriculum.

Intelligence Quotient (IQ)

IQ is a commonly used term, which was first suggested by Stern and Kuplmann in 1912. On individuals, Intelligence quotient is expressed as a ratio of mental age (MA) to the chronological age (CA).

$$IQ = \frac{MA}{CA} \times 100$$

The ratio is multiplied by 100 to remove the decimal. If the child has an average mental age, then a correlation of his mental age (MA) and the chronological age (CA) will form a straight line. In case the individual's mental age (MA) is higher than the chronological age (CA) then the curve will be different as shown in Figure 6.3.

An individual with an average intelligence has an IQ of 100. If the mental development falls behind the individual will have an IQ less than 100 and if the rate of development is faster the individual will have an IQ more than 100. If two children six and eight years old obtain a MA of seven years on an intelligence test then the younger child has a higher intellect.

If Child - A $\frac{MA\ 7}{CA\ 8} \times 100 = 88$

Child - B $\frac{MA\ 7}{CA\ 6} \times 100 = 117$

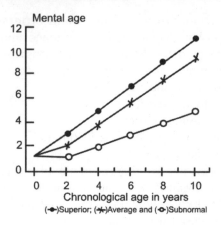

Fig. 6.3: Correlation of mental age and chronological age

Child A with an IQ of 88 is dull in comparison to child B who has superior intelligence with an IQ of 117. Descriptive terms are also applied to individuals whose intelligence test scores fall within the various bands under the normal curve (Atkinson et al. 1993). These are given in Table 6.2.

Table 6.2: Classification of IQ scores

IQ score	Descriptive term
130+	Very superior
120–129	Superior
110–119	Bright normal
90–109	Normal
80–89	Low normal
70–79	Borderline
50>~ 69	Mild mental subnormal
35–49	Moderate mental subnormal
20–34	Severe mental subnormal
0–19	Profound

These terms are used into determine what level of remedial treatment or care is required by those with mental subnormality.

Growth of Intelligence

Generally the growth of intelligence is rapid during early childhood and then slows down in teens (Fig. 6.4). Longitudinal studies using Wechsler's tests have shown that mental ability increases upto the age of twenty-six, after which it levels off and remains unchanged till late thirties. There is a gradual decrease in the intellectual ability after forty with a sharp decline after sixty. But it must be noted that decline in ability depends both on the person and the type of ability tested. Individuals engaged in active stimulating working environments with good physical health show little decrease in intellectual ability upto age seventy. Physical disabilities, particularly those resulting from strokes or progressive reduction of blood circulation to the brain usually result in a significant decrease in intellectual ability.

Mental abilities that require speed and short-term memory decline earlier than general knowledge. The rate of decline of specific abilities is related to one's occupation, like people in literary work or professionals do not decline in mental ability as early as others. Experience and accumulated knowledge compensates for diminished speed in old age.

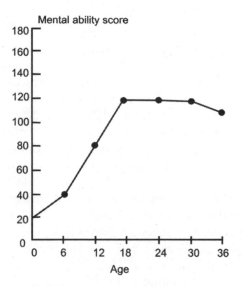

Fig. 6.4: Growth of intelligence

Stability of Intelligence

The stability of intelligence or IQ has received a great deal of attention from the educational psychologists because of its usefulness in education. There are two opinions. One holds that the IQ remains relatively stable over the years changing only very slowly. Another opinion is that if determined effort is made, a change in IQ can be obtained. There is a considerable evidence to indicate that stability in IQ is not absolute but only a small range of scores would change.

An extensive body of data accumulated, shows that intelligence test performance is quite stable. Studies have reported high correlations ranging from .72 to .83 on retest of intelligence scales. Bradway, Thompon and Cravens conducted a follow up on children originally tested between the age of 2 and 5.5 years as part of the 1937 Stanford Binet standardisation sample. Initial IQs correlated .65 with 10 years retests and .59 with 25 years retests. The correlation between 10-year retest mean age 14 years and mean age 29 years (25 year retest) was .85. If the initial assessment is done in late childhood or after that then the correlations are found to be very high. The instability of IQ may occur as a result of drastic environmental changes. It can increase with stimulation and training but can decrease due to prolonged or severe illness, head injury, brain damage, high fevers, epilepsy, meningitis and adverse environmental factors like conflict at home, death of parent, malnutrition. Instability of scores could also be due to fast or slow development of the child than that of the normative sample population. Generally children in continually disadvantaged environments tend to lose and those in stimulating environments gain in IQ with age. The relationship between IQ, educational attainment, and later occupational achievement is positive. Many highly intelligent people perform disappointingly, while many with average IQ may do remarkably well. This is because factors other than intelligence, such as drive, persistence, attention, useful social contacts, and highly-developed social skills, are of major importance in the achievement in later life.

Determinants of Intelligence

The question of relative importance of 'nature' and 'nurture' as a determinant of intelligence has been controversial. The role of genetics or heritability and environment has been extensively studied. Their comparative roles in determining intelligence are as follows:

Heredity

Evidence pointing to the influence of heredity on intelligence comes mainly from family and the twin studies. A heritability index shows the proportional contribution of genetic or heredity factors of a particular trait in a given population under existing conditions. A frequent procedure to compute heritability index is to utilise intelligence test correlations of monozygotic (identical) and dizygotic (fraternal) twins. Correlations between monozygotic twins reared together and between monozygotic twins reared apart in the foster homes, have also been used. Table 6.3 summarises the results of a large number of studies (Bouchard et al 1990), indicating that closer the genetic relationship, the more similar is the tested intelligence.

Table 6.3: Correlation of intelligence with heredity

Relationship	Correlation
Parents and natural children	.40
Parents and adopted children	.31
Dizygotic twin	.60
Monozygotic twin	
Reared together	.86
Reared apart	.72
Cousins	.15

Heritability estimates for intelligence have ranged from .40 to .86. The lower estimate is based on the assumption that a sizeable portion of variation in IQ scores can be attributed to a genetic environmental covariation. Parents can influence their offspring both by direct genetic transmission and by the kind of environment they provide.

Environment

Even though intelligence has a significant genetic component, environmental conditions can also be crucially important. The influence of the environment begins from the moment of conception. The development of the foetus, especially at critical times, may be affected by various physical factors including mother's diet, smoking, disease such as rubella and certain drugs. Subsequent environment especially during childhood, socioeconomic status, nutrition, health and educational influences of the family are very important determinants of IQ.

It has been recognised that children from lower social class families generally perform less well on intelligence tests than those from higher social classes. Studies of family influences suggest that greater parental attention received by children of smaller families and the first-born may result in higher scores. The use of media and the educational toys provide the right environment for intellectual stimulation. Similarly urban and rural set up, type of school attended lead to differential stimulation and type of experience which in turn affects the intelligence scores. Effect of education not only influences the test scores, but teacher's expectation may speed up or slow down the development of individual child.

One of the most convincing evidence for the influence of the environment comes from successful attempts, through intensive stimulation and education, to improve the IQs in high-risk children and mentally handicapped. Similarly IQ scores have been found to increase, when children are transferred from poor institutions to good foster homes.

To sum up, both heredity and environment play an important role in determining intelligence. These can be compared to land and seeds used to grow crop. Seed is like heredity and the land is like environment. If the land is not fertile, then even with good seed one cannot have a good crop. Similarly with a fertile land if poor quality seeds are used, the crop will not achieve good results. Thus just as for good crop, both fertile land and good quality seeds are required, similarly both heredity and stimulating environments are required for higher intelligence.

Extremes of Intelligence

Mental Subnormality

Mental subnormality refers to subaverage general intellectual functioning, which originates in the developmental period and is associated with impairment in adaptive behaviour. A person is regarded as mentally subnormal if: (i) the IQ attained is below 70 on standard psychological tests of intelligence; (ii) their adaptive skills are inadequate to cope up with the daily routines. Adaptation skills are those behaviours by which an individual makes adjustments and independent living in the society. In childhood these are the self help activities such as eating and dressing independently. Later on the adaptive behaviours are concerned with basic academic skills, coping skills such as telling time, using money and assuming social responsibilities. Slowness in intellectual development may be widespread and affect all aspects of cognition. Only rarely will a child's functioning be retarded to the same degree over the entire range of skills, but where such skills are significantly impaired, it is reasonable to think of the child as showing general mental subnormality.

In our country the problem of mental subnormality is quite significant. The studies have shown an incidence of 4-5 per 1000 individuals. Mental subnormality is categorised in four levels—mild, moderate, severe and profound. Table 6.4 gives the characteristics of each of these levels.

Clinical features: Mental subnormality may first be identified by delay in their motor milestones in the first few months of life. The child will be slow to obtain head control, sit unsupported. Large number of moderately retarded children however, shows normal motor development and present for the first time with language delay. The child may be thought to be deaf because he fails to take notice of sounds or shows lack of single words or word combinations at the appropriate age. Mildly retarded children may not be detected until they enter school when failure of educational progress may be found to be due to a general slowness of development rather than to a specific learning disability. Usually however, it will be found that the early development of the mildly retarded especially their early language development has been slow. Occasionally mental retardation arises as a result of some postnatal event, such as a head injury or cerebral infection. In these cases the time course of the condition will, of course be different.

Once diagnosed, the clinical features of children with mental retardation will depend more especially on:
1. The severity of the condition
2. The presence of associated physical and psychiatric conditions
3. The quality of care and education the child receives.

Management: Management should begin with an explanation to the parents of the diagnosis, its probable cause, the way in which the child can be helped, and the likely outcome. It is important to reassure parents that their behaviour has not produced the condition, though this does not mean that, in the future, there is not much they can do to help the child.

Table 6.4: Characteristics of persons with various degrees of mental subnormality

Description	Mild	Moderate	Severe
Preschool 0-5 yrs.	Can develop social and communication skills, minimal retardation in sensory-motor areas, often not distinguished from normal until late age.	Can talk, learn to communicate: poor social awareness; fair motor development, profits from training in self-help; can be managed with moderate supervision.	Poor motor development, speech minimal; general unable to profit from self-help; little or no communication skills
School age 6-20 yrs. Training and Education	Can learn academic skills upto approximately 6th grade level by late teens; can be guided toward social conformity	Can profit from training in social and occupational skills; unlikely to progress beyond 2nd grade level in academic subjects; may learn to travel alone in familiar environment.	can talk or learn to communicate, can be trained elemental health habits, profits from systematic habit training
Adult 21 and over social and vocational adequacy	Can usually achieve social and vocational skills, adequate to minimum self-support but may need guidance and assistance when under unusual social or economic stress.	May achieve self-maintenance unskilled or semiskilled work under sheltered conditions, needs supervision and guidance when under mild social or economic stress.	May contribute partially to self maintenance under complete supervision; can develop self-protection skills to a minimal useful level in controlled environment.

Retarded children take longer to learn new material and once they have learned something new, they usually forget more easily than the normal. Consequently they need more help, and more systematic help from parents, teachers, and other in the acquisition of skills. In particular, they often fail to learn by observation, and therefore, need more structured teaching. The help needs to be provided at an appropriate level for the child. It is useless to try and teach skills too far ahead of the child present mental age. Parents play an important role in training these children (also see Chapter 20).

In the preschool period the main role for professionals such as clinical psychologist, special educators, speech therapists, etc. is in helping parents to find ways to stimulate their child's development.

The Mentally Gifted

In distribution of intelligence, the right extreme of the bell-shaped curve represents the gifted or the genius (Fig. 6.5). These are the individuals with IQs of 140 or higher. About one out of every 100 children has an IQ of 140-160. Less than one out of every 1000 has an IQ above 160. In the early childhood, a gifted child is generally found to be misfit in his class because the level of teaching in a normal classroom is for an average child, whereas the gifted child is able to comprehend much faster. As a consequence, they often indulge in behavioural irregularities. They have been found to be gross under achievers and extremely unhappy. One problem seems to be that such extremely bright children find themselves intellectually misfit with children of their own age, and physically misfit with the older people who are their intellectual equals. But things improve by adulthood and they appear to be happier and better adjusted than most others of their age. These days there are separate schools for the gifted children. With the right type of training their superior potential is channelised in constructive tasks.

Clinical Applications

Assessment (see Chapter 18) and understanding of intellectual functions is helpful in your clinical work as with this knowledge, you can diagnose a patient with mental subnormality or with very superior intelligence. Assessment of intelligence is discussed in detail in Chapter 18. Your explanations or guidance to the patient would be according to his intellectual level. In some diseases like neuropsychiatric disorders, epilepsy, and psychiatric disorders and in some of the endocrinological disorders, assessment of intelligence is of great assistance in their management. Physical and/or mental ill health may temporarily impair intellectual performance. Distressing physical symptoms may obviously interfere with mental concentration, while great anxiety, deep depression or the thought disorder of schizophrenia may make it extremely difficult for a patient to respond adequately to test material.

The influence of motivation may be quite profound on performance on intelligence test. If the individual sees no relevance of the intelligence testing to his current situation or problems he may make little attempt to cooperate

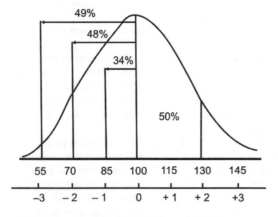

Fig. 6.5: Normal distribution of intelligence

with the tasks involved, and may then achieve a much lower score than would have been the case if he had been more highly motivated.

It is generally organic disease affecting the functioning of the brain that is likely to impair intellectual performance; so that it is in the field of neuropsychiatry particularly that intelligence testing may be of greatest assistance. Not only may there be evidence of a general falling off in intellectual functioning compared with an actual previous measurement, or an estimate based on past educational or occupational history, but more specific cognitive impairments may indicate lesions of particular parts of the brain.

The assessment of an individual's intellectual abilities can be of value in other clinical situations where psychological problems may be arising in an educational or vocational context.

Knowledge of intellectual functioning is also useful for yourself as a student and later as a teacher. Teaching method, content of the subject matter and expectations from students should be based on student's intellectual functioning.

SUMMARY

Intelligence is not a unitary concept, it is a global capacity of an individual to act purposefully, comprehend and think rationally. Various theories have been put forth to understand the nature of intelligence. Different theories have explained nature of intelligence. According to Spearman, intelligence has two factors, general and specific factors, the multifactor theories of Thurstone, provides seven primary abilities. Guilford has classified structure of intelligence in products, contents and operations; their combination produces 120 factors of intelligence, Guilford has also made distinction between convergent and divergent intelligence. Cattell has classified intelligence as fluid and crystallised intelligence acknowledging role of heredity and environment. Gardner has advocated seven types of intelligence. According to Sternberg, individuals can improve their experimental, contextual intelligence and componential intelligence by practice and effort.

Emotional intelligence is a term used for ability to control emotions and ability to handle interpersonal relationship. EI is considered important for success in later life. Scores are more or less stable, as the test scores of the early years have been found to correlate highly with the scores obtained in late adolescence. Heredity and environment both play an important role in determining the intelligence.

Intelligence can be assessed through verbal or performance test. Intelligence quotient is the ratio between mental age and chronological age. Average IQ scores range from 90 to 110 (obtained on standard tests of intelligence). Those having an IQ below 70 are considered as mentally subnormal, while those with an IQ above 160 are considered as mentally gifted. Knowledge of intellectual functioning and its assessment, is of a great importance in clinical practice, especially in neuropsychiatry, psychiatry, endocrinology and paediatrics.

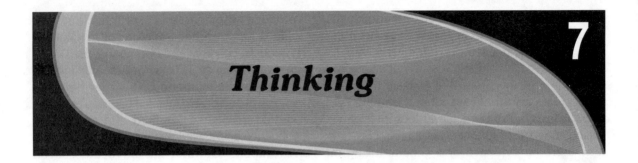

Thinking

Imagine yourself examining a patient in the emergency ward with an unusual to plan some treatment strategy immediately because if you do not deteriorate fast and he may even die. There is no other doctor in the casualty so you have to think, plan and start the treatment entirely on your own. Similarly, you can take another situation where you are driving home late in the night. You see a big crowd on the road due to some accident. Being a doctor you stop the car and go near the site of the accident. You find that the victim is lying in a pool of blood. What should you do? How should you do? These would be the common questions coming to your mind. You arrive at the solution for these problems based on thinking process.

Definition

Thinking is the mental activity that makes human behaviour complex and fascinating. It is some kind of ongoing mental activity with internal representation of the outside world of which the subject is aware but which is unobservable by another person. It must be inferred from the behaviour of the individual. It may or may not have been induced by an external stimulus and it may or may not result in some psychologist define thinking as a response to any stimuli. According to them thinking is more complicated than responding. For example, a mathematical problem at times can be solved by two different methods, with the same result. So thinking is not responding but a process by which one arrives at the solutions. These processes of solving problems can be different in different individuals and different situations.

Human thought process is like information processing sequences, building from basic information such as pattern recognition and perceptual analysis. Thinking is mental process of forming a new representation by transforming available information. Thinking involves attention, memory, reasoning, imagination, decision making and judging. Thinking has three characteristics—

- Thinking occurs in the mind but is inferred from observable behaviour.
- Thinking is a process that manipulates knowledge in a person's cognitive system.
- Thinking is directed toward finding solutions to problems facing the individual (Mayer, 1981).

How do we Think?

We store information from our experience with people and things; we make mental representation of these experiences in our minds. At times we generalise our experiences like learning is better early in the morning, all students who wear spectacles are studious. Thinking relies on a variety of mental structures to form a thought. These are symbols, concept, schema, imagery, cognitive maps and language.

Symbols

Thinking has also been defined as the manipulation of symbols. Symbol is an object that can represent other objects. For example, a triangle can represent family planning or × in a mathematical equation can stand for multiplication. Thus the red triangle and × are symbols. Though words form important symbols in our thinking, yet symbols are not limited to the familiar language of words. There are other symbolic languages, such as language of mathematics; Tangible symbols include such symbols as a stop sign, a cross on the church, a red cross on the ambulance. We think in symbols as verbal language is a rich symbolic process. A symbol conveys a meaning, it provides information about some object or event to which it refers and thereby suggests appropriate action to the persons who perceives it. Symbolic stimuli produce reactions appropriate to some stimulus other than themselves, e.g. sign DANGER alerts someone to take necessary action. Though thinking is private and invisible yet we can study the result of simple manipulation and then work backwards making guesses about what kind of symbols might have been manipulated and about how this manipulation is performed. The study of the process of thinking is dependent upon introspection and verbal report by the subject.

Concepts

When symbol stands for a class or group of objects with common properties, it refers to a concept, like green, women, injection. Concepts are labels one gives to a group of objects; it is the organisation of a variety of different objects or events into categories. Some concepts can easily be formed as they are basic, whereas other concepts are difficult to form. Concept learning is based on principles of generalisation and discrimination (see Chapter 5). A child learning the concept of dog may generalise all small animals as dog. Later with parental correction and with personal experience the child is able to discriminate dog from other small animals. Language ability helps us to form concepts from concrete to the abstract ones. Piaget's stages of intellectual development indicate that the child first learns object concepts and develops more abstract concepts only as he grows older (see Chapter 12). The inability to form abstracts is characteristic of certain disorders like, schizophrenia, mental subnormality and some neurological disorders. Normal individuals have capacity to treat new stimuli as familiar and remembered categories. This ability to categorise individual experiences is regarded as one of the most basic abilities of thinking organisms (Mervis and Rosch, 1981).

Psychologist have identified a level in concept hierarchies at which people best categories and think about objects. The basic level can be retrieved from memory, e.g. chair is identified as piece of furniture. The basic levels of concepts are the fundamental of thought.

Schemas

Schemas are general conceptual frameworks regarding certain people objects and situations one's life. You correlate 'exams' with studying most of the time, anxiety to finish the course, lots of books and cutting down on social activities. This visual representation provides expectation about the features likely to be found in a particular situation. Whenever incomplete or ambiguous information is available, we make inferences. Schemas are the primary units of meaning in the human information processing systems. We comprehend new information by integrating new inputs and what we already know.

We also have schemas of events; these are referred to as script. A script is a cluster of knowledge about sequences of interrelated, specific events and actions expected to occur in a certain way in particular settings. We have a script for going to a picnic, traveling in train, making presentations. Scripts may depend upon the culture, e.g. traveling in train in India is different from traveling in train in Japan.

Imagery

Supposing you have joined a hostel and you have an empty room. You are supposed to arrange the room. What will you do? How will you plan the places for your things like bed, study table, books, music system and other accessories? For this you need an imagery to plan the arrangement and setting of your things. Imagery is the mental picture which is usually not complete. Imagery is an important tool for solving many problems. Mental imagery is the ability, which varies between individuals, to experience 'internally' something resembling but not identical with a percept, visual, auditory, olfactory, etc. These mental images may be memories of previous events, scenes, etc. or apparently original as, for example, in the case of some creative artists. The ability to experience vivid and details images which are then projected into the environment and perceived as if external is known as eidetic imagery. The images may occur spontaneously in some situations, while on other occasions they may result from a conscious effort on the part of the individual. These may be referred to as autonomous and controlled imagery respectively. This difference may be extended to all thinking so that a distinction is made between what may be described as purposive and fantasy thinking—the difference depending essentially on the degree of control exercised by the thinker.

Cognitive Maps

A cognitive representation of a physical space is called a cognitive map. These are internal maps that guide future actions towards desired goals. Cognitive maps help people to visualise a situation like one draws a visual route to reach a particular destination. Visual thought and verbal thought differ in the ways information is processed and stored. Visual thought increases complexity and richness to our thinking. Visual thinking can be useful in solving problems related to special or geographical relationship.

Culture influences the cognitive maps due to the subjective impression of physical reality. The maps often mirror our personal or culturally egocentric perspective. If you are asked to draw a female figure that would be different in features and dress as compared to a figure drawn by an American.

Language

Thinking involves the manipulation of internal or covered representations of external and overt events or behaviour, but that is because of the existence of language. Language serves two major functions, it helps us to communicate with one another and it provides system of symbols and rules that facilitate thinking. Language like any other external behaviour may be represented internally, and much human thinking involves a kind of internal speech. There are also many examples of nonlinguistic thought as when composer 'hears' in his mind music that he is creating or an artist 'sees' a painting he will put on to canvas.

Neurological Basis of Thinking

Luria, the Russian psychologist, on the basis of studies of children, has regarded the internalisation of speech as the major factor in the development of thinking. He has also shown that patients with lesions of the frontal lobes may suffer from loss of speech control as well as more general disorganisation of behaviour, and presumably of the thinking process underlying it. Milner (1963) has also found that frontal lobe patients show impairment on a card-sorting task in which cards can be categorised in terms of colour, form of number. If the principle was changed (e.g. from form to colour), the patients continued to sort cards according to the original principle, showing preservation of behaviour. There are also other disturbances associated with frontal lobe damage, including motivational deficit, so that the association of frontal lobe and the process of thinking can only be regarded as tentative.

Types of Thinking

Thinking has been classified in number of ways. Some of the important types of thinking are discussed here.

Purposive and Fantasy Thinking

Our thought can go to extremes from purposive, realistic thinking to fantasy or autistic thinking. Autistic thinking is a personal, idiosyncratic involving fantasy day dreaming being in your own world. This type of indivisualised thoughts can be important for creative acts. But in extreme cases it can be abnormal as it generates delusions and hallucinations. Realistic thinking is logical, takes account of external reality and, clearly, is involved in reasoning and problem-solving. Autistic thinking in contrast, is primitive, non-logical in its association of ideas and is not subject to correction by reference to reality.

Convergent and Divergent Thinking

Another dichotomy between two forms of purposive thinking as suggested by Guilford (1956) and later developed by Hudson (1966). Convergent thinking applies to problem solving which involves focussing on to the one and only correct answer—the sort of problem that has commonly been used in conventional tests of intelligence (e.g. 'fat is to think as tall is to …..?') Divergent thinking requires the production of as many answers as possible (e.g. 'how many uses can you think of for a flower pot?) and has been considered to be important in relation to creativity.

Functions of Thinking

Thinking has various functions that help us in our day-to-day activities requiring reasoning, problem solving, and decision making and judging.

Reasoning

Reasoning is a process of realistic, goal directed thinking in which conclusions are drawn from a set of facts. In reasoning information both stored and collected from the environment are used according to the set rules. Reasoning is classified as deductive and inductive.

Deductive reasoning involves drawing a conclusion that follows logically established rules from two or more statements. Examples of this reasoning is that A has high blood sugar, so he has diabetes.

Inductive reasoning uses available evidence to generate a conclusion about the likelihood of something. For inductive reasoning one constructs a hypothesis based on available evidence and then test it against other evidence. Inferences are accomplished by integrating past experiences, weighted value of the importance of the evidence and creativity. Examples of this type of thinking are probing into a murder case.

Most scientific reasoning is inductive as often a medical diagnosis is made on the inferences drawn from the case history of the patient. Inductive reasoning plays a key role in our lives in solving many problems, like misplacing certain object and then trying to find that.

Problem Solving

Problem solving is thinking that is directed towards solving specific problems. This is the important part of our thinking that moves from an initial state to a goal state by means of a set of mental operations. Solving a problem implies that the organism is faced with a task the solution to which is not immediately apparent, but which it is able to solve after an interval during which the problem-solving activity including thinking or reasoning has occurred. In other words, problem-solving involves the acquisition of an appropriate response to a novel situation.

The ability to find an answer to the question that is to solve a problem is a cognitive ability which has a goal. Goal can be achieved by various methods for which the psychologists have explained on the basis of different theories. These are—learning theory, Gestalt theory and information processing theory.

Learning theory : The learning theory approach to problem solving is illustrated by work of Pavlov, Watson, Thorndike. According to Thorndike the cats placed in the puzzle boxes learned to pull the string that got them out of the trial and error process. Here the cats were only learning a new habit because of the reward and reinforcement of getting out of the box. The cats did not understand the mechanism of pulling the string led to the escape.

Gestalt theory : The work of German psychologist Kohler (1927) is an example of Gestalt approach where famous experiments of insight learning were conducted on the chimpansee, Sultan. The bananas were placed outside Sultan's cage, out of reach, and he was given a stick, he would use the stick to pull the bananas to him. Sultan's problem occurred when neither of the two sticks he had was long enough to reach the bananas. He tried to get the bananas with one of the sticks but was not successful and walked away. Suddenly, he went back and by chance combined the two sticks together, make a single long stick. With this he could immediately reach to the bananas. According to Kohler, Sultan used insight which is often known as an 'aha' experience. He came up with a completely new creative solution to his problem which he continued to use in the similar situations.

The Gestalt approach to solving problem is based on rearranging the situation to gain on insight into its fundamental nature. Here is a problem for you to answer.

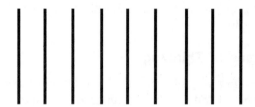

These are nine sticks, try to make them ten without adding another stick

Problem-solving occurs through a process of trial and error. You would have experienced many such incidents where the initial method to solve the problem was based on trial and error but later on the solution comes through insight. It may come suddenly to your mind while you were doing something different. The Gestalt view of problem-solving, is a more holistic one. Instead of a solution proceeding gradually by small steps as proposed by Thorndike, the Gestalt school considered that the problems are solved efficiently when organised into a good structure. This is also called reproductive thinking as it duplicates or reproduces old habits. The productive thinking.

Information processing : According to this approach problem-solving is a complex activity comprising several processes. These processes include—registering information, retrieving information from memory and using both kinds of knowledge in a purposeful way. The study of information processing has grown along with the use of computers and at times it has been equated to artificial intelligence.

Stages of problem-solving : Whenever you have to solve a problem try to think what all is required. Supposing you have been asked to make a research proposal, what necessary steps would you take ? Generally, whenever they have to solve a problem, we go through three hour stages, we prepare, we produce and we evaluate.

Preparation: The first step to problem solving is to understand the problem as our interpretation can be affected by the way the problem is presented. At times, there is a problem of fixed or rigid mental set which can interfere in understanding and thereby working on the problem.

Production: We need to generate possible solution. Simple problems may be solved just by collecting correct information either from long-term memory or from other sources like books, advice from others, etc. The more complicated problems require complex strategies. The two basic kinds of solution strategies are algorithms and heuristics.

An algorithm is a strategy that exhausts every possible answer till it comes up with the correct solution used diligently, it guarantees a correct solution. Algorithms are rarely used because they do not exist for many problems and they are very time-consuming. A heuristic is a "rule of thumb" that can lead to a very quick solution to no solution at all. Heuristics may involve planning that ignores some of the problem information while focussing on other information or it may involve means end analysis that tests for a difference between the state that currently exist and one that desired and doing something to reduce the difference. Heuristics may also involve working backward to review the ideal situations and then determining what steps will lead to the ideal situation.

Evaluation: We have to decide how good is our solution. It may be easy for some solutions but many problems have less precise goals and are harder to judge may have many solutions to the problem in which we have to decide which is the best solution. When a problem is solved by insight learning the evaluation is very quick but in information processing and association type of problem-solving one may move up and down and gradually come to the solution of the problem. Hence, the evaluation process is also different than that of insight.

Mental blocks can hinder problem-solving ability. Mental blocks are functional fixedness, i.e. one may find it hard to perceive a new function for an object that was previously associated with some other purpose. Some other factors like habitual strategy, past experiences or conditioning, actor-Observer bias and mental set may interfere with finding right solutions. Mental set is a tendency to respond to a new problem in the same manner used to solve previous problem. These factors function as "Black Box" in our thinking.

If you want to avoid pitfalls in problem-solving follow these guidelines—
- Formulate a plan by making a outline
- Work in a organised manner
- Begin working with easy options
- Mentally rehearse taking the right action
- Involve yourself completely in the problem, try to get maximum information on that
- Be enthusiastic, think positively
- Anticipate the challenge.

Decision Making

In our day-to-day living there are many incidents in which we have to make decisions. It may be a simple decision as to which dress to wear, or complex decisions like whether to join Paediatrics or to take up Radiology for postgraduation. Similarly, we have to take number of decisions related to patient care like diagnosis and treatment. Decision making is an important part of all science-based professions. This is a cognitive process leading to the selection of a course of action among alternatives, it produces a final choice and is an action or an opinion.

Decision making is a kind of problem-solving. In which we are presented with several alternatives among which we must choose. While taking decisions one tries to optimise utility—perceived benefit or psychological value. Most decisions are risky in the sense that we cannot be sure of the outcome for example, while treating a patient with intestinal carcinoma, you are not sure whether the patient would benefit with chemotherapy, radiotherapy or surgery. You take the risk of deciding one type of treatment that is to be given.

The problem arises when we have to decide and choose between several alternatives. When there are no fixed rules of deciding then there is a risk of making errors in decision making due to subjective bias. We often make use of the heuristic of representativeness to arrive at subjective probabilities, we decide whether the current situation is similar to one we have encountered before, and then we act accordingly. While in some situations it may be useful to decide according to the past experience, but this approach can at times cause problems as it may interfere with new way of thinking. While deciding one also considers availability of options and weighing the relative advantages and disadvantages of a particular decision.

Decision making style have been suggested by MBTI (Myers-Briggs Type Indicator).

According to this there are four dimensions—thinking and feeling, introversion and extroversion, judgement and perception, sensing and intuition. People high on intuition, judgement and thinking tend to take better decisions.

Decision frame is a structure of a problem presentation. Decisions are influenced by decision frame that is how the facts are presented for decision making. The oncologist in favour of radiotherapy as compared to chemotherapy may present morbidity rate with chemotherapy.

Personal Biases in Decision Making

There are several personal bias which interfere with correct decision making. These are:
- Selective search for evidence
- Premature termination of search for evidence unwillingness to share a view
- Experiential limitations
- Selective perception
- Wishful thinking or optimism
- Choice-supportive bias—when we distort our memories of chosen and rejected options to make the chosen options seem relatively more attractive
- Recency—tendency to place more attention on recent information and either ignore or forget more distant information
- Repetition bias
- Influences of initial information
- Inconsistency
- Role-fulfillment
- Faulty generalisations.

Judging

Judgement is a process by which we form opinions reach conclusions and make critical evaluations of events and people on the basis of available information. Sometimes we make spontaneous judgments based upon our attitude. Often decision making and judgement are considered as two sides of a coin. Judgements are based on inference, the reasoning process of drawing a conclusion on the basis of evidence or prior beliefs.

Blocks in Cognitive Process

"We may try to see things as objectively as we please. Nonetheless, we can never see them with any eyes except our own".

Sometimes we may make wrong judgements due to over-generalised stereotypes based on minimal or faulty information. There are several factors which cause mental blocks in our thinking.

The unconscious prejudice may bias our thinking due to which one may not arrive at impartial and neutral judgement. The past experiences hidden in our unconscious mind may interfere with our judgement. Prejudices like racism and sexism are commonly witnessed in the judgements.

Cognitive bias is a systematic error in inference, decision and judgement. Apprehension of bias is inevitable as decision making process depends on different experiences and perspectives. This can occur when we perceive random events and nonrandom, when we make short cuts to solve a problem, perceiving people as causing rather than being victimised by events, not exploring a range of possible solutions. The reasons for cognitive biases are first and last impression, self-esteem at stake, personal need, ego enhancing bias, beliefs and stereotypes. Often mental state of a person like anxiety, depression, frustration and irritability may lead to wrong judgements. Some psychologist have studied how complex judgements are made. They have suggested that there two main heuristics (mental short cuts) that are responsible for mistakes made in judgement. These are availability heuristic and representativeness heuristic. The availability heuristic means that we make judgement based upon how easily we can come up with a similar example. It is a cognitive strategy that estimates probabilities based on personal experience. You estimate the likelihood of an outcome based on how easily you can imagine similar outcomes. As example of this strategy recall that you were in a hurry, you decided to take a particular route to reach a particular destination. On the contrary, you had encountered more obstacles on this route or would have taken longer to reach your destination. The representativeness heuristic is a cognitive strategy that assigns items to categories based on whether they possess some representative characteristics of the category. The danger of this strategy is oversimplified thinking.

We look for common features found in a typical category member for example; we assume certain characteristics for vegetarian people.

Clinical Applications

In recent years, with the development of computer technology in clinical decision-making the process of diagnosis, prognosis and treatment may be represented in the form of 'decision tree'. The decision is taken based on elements of evidence or 'indicants', such as answers by the patient to a question, the presence of a physical sign on examination or the result of a laboratory test. Later, a comparative evaluation is done of the computer programme of the diagnostic programme with diagnosis formed by clinicians. A similar procedure is used in the experimental study of thinking by computer stimulation, but it has been shown that clinicians themselves differ widely in their diagnostic behaviour. A further application has been the construction of computer programmes actually to aid diganosis in specific clinical areas such as congenital heart disease and thyroid disease.

Disorders of thinking are one of the prime concerns in psychiatric patients. Many psychiatric disorders specially schizophrenia and some neurological disorders like dementia, delirium cause disorders of thinking, the examples, lack of association, neologisms (coining new words), circumstantiality, flight of ideas and delusions. In depressive illness aim of cognitive therapy is to modify negative thinking in terms of not being liked by others, rejection by others and bleak future.

Decision making is not only important for the physician who is treating but is also important for the patient and his relatives. Imagine a situation where a patient is on the ventilator for two months and the doctor provides the options to the family to continue or to wean off the patient from the ventilator. Similarly, the patient might have to decide whether he wants to be treated for angina by pharmacotherapy or he should undergo surgery. Similarly while dealing with patients with substance abuse decision to stop abuse of the substance is entirely patient's responsibility. To help individuals who are poor in making decisions, programmes have been developed to provide skills training, which is based on cognitive and behavioural theories.

SUMMARY

Thinking is a mental activity in which one responds to the problem by cognitive rearrangement or manipulation of both information from the environment and the information stored in a long-term memory. We think by means of symbols, concepts, schema, scripts, imagery and cognitive maps. Thinking has important function in problem solving, decision making and judging. Problem-solving has been explained on the basis of learning theory, Gestalt theory and information processing. To solve a problem generally we take three steps like we prepare or plan, we produce and we evaluate the solution. Decision making is important in clinical practice for the physicians as well as the patients. Cognitive bias may interfere with impartial rational judging. Problem-solving and decision making are used in every step in patient care.

Motivation

8

Mansi, a singer has developed hoarseness of voice and is not able to sing. The doctors treating her feel that it will not be possible for Mansi to sing again. Music is Mansi's life and without being able to sing there is no meaning in life for Mansi.

The sheer motivation helps Mansi to sing again which is surprising to the doctors. You will come across many patients in your medical practice who fight with the illness and survive due to their motive to live.

Definition

Motivation means 'to move' and is defined as an internal process that provides energy for behaviour and directs it towards a specific goal. Motive in a person helps to infer, explain and predict his behaviour. Motivation is a general term for all the processes involved in starting directing and maintaining physical and psychological activities, it can be understood by studying the underlying urges, wants, needs, desires and goals. Drive refers to biological motivation like hunger. Motives refer to psychological and social needs that are assumed to be learned through personal experience.

Indicators of Motivation

The following are some of the measurable qualities and events that indicate motivation underlying behaviour:
- The more motivated an organism is, the higher will be its level of activity.
- Strong motivation increases an individual's rate of learning.
- Motivation enables one to attain a higher level of performance.
- Once learned, a motivated response will be more resistant to extinction.
- Being motivated in one task can disrupt efforts in other activities.

Models of Motivation

Various models have been proposed to understand motivation. Some of the important models are drive and homeostatic model.

Drive Model

It is assumed that each organism is born with or later develops a variety of biological needs. A need is something that is required physiologically, for example, the need for food, water, and the elimination of bodily wastes. When a sufficient amount of time passes during which a need is not satisfied, a relevant drive is aroused. Subjectively, we decide that we are hungry or thirsty and are directed to act in order to overcome the unpleasant state.

Once the individual is in a high drive state, there is a readiness to respond to external stimuli that are related to the aroused drive. These stimuli are known as incentives. When our drives are activated, we move toward such incentives as the food or water, in the refrigerator or the kitchen. Much of our behaviour is directed by incentives. An incentive may be thought of as an appropriate object or activity for satisfying a need. Once the incentive has been obtained, the individual engages in consummatory behaviour. That is, he eats or drinks. Such activity satisfies the need in question and is said to be the goal of the motivated behaviour. Obtaining such a goal reduces the aroused drive, and this drive reduction acts as a reward or positive reinforcement. Once a need is satisfied, the organism becomes relatively inactive again. The general cycle of events is illustrated in Figure 8.1. It may be seen, then, that motivation energises the organism to seek an appropriate goal by approaching relevant incentives. Motivation also accounts for the tendency to be persistent in this behaviour until the need is satisfied.

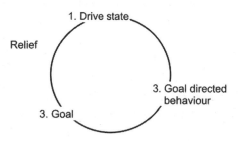

Fig. 8.1: Drive cycle

Within this general model, drive is often said to be a stimulus for behaviour. That is, when a need is unsatisfied, various internal stimuli are activated, and these stimuli lead to responses. Any strong, persistent stimulus can have properties to be a drive for example, a very brightlight or an unpleasant loud noise will cause an individual to close his or her eyes or cover his or her ears, and if possible to move away from the annoying stimulus. In such instances, there is no need deprivation in the usual sense but rather an external stimulus that acts as a drive. It has been suggested that individuals act to avoid intense external stimulation are motivated by the 'need to avoid pain'.

The Homeostatic Model

Homeostasis refers to the regulatory process that impels us to eat when we are hungry and to stop eating when we have had enough, to drink when we are thirsty and to stop drinking when that need is satisfied, and so on. There is a natural tendency toward balance that serves to keep our internal environment at a relatively constant state with respect to the various needs.

Both the drive model and the homeostatic model are based on a common assumption, namely that an organism when aroused strives to return to a quiet, stable state. A more inclusive view suggests that drive induction and drive reduction can each be reinforcing under appropriate circumstances.

Anxiety as a drive The concept of anxiety as a drive was based on the assumption that this is a relatively stable characteristic in which individuals differ. Anxiety has been classified as a trait and as a state. Trait anxiety is considered as a personality variable. Those who were anxious would be expected to experience anxiety in a variety of situations. State anxiety refers to a temporary condition of arousal in response to particular situations. For example, even if you are not a particularly anxious person (trait), you might feel very upset as you sit in a dentist's waiting room (state).

It has been proposed that individuals who are characteristically anxious and tense must ordinarily experience a higher drive level than calm, placid individuals. If so, those high in anxiety should, when compared with those low in anxiety, demonstrate greater response strength with respect to various habits. As an example of such effects, consider what happens when an experienced driver sees a small child suddenly coming in front of his car. The well-learned, well-practiced habit of stepping on the brake is much stronger than any competing habit, so it is very likely to occur. If such a driver were extremely anxious, the braking response would be even more likely to occur—more quickly and with greater force. Imagine the same situation with someone who is just learning to drive. Many new habits are being learned, and they are about of equal strength. If a child dashes in front of the car, a new driver may be equally inclined to step on the brake, step on the accelerator, or honk the horn. If that person were highly anxious, it would only complicate matters since all of the responses (both appropriate and inappropriate) would be strengthened by such a drive state. Extremely bright individuals do well even if they are anxious. Those who are extremely dull do badly even if their anxiety is low. In the middle range, though, it is clear that highly anxious students do less well on exams, obtain lower grades and are more likely to leave school (Spielberger, 1966). Students with high anxiety can be helped by assessing the severity of anxiety and then providing therapy to reduce their anxiety (see Chapter 20).

Humanistic Model

Some theorists have proposed more complex system of categorising needs. Abraham Maslow (1970) has classified motivation into a hierarchy consisting of seven separate needs. As shown in Figure 8.2, these range from the most necessary requirements for survival to the most important expressions of the human potential. Let us look briefly at each of the five levels.

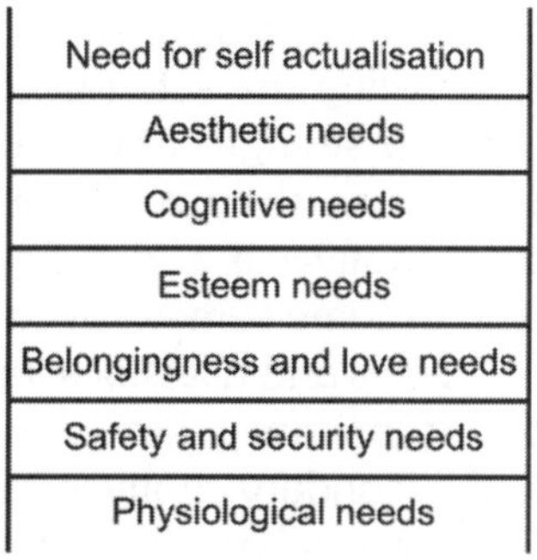

Need for self actualisation
Aesthetic needs
Cognitive needs
Esteem needs
Belongingness and love needs
Safety and security needs
Physiological needs

Fig. 8.2: Hierarchy of needs

Physiological needs: These are the primary motives that serve to keep the individual alive and to permit the continuation of the species.

Safety needs: In addition to mere survival, there is the need to avoid pain, to obtain bodily comforts, and to be free from fear and insecurity. These are said to be powerful, lower-order needs.

Need to belong and to love: The higher-order needs begin with the desire to obtain security by means of identification with a group? For this reason, we seek to identify with our families, with our school, our organisation, our religion, our nation, our race, and so forth. Somehow, we feel better about ourselves as individuals when we are able to find our roots in a larger body of people, i.e. experience love. Besides, having a lower-order need for sexual release, we have a higher-order need for the feelings of affection and love - both to give and to receive. Establishing at least a loving relationship with one individual.

Esteem needs: Each of us wants to feel that he is a worthwhile individual who counts for something. This includes the feeling of competence or mastery of the environment, and also the need to accomplish and achieve. In addition, self-esteem is said to be highest if we can be independent and free.

Cognitive needs: Individuals have an innate need to make sense of various aspects of their external environment. This forms the need for knowledge and understanding.

Aesthetic needs: These constitute the needs for order and beauty, which individuals strive for in their lives and external environment.

Self-actualisation needs: The highest of all needs are met if an individual can achieve self-actualisation. This is a rather complex concept involving the need to know all that we can, about ourselves and about the world around us, the need to create and to appreciate beauty, and the tendency to be a spontaneous and inner-directed achiever.

In Maslow's view, each of us would progress smoothly up this hierarchy as each set of lower needs is met. We would each become secure, creative 'self-actualisers'. However, harsh environmental conditions can force people to spend their entire lives working very hard just to meet the lower-order needs.

In addition, changes in the solution can very quickly propel an individual back down the hierarchy. Many times, a person will have a lower-order need that is not met, and higher-order needs will be ignored as the person is strongly motivated to eat, to obtain sexual gratification, or to find a bathroom. There also can be a serious disruption of one's life that can force a total concentration on the basic needs. For example, a painful illness or some natural or man-made disaster can turn even the most creative, self-actualised person into an individual concerned only with safety and survival. In the recent past many well-established Kashmiri immigrants both intellectuals and businessmen were seen to be having such basic survival problems.

Social Cognitive Model

Social cognitive model of motivation share the concept that human motivation comes not from objective realities but from our subjective interpretation of them. You often experience that if you think that achieving a particular goal is important for you then under any circumstances you work to reach that goal. That means what we do is controlled by what we think is responsible for causing our action, what we believe we can do and anticipate the outcome of our efforts. Social cognitive model gives importance to higher mental processes that control motivation rather than physiological arousal or biological mechanism. Locus of control is another concept given by Julian Rotter to understand social learning model. According to this model an individual will engage in a given behaviour is determined by two factors. One is expectations of attaining a goal and the other is the personal value of that goal. Expectations of a future occurrence are based on our past experience, which helps in developing a personal sense of locus of control. Often we find that student's who are poor in studies do not have motivation to study because they do not anticipate a positive outcome of their studies. Locus of control can be internal or external. When a person thinks the outcome of our actions can be controlled by our efforts that is internal control. On the contrary, if one believes that the outcome is controlled by external factors for example, a student thinks that his poor marks are due to teacher's bias that is called external control.

Classification of Motives

Needs are often an important component in studying motivation. They are classified into primary and secondary motives, the primary or physiological necessities are: hunger, thirst, a desire for sex, temperature regulation, sleep, pain avoidance and need for oxygen. The secondary or learned, acquired desires are: achievement, power, affiliation, aggression, autonomy, nurturance and play. The secondary motives are also called as social motives because they are learned in social groups, in the family, in the school, and with peer group. The social motives are general, persisting characteristics of a person and they differ in strength from individual-to-individual because they are learned. This classification of motives is a useful one, but the distinction can become somewhat blurred. That is, learned appetites and aversions influence the satisfaction of primary motives, and the satisfaction of secondary motives can become closely tied to biological processes. For example, does your desire to earn money involve the instrumental use of money to buy something basic such as food? Is it used instead to buy some product that would provide you instant popularity in the hostel? Or, is the money to be acquired purely for its own sake, because you have learned to enjoy a huge bank balance. It seems that much of what we do can be identified as a mixture of primary and secondary motivation.

Hunger Motive

While most of us take for granted the daily activity of eating, food means more than fuel for the body with symbolic associations. Food may symbolise love, social bonding, and the display of affluence. The way we eat may reflect our attitudes toward our families, our society, and ourselves.

How does our body tell us we need food? We are more likely to feel the stirrings of appetite, but very poor persons have the pangs of a body depleted by hunger. In either case, however, the underlying mechanism is probably the same. A basic signal for hunger is the presence of stomach contractions. When the stomach is empty, contractions occur and are sensed. More recently the research in this field has indicated that levels or rates of use of dissolved nutritive substances circulating in the blood are crucial for the activation of feeding. Low level of glucose (sugar) in the blood is now believed to be an important cause in the initiation of hunger motivation. Hypothalamus is also involved in hunger motivation, as indicated by some experiments. However we all are aware that hunger motivation is not entirely governed by the internal stimulation. A host of external factors are also responsible in initiating hunger motivation.

Achievement Motive

People are very different from one another in their desire to compete and to win at whatever they undertake. It has been proposed that differences reflect variations in the learned motive to achieve (Atkinson, 1977). Achievement is task-oriented behaviour that allows the individual's performance to be evaluated according to some internally or externally imposed criterion. Achievement motivation can be seen in many areas of human endeavour such as school, job, sports or art performance such as painting, singing, dancing. Achievement motivation is learned, children copy from their parents and other important persons in their lives. The expectations of the parents from their children are important in development of this motivation. It has been found that high achievers generally have high achieving mothers.

Achievement motive has been associated with the behaviour. High achievement oriented behaviour expresses in many ways such as, persistence, taking challenges, high aspirations, constant need for feedback and control over the environment. These individuals are generally most successful in their profession provided their need for competition is not very strong.

Aggression Motive

An aggression is intended to hurt someone or something. In most places aggression leads to violence, destructive action against people or property. At other times the aggressive impulse is confined to competition, verbal attack, or some other expression of hostility short of physical injury. When we talk about aggression, then, we are talking about behaviour that the doer engages in with the intention of doing harm. It could be in the form of verbal attack, physical injury, violence or destructive action against people or property only.

Hormones and chemicals do not produce aggressive behaviour itself. What they do is to lower our threshold for expression of aggression. Very often aggression is the response to frustration (the thwarting of some goal directed behaviour), insults, and negative evaluations. Frustration does not always bring about aggression; however, it is likely to lead to aggression only when it is intense and unexpected or arbitrary. You are less likely to become angry when you are refused a job if you had not counted on getting it and if you think the interview was fair. Furthermore, frustrated individuals are not likely to become aggressive, no matter how angry they get, unless the stage is set for aggression. This stage setting may consist of cues for aggression, such as an atmosphere that promotes violence (communal riots, setting fire to religious places), the presence of weapons that remind you how they can be used to hurt someone, or a previous dislike for the person who frustrated you (Berkowitz, 1967).

Children learn from an early age that calling people names is almost sure to make them angry, and laboratory researchers have confirmed the aggression-eliciting power of insults by acting rudely toward subjects, sometimes questioning their intelligence. Negative evaluation given by teachers has often resulted in frustration in the students.

How do we learn to be aggressive? We learn aggressive behaviour from the people around us. Parents usually teach their children not to hit other children especially smaller children, and other adults. But when parents themselves behave aggressively, they become role models for their children. Parents exert a great deal of influence over children's aggressiveness. One major study found that the parents of children who were aggressive in school were less nurturant and accepting, punished their children for aggression at home, and, in general, gave them little support (Eron, 1980).

We learn aggression from television serials. At present there are many programmes both meant for adults and children like WWF in which children see lots of aggression and violence. Later they try to imitate these aggressive stunts. While some people argue that viewing aggression or even acting it out to a limited degree helps to drain off aggressive energy. But acting aggressively is likely to make someone more, rather than less, aggressive. And the bulk of the research on viewing aggression indicates that children who watch a lot of television learn that we live in a society that condones aggression in many situations, and they learn what to do when they feel aggressive themselves (Bandura, 1973). But when parents let their children know that violence is not an acceptable means of settling disputes, then watching TV does not lead to more aggression.

Arousal and Curiosity

Most psychologists believe that a basic motivational system underlies exploratory behaviour and curiosity and arousal are related in important ways. Anyone who has ever spent much time in the company of a three year old knows that human beings are very curious creatures from a very early age. We want to know about everything in our lives—why people act as they do, why events occur, how things work, what is on the other side of a hill, a mountain, and an ocean. To satisfy our curiosity we begin as infants to touch, to put new objects in our mouths. As we grow older, we continue to process the information that comes in through all our senses, we explore our surroundings, we ask questions, we study, we think. We seem to do many things for no intrinsic reward other than satisfying our curiosity.

Motives and Conflict

You would have experienced some time in your life that you have to choose one between two attractive offers, both of them being motivating to some degree. Motivation researchers have classified such competing motives into the following four categories.

1. *Approach approach conflicts* occur when you are simultaneously attracted to two desirable outcomes or activities, as in a situation when you are trying to decide which of two good courses you should take up for career.
2. *Avoidance avoidance conflicts* arise when you are repelled by two or more undesirable outcomes or activities. Suppose there is a required course in computers that you have to take and that clashes with your most important clinical posting or clashes with your exam time. Still, you know that if you want to graduate, you have to choose one of these unwanted alternatives.
3. *Approach avoidance conflicts* come up when a single option has both positive and negative elements. Suppose you are asked to speak to a group that can be influential in helping you to get a good job, but you are terrified of speaking in public. In this kind of conflict, individuals sometimes adopt unhealthy means to combat anxiety.
4. *Multiple approach avoidance conflicts* are the ones we most often face in life. These involve situations in which several options exist, with each one containing both positive and negative elements. Not surprisingly, these are the hardest to resolve, and the most stressful.

Clinical Applications

There can be two major applications of knowledge of motivation to clinical field. First, it can be of help in understanding the wide range of behaviours of patients in relation to their illness and treatment. Psychological response of patients to their disabling illness is likely to differ according to the degree of dependency or dominance needs of the patient. Second, it is concerned with the problems, which arise directly from abnormalities of drives of their goals. The aggressive drive appears to be expressed to a pathological degree in some individuals, who may thereby be a danger to others a so-called aggressive psychopath. Sexual deviations occur in which the aim of the sex drive departs to varying degrees from the usual goal of heterosexual intercourse, sometimes with an admixture of aggression as in sado-masochism. Such abnormalities are seen in patients having psychological disorders. One of the explanations for such behaviour is based on approach-avoidance model where, possibly owing to earlier experience, the 'normal' sexual object is both attractive and frightening, so that either an intermediate position between approach and avoidance is chosen, (e.g. voyeurism or indecent exposure) or a less aversive object (e.g. small girls instead of adult women).

Importance of motivation is of prime importance in psychiatric disorders. Schizophrenia, a common feature, particularly in the later stages of a chronic illness, is a loss of motivation so that the patient becomes apathetic and generally inactive. Current trends of treatment are focussed on enhancing motivation in these patients. Seligman (1975) has given a concept of 'Learned Helplessness', which has been applied to aetiology of depressive disorders. Learned helplessness means that the depressed person is convinced that he is out of control, nothing he can do would make any difference in changing an important feature of his life. Since they believe they can't do anything to change a situation, they don't have any motivation even to try. Learned helplessness is a traumatic experience as one who feels powerless to escape from stressful situations often gives up and die. Learned helplessness is also reported at times by patients with chronic illness, elderly and institutionised persons.

Other disorders of motivation are found in such conditions as alcohol and drug dependence and over-eating leading to obesity. Since these disorders are on the increase thus shall be discussed at length later in this section. Motivation for apparently self-injurious behaviour can be understood in terms of the needs that it satisfies or the rewards that it brings—though often in the short term. The child who repeatedly gets into trouble, through 'misbehaviour' knowing fully well that he will be punished, may be motivated (though without being aware of it) by the fact that only by so doing will he receive more attention from others.

The degree of control exerted over the overt expression of basic drives—such as sex and aggression may be weakened by organic disease affecting the functioning of the brain. The first signs of such disease may sometimes be the appearance of behaviour quite 'out of character for the individual. Such a change of personality may therefore, be an important in dictation for clinical assessment for neurological disease.

Motivational Basis of Addictive Behaviour

Alcoholism is a condition in which heavy drinking interferes with an individual's ability to function effectively in dealing with other people and in working. Similar problems are also present in patients with drug addiction. There has been a great deal of research directed to discover the way in which we acquire this powerful and often dangerous motive. Three major factors seem to be involved.

First, there are the basic learning processes that underlie the acquisition of any motive. If an individual grows up in a society in which adults drink whenever they want to celebrate something and whenever they want to relax and have fun, such activity clearly is associated with positive feelings. Individuals tend to model their behaviour after that of others. Experimental subjects have been found to drink more when exposed to a stranger who drinks heavily than when the stranger is a light drinker or does not drink at all. In addition, by adolescence there are often strong peer pressures to drink.

Second, in addition to external sources of rewards for drinking, alcohol itself can provide a powerful reinforcement. It is a depressant drug that acts on the central nervous system to bring feelings of relaxation and reduced anxiety. The fact that a few drinks can very quickly relieve tension and fears means that drinking is easily learned as a method of dealing with stress.

Third, 'alcoholic' individuals may have a special physiological weakness that results in a craving for alcohol. Several biological differences between alcoholics and nonalcoholic have been identified. For example, problem drinkers feel less physical pain when they consume alcohol, but social drinkers actually feel more pain after a few drinks. The fact that it is possible to breed animals that drink alcohol readily while others of the same species avoid it suggests that a genetic factor is involved.

A complex combination of cultural, psychological, and physiological factors contributes to drinking behaviour and to alcoholism.

Eating Disorders

Raju aged 12, weighing 88 kgs was referred from endocrinology OPD. All his investigations were normal; no physiological or endocrinological cause for his abnormal weight could be elicited. During psychological assessment his father's motive to get the child's name in Guiness Book of World Record was noted. Through this he wanted to get a large amount of money. Father always reported that the child has normal appetite and a small amount of food was given to him, but in reality the child was always overfed. This is an example of motivation for one type of problem related to eating. In India obesity has always been present but was not considered a problem. Now with awareness about its harmful effects, as it prevents a normal life and is a menace to health, people have become concerned about it and more and more people are seeking treatment for obesity.

It is not uncommon to find that the excessive intake is due to actual feelings of hunger than to eating, becoming associated with needs other than the food itself to reduce feelings of anxiety or unhappiness, for example in a depressed state people tend to eat more.

Two other kinds of eating disorders, which seem to have become more common in recent years, especially among young women, are anorexia nervosa, a form of self-starvation that can actually lead to death, and bulimia, in which an individual regularly eats vast quantities of food and then purges the body of them either by induced vomiting or laxative use.

Losing Weight by Applying Motivational Principles

1. Eat only at one place at regular times: This will help you cut down on snacking, by limiting the number of places and times that have associations with eating.
2. Eat slowly: This helps you get the most pleasure from the least amount of food, helps you fool yourself into thinking you are eating more than you actually are, and gives your body time to give you feedback on when you have had enough.
3. Do not do anything else while you are eating such as reading or watching television, so that you can concentrate on your food and be more responsive to your body's internal cues.
4. Reduce the availability of fattening foods. If you cannot resist seine high calorie food of your choice, do not bring them home. If you buy nuts, buy them with their shells on so you will have to expend more effort to eat them, you will eat less.
5. Allow for some variety in your diet, if you deprive yourself of all the foods you love, you will binge when you get the chance so it is better to incorporate a small serving of high-calorie food into your menu plan instead of avoiding it completely. However, since people eat more food when faced with a large variety, limit your meals to a few basic dishes instead of wide choice.
6. Avoid fatty and rich-tasting foods as the look; smell, and taste seem to stimulate the appetite.
7. Eat in the company of other people who are moderate eaters themselves, you will be inclined to eat more moderately when other people are witnesses to what you eat. Also you will be able to guide your intake by theirs.
8. Use small serving plates; food heaped on a small plate looks more than the same amount on a large plate. Take advantage of this visual illusion to fool you into eating less.
9. Incorporate exercise into your daily schedule. Aside from the direct expenditure of energy in the activity itself, exercise seems to reduce appetite. Programmes that combine dieting, changes in behaviour, and exercise result in more weight loss than any one of these changes alone. The most effective exercise schedules include sessions of at least 20 minutes each, three times a week, of activities that are strenuous enough to expend 300 calories per session or to raise the heart rate to 60 to 70 per cent of its maximum (Thompson et al 1982). This generally means like swimming, running, bicycling, dancing, or some other kind of aerobic activity (requiring high consumption of oxygen for a sustained period of time) rather than a more static exercise like weight lifting or sit-ups.

SUMMARY

Motivation is the force that energies and gives direction to behaviour and that underlies the tendency to persist. According to drive model, once the individual is in high drive state, there is a readiness to respond to external stimuli that are related to the arousal drive. Once the incentive is achieved that satisfies the drive. Among the models, the homeostatic model discusses a natural tendency of the body towards maintaining balance that serves to keep our internal environment at a relatively constant state with respect to various needs. It proposes that individuals who are characterised anxious and tense must ordinarily experience a high drive level than calm, placid individuals. Maslow has given humanistic model of motivation, wherein five stages are given namely—physiological, safety needs, belongingness, esteem needs and self-actualisation. The cognitive social model emphasises on the expectations an individual has about himself to reach to goal and the meaning of that goal for the individual. Locus of control can be internal (conditions are within the control of the person) or external (Conditions are controlled by other people or situations).

Motives are classified as primary motive, the physiological secondary motive, the learned or acquired desires. A low level of glucose in blood does not only indicate hunger motives but also include symbolic content of the food as love and sharing. People are different from one another in their desire to compete and win at whatever they undertake. Achievement motivation may be learned, there may be a dominant pattern with high achieving motives and is also associated with individual's behaviour as being persistent, challenging, high aspirant, etc.

Aggression motive is inclusive of the behaviour that the doer engages with an intention of doing harm in form of verbal attack, physical injury, violence or destructive action against people or property. Very often aggression is a response to intense frustration. We learn to be aggressive by observing our parents, the attitudes prevalent in the society and by observing television. Most psychologists' believe that a basic motivational system underlies exploratory behaviour and curiosity and arousal being related in important ways.

Frustration is the result of conflict between the competing motives. The conflicts are classified as: approach- approach, approach - avoidance, avoidance - avoidance, and multiple approach - avoidance conflict.

The shady of motivation has two major clinical applications: firstly, it can be of help in understanding the wide range of behaviours of patients in relation to their illness and treatment. Secondly, it is concerned with the problems, which arises directly from abnormalities of drives (sexual deviations and aggression). Motivation enhancement is becoming an important aspect in all treatments regimens as it relates to compliance. The outcome of some treatment intervention depends to some degree on the motivation of the patient.

Emotion

Bharati aged 48 years, is married and has two children. Bharati has been referred for her asthmatic attacks, which have recently become very severe and also occur more frequently. Her medication has been increased but Bharati has not got any relief. Bharati and her whole family are very upset due to her severe attacks, which at times even require hospitalisation. What could be the reason for Bharati's problem? One of the common causes in such situations is emotional distress. A detail history of psychosocial factors revealed that lately Bharati has been very upset, as her young daughter wanted to marry a boy from other caste. Bharati had tried to dissuade her daughter, but the daughter had her own perspective. Bharati has been worrying about this, has not been able to sleep, and has not discussed her problem with any one else. It is well known that the emotional state of the person has a great impact on the physical health; emotions can precipitate or aggravate an illness.

Emotion is one of the important aspects of human relationship. Emotions have a psychological aspects also related to behaviour and cognition, which influences the physiological aspects of the emotion. When you are screaming at someone's behaviour, it arouses sympathetic nervous system and your body reacts accordingly. An emotion involves a subjective awareness of a particular state of mind, which is recognised as happiness or fear, and an objective physiological change, like change in heart rate, and expressive motor behaviour (over activity, running away), which is observable and can be measured. Emotions are closely associated to health and sickness, thus an understanding of emotions is of great importance.

Definition

The dictionary gives many definitions of "emotion", most of which have to do with agitated movement of some kind. And most of this "agitated movement" has to do with goals. You often feel joy and happiness, when you reach a goal. You often feel angry and frustrated, when you perceive a barrier between you and a goal. And you may experience pain and depression, when you believe you cannot possibly get what you want or need. The emotional experience has not been much emphasised in the scientific definitions of emotion.

According to biologically oriented psychologists, emotion is primarily a physical reaction that involves rather special parts of your nervous system. The purpose of emotions is to arouse body for some kind of specific action (such as fighting), or to depress physical responses, so that body can regain itself.

To other psychologists, emotion is primarily an intrapsychic experience that involves "inner feelings" rather than physiological reactions (for overt behaviours). Some of these experts divide emotions into various types of mental experiences such as fear, anger, love, hate, and lust. Other intrapsychic psychologists view feelings as being bipolar either "pleasant" or "unpleasant". Still other group of psychologists perceives emotions as being behavioural responses. They are concerned with fearful reactions, rather than fears, and of inactivity or unresponsiveness rather than depression.

Cutting across this debate about what emotions are, is the age-old controversy about where emotions come from. Some psychologists believe that all cultures share similar emotional reactions. Other behavioural scientists view the emotions as being mostly learned reactions acquired through experience. These psychologists believe you had to be carefully taught to love the things you love, and to hate the things you despise.

The Physiology of Emotions

Emotionality has been viewed by some physiologists as primarily a biological event, and they tend to focus on arousal and depression. Emotional reactions are perceived by them as being one's way of preparing to respond to some kind of physical or psychological challenge. Imagine you are about to be attacked by some robbers. Then you must prepare yourself either to fight or to get out of the threatening situation. Your physiological emotional responses will take place without your conscious volition or desire; you do not have to "will" your sweat glands to secrete water or your teeth to start chattering, when you are frightened or cold. These activities are handled for you automatically by the unconscious parts of your brain and nervous system.

Autonomic Nervous System

Autonomic nervous system is that part of body which controls emotional reactions. It is connected to most of the glands and many of the muscles in the body. Autonomic nervous system has two major parts: (1) the sympathetic nervous system, whose activity tends to excite or arouse and (2) the parasympathetic nervous system, which tends to depress or slow down many of the bodily functions. Both parts of the nervous systems work together in a coordinated fashion to control bodily activities. When one needs to relax, parasympathetic system increases its neural activities, while sympathetic system slows down. It is the joint action of the two systems, which allows responding appropriately to most of the physical and psychological challenges one meets in life.

Sympathetic Nervous System

Your sympathetic nervous system consists of a group of 22 neural centres, lying on or close to your spinal cord. From these 22 centres, axonic fibers run to all parts of your body, to the salivary glands in your mouth, to the irises in your eyes, to your heart, lungs, liver, and stomach, and to your intestines and genitals. Your sympathetic nervous system is also connected with your sweat glands, your hair cells, and with the tiny blood vessels near the surface of your skin.

Whenever you encounter an emergency of some kind—something that enrages you, makes you suddenly afraid, creates strong desire, or calls for heavy labour on your part, your sympathetic nervous system swings into action in several ways:
- The pupils in your eyes open up to let in more light.
- Your heart pumps more blood to your brain, muscles and to the surface of your skin.
- You breathe harder and faster.
- Your blood sugar level is elevated.
- Your digestion is slowed down to a crawl.
- Your skin perspires to flush out the waste products created by the extra exertion and to keep you cool.
- The sympathetic nervous system also controls orgasm and ejaculation during sexual excitement.

In short, activity in your sympathetic nervous system prepares you for fighting, fleeing, feeding, or sexual climax.

Parasympathetic Nervous System

Your parasympathetic nervous system connects to most (but not all) parts of your body, as does the sympathetic. In general, parasympathetic stimulation produces physiological effects that are the opposite of those induced by sympathetic stimulation. Activity in your parasympathetic system does the following things:
1. It closes down or constricts the irises in your eyes.
2. It decreases the rate at which your heart beats.
3. It slows down your breathing.
4. It lowers your blood sugar level.
5. It increases salivation, stimulates the flow of digestive juices, and promotes the processes of excretion.
6. It retards sweating.
7. It induces penis erection in the male and nipple erection in the female during sexual activity.

Generally speaking, activity in your parasympathetic nervous system conserves or builds up your body's resources.

Homeostatic Balance

Increased neural excitement in the sympathetic system tends to inhibit activity in the parasympathetic, and *vice versa*. But the two systems are not really antagonists or competitors. Rather, they function together smoothly in a coordinated fashion to maintain an optimum balance between over-arousal and under-arousal. The sympathetic system gears the organism for energy output. As the emotion subsides, the parasympathetic system, the energy-conserving system, takes over and returns the organism to its normal state.

An example of joint activity of these two systems is the sexual act, where parasympathetic stimulation is necessary for erection to occur. However, orgasm and ejaculation are controlled by sympathetic excitation. Thus, sexual activity must begin with relaxation (parasympathetic stimulation) but typically goes on to arousal and climax (sympathetic stimulation). Too much sympathetic arousal or inhibition early in the sex act, leads to impotence in the male and disinterest or frigidity in the female. And too much parasympathetic stimulation will prevent orgasm in both sexes. Under normal circumstances, in most of the activities there is a normal balance between parasympathetic and sympathetic stimulation. On the contrary, individuals who are under stress or are angry, agitated, the balance between the two systems is disturbed and the sympathetic nervous system becomes more active.

The Adrenal Glands

There are two adrenal glands, one sitting atop each of the kidneys. Adrenals produce hormones that influence sexual development and that monitor bodily functions such as urine production. But these glands also produce two chemicals that are referred to as the "arousal" hormones. Earlier, these two hormones were called as adrenalin and noradrenalin, now these are more commonly referred as "epinephrine" and "norepinephrine."

When epinephrine and norepinephrine are released into the bloodstream by adrenal glands, these hormones bring about all of the physiological changes associated with strong emotions such as fear, anger, hostility and sexual aggressiveness. These two hormones act to prepare blood pressure and heart rate, speeding up breathing, widening the pupils in eyes, and increasing perspiration. The release of epinephrine and norepinephrine is under the control of sympathetic nervous system, whose activities are imitated by the hormones. When you encounter an arousing situation, your sympathetic nervous system goes into action first, mobilising your body's energy resources and also causing the secretion of the two "arousal" hormones. As you secrete epinephrine, the arousal process by chemically stimulating the same neural centres that the sympathetic nervous system has stimulated electrically.

But the hormones also increase the firing rate of the nerve cells in the sympathetic nervous system itself. This stimulation causes you to secrete more of the hormones, which increases activity in the sympathetic system, and so on until the emergency has passed or you collapse in exhaustion.

General Adaptation Syndrome

Hans Selye (1976) outlined the three states that body seems to go through when its resources must be mobilised to meet situations of excessive physiological stress. According to Selye, biological reaction to stress almost always follows the same adaptive pattern. Selye calls this pattern the General Adaptation Syndrome, or GAS and has three main stages or parts: (i) Alarm stage, (ii) resistance or counteraction and (iii) exhaustion. Suppose you suffer from a severe physical or emotional trauma. Your body will immediately respond with the alarm reaction, which is the first stage of the General Adaptation Syndrome. During this stage, your body and mind are in a state of shock. Your temperature and blood pressure drop, your tissues swell with fluid, and your muscles lose their tone. You may not think clearly and ability to file things away in long-term memory may be disrupted.

The second part of the GAS is the stage of resistance, or countershock. During this stage, your body begins to repair the damage it has suffered, and your mind begins to function more clearly. ACTH hormone is released by the brain, which acts on your adrenal glands, causing them to release their own hormones. These adrenal hormones counteract the shock in several ways, primarily by raising temperature and blood pressure. However, you pay a price for resisting the shock, for your body uses up its available supply of ACTH and adrenal hormones at a rapid pace. If the stress continues, your adrenal glands will swell as they strive to produce enough hormones to neutralise the stress.

During the first two GAS stages, your sympathetic nervous system is intensely aroused. However, if the emergency continues for too long, an overwhelming counter-reaction may occur in which your parasympathetic system takes over. You may fall into the third state— the stage of exhaustion. During this stage, you go into shock again because your body has been over-stimulated for so long, that it is depleted of ACTH and adrenal hormones. Further exposure to stress at this time can lead to depression, psychophysiological disorders or even death.

Theoretical Explanation of Emotion

Psychologists and physiologists have tried to formulate some general principles to explain emotions. These theories are concerned with the relationship between individuals' bodily states the emotions they feel, and how emotions are involved in behaviour.

The James-Lange Theory of Bodily Reactions: The most famous physiological theory of emotionality was proposed by William James in 1884. According to James, body always takes the lead in emotional situations; "feelings" are merely mental responses to the changes that have occurred in nervous system, muscles and glands.

An example of this could be, suppose you are walking through the woods one day and you almost step on a huge rattlesnake. Chances are, you will momentarily go into shock. Then, almost immediately, your heart will start pounding, your hair will stand on end, and you will breathe more rapidly. And if you are wise, you will slowly back away and then run for your life. Moments later, usually after you are out of danger, you will notice these physiological reactions and realise that you are scared.

You may think that you saw the snake, became frightened, and then ran. But according to James, this is not the case. For he presumes that your bodily reactions precede and thus cause your feelings. According to this theory, we are afraid because we run; we do not run because we are afraid. Later, similar explanation was given based on independent research by Lange and this is often called the James-Lange theory of emotions.

The Cannon-Bard Theory of Central Neural Processes: Some objections were pointed out to the James-Lange theory by the physiologist Walter B Cannon. First, James-Lange assumed that feelings are dependent upon activity in the sympathetic nervous system. However, people who (through accident or disease) have lost use of their sympathetic systems still feel emotions and show emotional behaviours. Second, the bodily changes associated with emotions generally occur after the "feelings and behaviours" have started, not before they take place. Third, the same physiological changes occur in very different emotional states and in nonemotional states as well.

Cannon believed that emotional inputs were processed almost simultaneously by two different parts of the brain, the thalamus and the hypothalamus; the thalamus controlled emotional feelings, while the hypothalamus controlled bodily responses. You would experience conscious *"fear"* of a snake, even if your body were totally paralysed because "fear" and "running" are mediated by different centres in your brain. Bard advanced almost the same viewpoint later in 1937, since then this approach to the explanation of emotionality is called the Cannon-Bard theory.

The Lasarus-Schachter Theory of Emotional Arousal

Sensory experiences lead to emotion only when the stimuli are cognitively appraised as having personal significance. Richard Lasarus (1984) advocated cognitive appraisal view, that emotional experience 'grows out of ongoing transactions with the environment that are evaluated'. According to Stanley Schachter (1971) the experience of emotion is the joint effect of the physiological arousal and cognitive appraisal. All arousal is assumed to be general and undifferentiated and it comes first in the emotion sequence. Cognition serves to determine how this ambiguous inner state will be labeled. This theory is also known as two factor theory of emotion. This approach has been challenged, as awareness of once physiological arousal is not a necessary condition for emotional experience.

Other Physiological Viewpoints: Karl Lashley (1960) noted that people with damaged thalamuses still experienced emotional feelings, and people with damaged hypothalamuses still showed emotional responses. At about the same time, other scientists showed that both the limbic system and the right hemisphere were involved in mediating emotional feelings and behaviours.

The recent theorists have pointed out that bodily reactions do play an important role in creating and sustaining emotions. However, our feelings are so frightfully complex, that we simply cannot reduce them to mere hormonal neural activity. To gain a more complete understanding of emotionality, therefore, we must look at intrapsychic variables as well.

Intrapsychic Aspects of Emotionality

Intrapsychic psychologists believe contrary to the biological psychologists that how you perceive and feel about a situation determines your bodily reactions. An intrapsychic viewpoint emphasises the reverse.

For example, you can tell the difference (subjectively) between your emotions and you differentiate between such emotional states as hunger, fear, and anger. You apparently do so on the basis of intrapsychic cues rather than biological states. The physical changes that occur in your body are pretty much the same, no matter what type of emotional upheaval you are undergoing.

There is some recent evidence that adrenal glands produce more epinephrine when you are afraid, but secretes more norepinephrine when you are angry. However, both hormones are released to some degree in all arousal situations. Thus, we cannot tell objectively whether you are angry or afraid just by measuring the relative amounts of epinephrine and norepinephrine floating around in your bloodstream.

The importance of psychological factors in emotions has been supported by a study, in which human volunteers were injected with large amounts of epinephrine or norepinephrine, they often reported feeling as if they were "about to become emotional", but they could not say why. The "arousal" they experienced did not seem "real" somehow, because it was not focussed or directed toward any given object. Many of the volunteers described the experience as "cold rage".

Cognitive Factors in Emotion

Bodily sensations, particularly the activity of the autonomic nervous system, are important to feelings of emotion, but different emotions show pretty much the same physiological patterns. People are usually aware that something is going on internally when they are angry, or excited, or afraid, but they do not discriminate their heart rate or blood pressure or what is happening in their stomach very well. The individual identifies and labels his state of physiological and psychological arousal in terms of the immediate circumstances, what angered them, or pleased them or frightened them. They go on to describe some of their bodily reactions and this determines whether he is, angry, fearful or happy. They do not define the emotion solely in terms of their own internal feelings.

These results support cognitive-physiological theory of emotion. According to Schachter (1971), emotion is internal physiological arousal in interaction with cognitive processes. Feedback to the brain from physiological activity gives rise to an undifferentiated state of affect, but the felt emotion is determined by the "label" the subject assigns to that aroused state. The assignment of a label is a cognitive process; the subject uses information from past experiences and his perception of what is going on around him to arrive at an interpretation of his feelings. This interpretation will determine how he acts and the label that he uses to define his emotional state. According to Lasarus (1966), the individual cognitive appraisal of any situation determines the emotional response, including its accompanying physiological changes. Appraisal is influenced by past experience and current availability of strategies for coping with threat.

Learning to label bodily sensations in terms of emotional tone (i.e. as pleasant or unpleasant) is relevant to some of the differences observed between experienced and inexperienced users, of alcohol, marijhuana, and other drugs. First, sensations are often unpleasant but much of the pleasure associated with the use of such drugs comes from cognitive and social factors. Initial users have to learn to label the physical sensations as enjoyable.

Modifying Arousal by Altering Cognitions: If our state of emotional arousal is determined by our cognitive evaluation of the emotion-producing situation, then it should be possible to alter arousal level by changing one's cognitions.

Indeed, you can think of instances where initial emotional responses to stimuli change as the situation is reappraised as threatening or benign. You are awakened by the telephone at midnight. Your initial fear reaction aroused by the thought that some catastrophe has happened to a loved one changes to relief as you discover it is a wrong number. A potentially emotion-producing situation has become neutral because of a change in your appraisal of it.

Types of Emotions

How many different types of emotions have you experienced? You would include love and hate, joy and sadness, anxiety and calmness, guilt and relief, anger and friendliness, fear and security, elation and depression. There are various classifications of the emotions. There are three basic innate emotions: fear, rage and love. From these, all other emotions are derived through conditioning process. McDougall (1908) listed seven primary emotions: flight-fear, repulsion-disgust, curiosity-wonder, pugnacity-anger, self abasement-subjective, self-assertion-elation and parental care-tenderness. There are complex emotions such as admiration, envy and sentiments (e.g. love, hate, respect). Sentiments are regarded as habitual responses to an object, involving a persistent disposition to respond in a particular way.

Emotions are generally measured on the scale with two extremes on either side; it may also be referred as positive pole or negative pole. An illustration of this would be—

Positive	Negative
Arousal	Inhibition
Joy	Sadness
Love	Hate

Verbal descriptions of emotions are at best poor descriptions of complex psychological processes. Is your love for material things, the same sort of intrapsychic experience as your love for your mother or for your country? And when you say, you are "somewhat afraid of lizards", is that merely a weaker form of the fear someone else feels when he says, "I despise those creepy-crawly things." We seldom experience emotions in a vacuum. Rather, emotions are tied to specific events, situations, and objects. Thus, it seldom makes much sense to talk about "love" in abstract terms. Rather, we should probably speak of "love of" something, or "the love for" something.

Some emotions are not only positive and arousing, they give us a pleasant feeling as well.

Other emotions are not only negative and depressing, they are also downright unpleasant. But again, things are not as simple as they seem. Some love makes us happy, whereas others are frustrating and unrewarding. Some hatred is depressing, while others stimulate us to pleasurable accomplishments.

Karl Pribram has attempted to explain the concept of "feeling tone". He believes that there are two types of positive affect: gratification and satisfaction. There are also two types of negative affect or feeling tone, which Pribram calls distress and dissatisfaction. You experience "gratification", whenever your needs are satisfied or your physiological drives are reduced. The feelings that accompany this gratification are relief, calmness, and tranquility. "Satisfaction" goes beyond mere calmness, it occurs when you reduce your uncertainty about things. The feelings associated with satisfaction are those of delight, relish, joy, and exhilaration.

Role of Learning in Emotional Arousal

Some situations appear to be innately emotion producing. Anger tends to be provoked by restraint against the carrying out of a motivated sequence of behaviour. Fear can be aroused by pain, a loud noise, or sudden loss of support in any young individual. The fear-arousing element seems to be strangeness, and we can postulate that the important factor is the ability to discriminate the new from the familiar.

Fear of something strange seems to be largely innate, but maturation and learning may be required as a background. At about eight months, human infants show an intense fear of strangers. No matter how sociable the child has been prior to this time, or how many different people he has been exposed to, the onset of "stranger shyness" is usually abrupt and intense? The most plausible interpretation is that maturation of perceptual abilities has enabled the child to discriminate familiar from strange adults.

Emotions may also be associated with new objects or situations by learning. In the classic experiment by Watson, the founder of Behaviourism, a boy named Albert was conditioned to fear, a previously neutral object, a white rat. When eleven-month-old Albert was shown a white rat, he reached for it, evidencing no fear. But every time he touched the rat he was frightened by a loud sound. He soon became afraid of the rat. The originally neutral rat became a "conditioned stimulus" to fear. Albert also showed fear of his mother's fur neckpiece and of other furry objects. Albert's fear generalised to objects that were similar in some respect to the rat but not to toys, such as rubber balls or blocks, that were unlike rat in appearance (Watson and Rayner, 1920).

It is probably that some irrational fears are acquired in this relatively automatic way. You would have experienced that children are very fearful of the hospitals because of their association of hospital with injections. Similarly, fear of thunder can be understood because lightning precedes thunder, the child may come to fear the lightning as much as the thunder, although the loud sound of thunder is the primary reason for fright. But most fears are probably learned in a more complex way, some through actual contact with harmful objects, but more through imitation of parental fears.

Emotional Expression

How emotions are expressed? Are there individual differences in expression of emotions? The different research finding have pointed out that there are some emotions, which are universally expressed in the similar way, these have been termed as innate emotional expression. There are some emotional expressions, which are influenced by learning, culture and individual style.

Innate Emotional Expression

The basic ways of expressing emotion are innate. Children all over the world cry when hurt or sad, and laugh when happy. Studies of children blind and deaf from birth, indicate that many of the facial expressions, postures, and gestures that we associate with different emotions develop through maturation, they appear at the appropriate age even when there is no opportunity to observe them in others. Certain facial expressions do seem to have a universal meaning regardless of the culture in which the individual is raised, like facial expressions of happiness, anger, sadness, disgust, fear, and surprise.

Hole of Learning in Emotional Expression: Although certain emotional expressions may be largely innate, many modifications occur through learning. Anger, for example, may be expressed by fighting, by using abusive language, or by leaving the room. Leaving the room is not an expression of emotion that is known at birth, and certainly the abusive language has to be learned. Certain facial expressions and gestures are taught by one's culture as ways of expression emotion. As you would have observed that laughter is restrained in some cultures.

Even gender differences in expression of emotions are seen, females are supposed to suppress expression of emotions. Thus, superimposed upon basic expressions of emotion, which appear to be universal, are conventional or stereotyped forms of expression, which become a kind of 'language of emotion', recognised by others within a culture. Skilled actors are able to convey to their audiences any intended emotion by using facial expressions, tone of voice, and gestures, according to the patterns the audience recognises.

Arousal Level and Effectiveness of Performance: A mild level of emotional arousal tends to produce alertness and interest in the task at hand. When emotions become intense, however, whether they are pleasant or unpleasant, they usually result in some decrement in performance. The curve in Figure 9.1 represents the relation between the level of emotional arousal and the effectiveness of performance. At very low levels of arousal (for example, when one is just waking up), the nervous system may not be functioning fully and sensory messages may not get through. Performance is optimal at moderate levels of arousal. At high levels of arousal, performance begins to decline. Presumably, the central nervous system is so responsive, that it is responding to too many things at once; thus, preventing the appropriate set of responses from dominating. Individuals differ in the extent to which their behaviour is disrupted by emotional arousal. Observations of people during crises, such as fires or sudden floods, suggest that about 15 per cent show organised, effective behaviour. The majority, 70 per cent, shows various degrees of disorganisation but are still able to function with some effectiveness. The remaining 15 per cent are so disorganised that they are unable to function at all. They may race around screaming or exhibit aimless and completely inappropriate behaviour.

Emotions, when sufficiently intense, can seriously impair the processes that control organised behaviour.

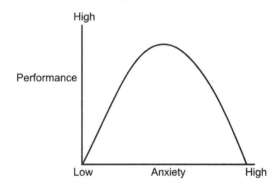

Fig. 9.1: Arousal and performance

Clinical Applications

Emotions according to their intensity can be adaptive or disruptive. Here, emotions are related to stress and individual's ability to cope with stresses. Sometimes emotions are not quickly discharged but continue to remain unexpressed or unresolved. Perhaps, the situation that makes one angry (e.g. prolonged conflict with one's employer) or mat makes one fearful (e.g. worry over the chronic illness of a loved one) continues for a long period of time. The state of heightened arousal can take its toll of the individual's ability to function efficiently. Sometimes, continual emotional tension can impair physical health. In a psychophysiological disorder, the symptoms are physical, but the cause is primarily psychological. A number of different types of illness, e.g. ulcers, asthma, migraine headaches, chronic fatigue, high blood pressure and skin eruptions, are related to emotional stress. Long-term emotional stress can impair a person's physical health as well as his mental efficiency.

The physiological changes accompanying intense emotions are the basis for use of the polygraph, commonly known as the "lie detector", in checking the reliability of an individual's statements. The polygraph does not detect lies; it simply measures some of the physiological accompaniments of emotion. The measures most frequently recorded are alternations in heart rate, blood pressure, respiration and the galvanic skin response, or GSR (the GSR is a change in the electrical conductivity of the skin).

Feelings involve the expenditure of physical, mental, or behavioural energy. Learning to cope with emotions, therefore, requires learning how to handle the stresses and strains of life. Anxiety and phobias are result of intense emotional experience. Apprehension of panic attack or anxiety is related to the James-Lange theory. Even if the autonomic changes are not the cause of the emotional state, awareness of them, acts like a positive feedback to many patients. Another clinical condition of interest in relation to emotions is epilepsy originating in the temporal lobes. The electric discharge in that part of the brain may give rise to a transient state of intense fear.

Emotions and the accompanying physiological changes are considered by many to be of great importance in relation to psychosomatic medicine. The psychosocial factors may contribute to the causation of, or affect the course and prognosis of, organic disease.

In psychopharmacology, study of emotions has become important, as many factor influence the effect of a drug on behaviour such as dosage, route of administration and the presence of multiple effects. Even the placebo effect is due to the psychological influences arising from the patient's perception of the situation in which the drug is administered.

SUMMARY

Emotion is an important aspect of human relationship. Emotions have a psychological aspect related to behaviour and cognition, which influences the physiological aspect of emotion. It is a subjective awareness as happiness or fear, and an objective physiological change like heart rate and expressive motor behaviour.

Emotion has been viewed as a biological event. Emotional reactions are controlled by autonomic nervous system, which has two parts: sympathetic nervous system and parasympathetic nervous system. It is the joint action of the two systems, which allows one to respond appropriately. When the individual is in a relaxed state, the parasympathetic nervous system increases its neural activities, while sympathetic nervous system slows down. A homeostatic balance is maintained between over arousal and under arousal. The physiological changes due to strong emotions are associated with arousal hormones produced by adrenal glands, namely, epinephrine and norepinephrine. The release of epinephrine and norepinephrine is under the control of sympathetic nervous system. General Adaptation Syndrome theory advocates that during excessive stress, the body goes through three stages mobilising its resources for an emergency. These three stages are the stage of alarm, the resistance and exhaustion.

James-Lange theory of emotion states that the emotions we experience result from our perception of the changes taking place in the body during emotion. However, the Cannon-Bard theory believes that emotional inputs were processed almost simultaneously by two different parts of the brain, the thalamus and the hypothalamus. The emotional feelings were controlled by the thalamus and the hypothalamus controlled bodily responses. Other physiological viewpoints do not agree with Cannon-Bard theory as the individuals with damaged thalamus also experience emotions. Thus, psychologists have given intrapsychic explanations; they view emotions as experiences that involve inner feelings, than physiological reactions. The cognitive-physiological theory of emotion states that the individual's cognitive appraisal of any situation determines the emotional response, including its accompanying physiological changes. Appraisal is influenced by past experience and current availability of strategies for coping with threat. Though emotional reactions are shared by all cultures, but some emotional reactions are also learned through experience. Different research findings have pointed out that there are some emotions, which are universally expressed, these are termed as innate expressed emotion. There are some emotions, which are learned through culture and individual styles. The relationship between the arousal level and the performance determines its effectiveness. Performance is optimal at moderate levels. At low levels, the nervous system may not be fully functioning, and at high levels the performance declines.

Sometimes, continual emotional tension can impair physical health. In a psychophysiological disorder, the symptoms are physical, but the cause is primarily psychological. A number of different types of illness, e.g. ulcers, asthma, migraine, headaches, chronic fatigue, high blood pressure and skin eruptions, are related to emotional stress. Long-term emotional stress can impair a person's physical health as well as his mental efficiency. Emotions and the accompanying physiological changes are considered by many to be of great importance in relation to psychosomatic medicine.

Negative emotions can be quite stressful; learning to cope with emotions requires learning how to handle the stresses and strains of life.

Stress and Coping

Vijay, 45 years old, is a company executive in a multinational firm. Being in the top position, Vijay leaves home at seven thirty every morning and returns back late in the evening. He has no time to rest, or able to enjoy leisure time activities. Every day he has to meet dead lines in work, attend official meetings and take decisions. He has not been able to take off from work even for a single day for the last two years. However, lately Vijay has been having some physical problems, like he never feels fresh, is tired all the time, is not able to have sound sleep, has often indigestion of food and his appetite has reduced. All the laboratory test has failed to get a cause for his problems. Such physical problems do occur as a result of persistent stress.

We all experience stress in some or the other form, such as meeting time-bound targets, competitions, getting stuck in a traffic jam while on the way to attend an urgent task, noise, social pressures, etc. We differ in the extent to which we get affected by stressors as we all have different ways of dealing with these situations.

Definition

Hans Selye (1974), the pioneer in stress research, defined stress as a stimulus event of sufficient severity to produce disequilibrium in the homeostatic physiological systems. We feel stress when our responses to even disrupt or threaten to disrupt our physical or psychological functioning. Positive stresses called 'Eustress', like shifting to a new house, promotion in job. When stress has negative effect on the individual, it is distress, for example, failure in examination, chronic illness, break-up with loved ones. The stimulus that evokes a stress response is called a stressor. A stimulus becomes a stressor by virtue of the cognitive interpretation or meaning that the individual assigns to the stimulus or by virtue of the fact that the stimulus affects the individual by way of same sensory or metabolic process, which is in itself inherently stressful. In physiological terms stress is the body's response to any stressful demand. Lazarus defined it in psychological terms as an Individual's cognitive judgement that his or her personal resources will be taxed or incapable of dealing with the demands posed by a particular event. According to Reuben Hill a stressor event is one that makes demands on the family system, rather than on the individual.

Components of Stress

Stress comprises of stressor, the sources causing the stress and stress response, which is how the individual copes with the stressful situation, his coping resources like person's skills and social support systems (Fig. 10.1).

Stressor represents stimulus events requiring some form of adaptation or adjustment. Stressor can be internal stimuli like cognitions or thoughts or external stimuli like crowd, noise, and interpersonal difficulties. The stressed person

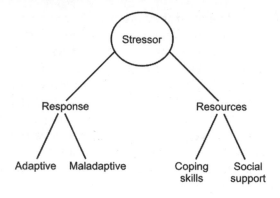

Fig. 10.1: Components of stress

shows several stages: (i) Stage of alarm, (ii) Stage of appraisal, and (iii) Stage of reaching for a coping strategy.

The stress response is a complex reaction pattern that consists of physiological, cognitive and behavioural components. The physiological component of the stress response activates the sympathetic and parasympathetic autonomic nervous system and elicits a set of physiological reactions. The stress response has three components namely the tonic—the resting or basal level of activity, the phasic—the reaction to the given stressor and recovery—return to the tonic level.

Sylve had described a three-stage reaction to stress consisting of alarm, resistance and exhaustion known as general adaption syndrome (GAS). The three stages are as following:
a. Alarm reaction, subdivided in two phases, shock and counter-shock. Shock phase is initial and immediate response. Counter shock is how the body rebounds to mobilise its defenses.
b. Stage of resistance: This is adaptation where you try to fight back.
c. Stage of exhaustion: This is extreme fatigue one feels after fighting against stress.

As an example imagine you are in a building, which has caught fire. The place is full of people and there is only one exit door. Your first reaction would be of shock. For some time you are numb, but in no time you try to size up the situation. According to the second stage of resistance, you look for an alternative way to get out; you break open the window glass, jump into the balcony and finally get out of the building. In the process of getting out you may also help others to escape from fire. Finally when you are out from this stressful situation then there is extreme exhaustion and fatigue.

The first two phases of GAS prepare one's body to respond to stress in one of the two ways—either attacking the threatening force (fight) or escaping to safety (flight). These physiological responses result from the action of the adrenal gland which has been stimulated to increase the body's production of adrenalin hormone that gives body the required energy needed to adapt to the demands of the stressor.

The cognitive components of stress response represents the conscious appraisal of the stimulus, the individual's evaluation or perception of the situation. This also includes mood state, ranging from elation to tension, depression, difficulty in concentration and fatigue. Coping styles are also an example of cognitive coping. The behavioural component represents overt behavioural response to the stressor. Behaviour can range from withdrawal to aggression, and violence. Facial expressions also indicate behavioural reactions. Frequent outbursts of anger, competitiveness and sexual dysfunctions are manifestation of stress response.

Types of Stress

Stress is not only desirable but also essential to life. A certain amount of stress is essential for normal health. Stresses can be positive or negative. The positive stress is called 'eustress', and the negative stress is termed as 'distress'

(Selye 1974). Some events are associated with positive emotions, while others are associated with negative emotions, which in turn determine the quality of the stress experiences. We usually think of negative events or situations as the causes of stress. Some positive changes like constructing a house, a new job, promotion, marriage or becoming a parent may be stressful due to increased pressure and responsibilities. As these are associated with positive feelings like excitement, happiness, love and joy, they increase our resistance to stress. On the other hand, negative situations such as death of the spouse, parents illness, interpersonal problems, difficulty at the place of work, financial losses, etc. are all associated with negative feelings such as sadness, dissatisfaction, conflict, irritation and confusion. These feelings lower our resistance to stress and make us more vulnerable to mental disturbances and diseases. The negative aspects of stress can produce harmful effects on the body especially if they are continuing for a long time. Stress produces tension and exerts a great pressure on the body systems. It is like the body being in a state of constant preparedness to meet a challenge. This tension disturbs the mental and the physical health. Stress can also prevent healthy and smooth functioning of different organs of the body and accelerates the aging process.

Stressful Life Events

Research suggests that experiencing an excessive number of 'life events' in a particular period of time can lead to increased ill-health. Holmes and Rahe (1967) have indicated the relation of life events to our health. These events are normal events that occur in everyone's life over a lifetime—birth, death, marriage, divorce, new job, retirement, moving house or going for a holiday. The important factor is how often you experience these changes, whether they occur together at the same time or in a short span of time and whether they are positive or negative. The greater the amount of social readjustment required, greater the likelihood of developing an illness. Paykel showed that loss events such as loss of job or death are more likely to be associated with illness than gain events such as new addition in the family or buying a new house. The variety of illnesses that have been linked with life events range from heart disease, cancer and depression to the less life-threatening common cold or migraine.

Daily Hassles

Major life events are rare occurrences for most of us. One does not generally get married more than once or have more than two or three children, or change jobs frequently. Usually most of us are able to cope with these events quite effectively without being under too much pressure.

What could actually be more stressful are the small daily hassles or events which appear trivial, like standing in long bus queues, getting stuck in a traffic jam, arguments and fights with an uncooperative colleague at work, tension between family members or a very sick, aging parent. These daily tensions can produce a cumulative effect and may result in your having a breakdown one day.

Chronic stress from such daily hassles or stressors can cause physiological damage and also lead to the development of certain psychosomatic illnesses such as arthritis, irritable bowel syndrome, bronchial asthma, hypertension, migraine and other chronic illness.

Stressful Life Events in Children: Children also experience stress and they have different stressful events than those of adults. An excess of life events was noted in adolescents attending outpatient clinics with recurrent abdominal pain (Green et al 1985). Children tend to report pain that is associated with tension and worry about specific situations—usually academic tests or new situations. Vulnerable children who develop psychiatric symptoms, especially those having psychogenic pains, demonstrate a direct association of a traumatic loss and illness event (Mehta et al 1993).

Singh et al (1994) studied the relationship between stressful family life events and somatic complaints in 77 school children, and found a significant association between life event and somatic complaints, these increasing in almost direct proportion to the number of stressful family life events. Occurrence of symptoms was more in girls. The most frequent stressful life events were financial problems, moving house, death of a relative, chronic illness in the family and frequent change in job of parents.

Robinson et al (1988) studied adolescents with functional somatic complaints (chest pain, recurrent abdominal pain, limb pain, and hyperventilation syndrome). Patients reported significantly more negative life events, a lower self-esteem, more psychophysiological symptoms and a lower self-evaluation than controls. They suggested that functional somatic complaints in adolescents might be associated with poor psychosocial adjustment and reaction to negative life events.

Maloney (1980) stressed that grief reaction is often an important precipitant of symptoms. Pantel and Goddman (1972) studied 100 adolescents with recurrent chest pain. 31 per cent subjects reported occurrence of significant negative life events within 6 months of onset of pain.

Scharrer, Ryan-Wenger and Nancy (1991) found that children with RAP had higher mean stress under the parameters of frequency, severity and total stress. Stresses included parental arguments, not spending enough time with parents and falling sick. Mean scores for coping efficacy and total coping were higher in non RAP group.

Rangaswamy and Kamakshi (1983) studied the role of stress in 30 adolescent hysterics aged 13-17 years using the social readjustment rating scale of Coddington for 12-16 years old. This study was the first systematic study in the field of life events in children in India and reported that the majority (85%) of hysterics had a significant life stress before the onset of symptoms. Malhotra et al (1992) found that sick children (hysteria/emotional disorders, hyperactive/conduct disorders, enuresis and miscellaneous category) scored higher on life events and stress scores when compared to normal children.

Daily hassles often have more adverse effect than major stresses. Mehta and Singh (1995) reported that the relatively minor life events, i.e. daily hassles and major life events were significantly associated with persistence of recurrent abdominal pain (RAP). These children experienced greater incidence of stressful life events like change in school (66%), beginning a new level in school (50%), increase in arguments between parents (43%), change in financial status of parent (33%), change in father's occupation (23%), loss of a job of a parent (20%), hospitalisation of sibling (16%), death of grandparent (10%), hospitalisation of a parent (6%), and mother beginning work (10%). RAP children and control had more or less similar problems but the appraisal (how much an event disturbs) was different in the two groups. Due to poor coping strategies RAP children perceived greater negative impact of stressful events. Children's perception of stressful events was different than that of their parents. Problems related to the personal lives in school as well as in the family had more negative impact on them.

Family Stress

All of us who live in families, however, have also experienced the kind of stress that we share with others in our households. Family stress can take many forms. Many stressors obviously affect the entire family—such events as theft, sickness, marriage or childbirth. In India we have a large number of extended families and joint families thus family stress is the common problem. If one member of the family has chronic illness or financial loss, the rest of the family members are also affected.

Executive Stress

The office culture at all levels causes lot of problems related to stress. Number of organisations are experiencing that at higher ladder people have more and more of stress-related problems, often manifesting in physical problems like high blood pressure, short temper, insomnia, chronic fatigue syndrome, low back pains, headaches and migraines and increased consumption of alcohol and smoking. These problems are now known as executive stress as besides long hours of work, these people are involved in decision making, given lot of responsibilities and have result-oriented tasks. They have to meet competitions and challenges. A study conducted at NIMHANS (1996), on the police officers revealed that police officers in certain cadres have 'burnt out' syndrome—emotional exhaustion, depersonalisation and reduced personal accomplishment. Many established organisations have expressed their concerned and have started stress management programmes for their employees.

Test Anxiety

Test anxiety is stress-related factor commonly seen in students. Virtually all students experience some anxiety before a test. But students with excessive test anxiety feel 'frozen up' and panic before exams. Due to high level of anxiety their academic performance is also affected, even with hard work and high intelligence they are unable to get good results.

Stress-esteem

Pearlin (1989) has observed, that coping style and social support have effect on stress outcomes. Self-esteem has been linked to elements of the stress process. According to Rosenberg (1965, 1986), self-esteem is "the evaluation which the individual makes and customarily maintains with regard to himself or herself: it expresses an attitude of approval or disapproval toward oneself". The process of self-esteem formation is said to involve the principles of "reflected appraisal", "social comparison", and "self attribution". Reflected appraisal involves the individual's interpretation of how he or she is viewed by others, whereas social comparison holds that "in the absence of objective information about themselves people judge themselves on the basis of comparison with others". Self-attribution refers to the tendency to draw conclusions about oneself from observing one's own actions, including the success or failure of efforts. It is clear that self-esteem is potentially modifiable by future social experience. Accordingly, to the extent it is relevant to psychological distress and disorder, it represents one obvious target for prevention and early intervention efforts in the service of mental health. The goal of such efforts would be to increase the individual's capacity to maintain self-esteem in the face of adversity and, especially, loss events.

A positive and resilient self-image (in contrast to a negative or labile self-esteem) represents a crucial resource for combating the negative implications for self that are the frequent accompaniments of stressful events. Presumably, the stability and extent of self-esteem is determined by the nature and consistency of one's cumulative experiences of reflected appraisals, social comparisons, and self-attributions.

Self-esteem and Psychological Distress: It has been noted that poor self-esteem can lead to depression. Low self-esteem represents a vulnerability factor that increases risk of depression three-fold in the presence of stress. The significance of self-esteem as a mediator of the impact of unemployment on psychological distress has been demonstrated by studies involving diverse populations and designs. It has been reported that individuals high in self-esteem appear to be more resistant to the negative effects of unemployment than individuals low in self-esteem.

Low self-esteem is generally taken as a key-defining characteristic of depression. This view is associated with the cognitive theory of depression, which suggests that low esteem may be state dependent, arising out of depressive affect rather than contributing to it. Thus, it can be concluded that some important part of the causation involved in the self-esteem-depression relationship goes from esteem to depression, and that self-esteem may be especially significant among the disadvantaged and in high-stress circumstances. One implication of this conclusion is that prevention or intervention efforts should be made to enhance self-esteem to reduce the risk of psychological distress.

Personality and Stress

Certain personality types are prone to specific illnesses. This understanding helps us to modify a behavioural pattern to prevent the onset of related illness. People who are perfectionists, self-sacrificing, conforming, self-conscious, inhibited, shy and nervous, sensitive, get easily worked up, are more prone to get physical diseases if exposed to prolonged and severe stress.

Type A personality has often been associated with stress and illness. As you will read in Chapter 11, that these people are intensely ambitious, competitive and impatient. They are always pre-occupied with deadlines and want to achieve things in the shortest possible time. Type A person expends enormous energy in pursuit of his goals. Migraine and tension headaches are also associated with this personality type.

COPING WITH STRESS

There is no way that we can escape stress throughout life. Stress whether good or bad, is an all-prevailing facet of life. It is unavoidable and inescapable. So, what everyone attempts is to cope with stress and maintain it at manageable levels. We all learn to cope with tensions.

Coping strategies in managing stress require change in yourself, others and the environment. You may have to use one of these according to the problem or situation. Coping means the ways and means you adopt to keep stress at manageable levels. If you are getting stressed because of overwork, you will need to learn to relax, change your working style, bring about certain changes in yourself, so that you perceive the stressor as not so threatening, or find ways to convert it into a motivating or driving force. If the stress is due to interpersonal problems then one can discuss with colleagues, similarly environment can be modified by reducing noise level, rearranging the things or going for a short holiday.

It is our reaction to stress that determines the effect of stress on our life. Cognitive appraisal or our perception of a stressor is the most important aspect of our coping ability, for example, for some people frequent travelling is pleasurable whereas a person with negative cognitive appraisal would think travelling as very tiring, monotonous, and waste of time. The way we feel depends to a great extent on the way we think about the events in our lives. Lazarus sees stress as a result of a transaction between person and environment. The way people appraise or construe their relationship with the environment is a function of cognition, or thought. These thoughts influence the way people feel. On the contrary individual's emotions affect the way they make sense out of the world around them. Thus, emotion (feeling) follows cognition (thought), and *vice versa*.

The way we all feel, think and act is a product of the way we as individuals interact with events. All experiences—the good and the bad: are filtered through one's unique personalities, personal histories, and viewpoints on life. By and large, we determine which of these experiences will be uplifting and which will be degrading. We do this partly in the way we act to shape our own lives and partly in the way we react to the shapes our lives assume.

Coping skills are an individual's attempt to resolve life stressors and emotional pain. Coping can be thought of as having two components, the methods used and the focus of the coping response. In terms of method of coping, the individual can utilise either an active response to resolve the stressful event or choose to avoid the stressor. The focus of the coping response may be directed at the problem itself (problem-focussed) or the emotional consequences of the stressor (emotion-focussed). Active cognitive coping responses manage one's appraisal of the stressfulness of the problem itself or its emotional consequences. Avoidance cognitive coping responses include those attempts to avoid having to confront the problem, like denying a heart attack, and claiming it to be just a severe case of indigestion.

Coping can be positive and negative. Some of the negative coping techniques are drinking alcohol, taking drugs, escaping from the stressful situation. There are certain ways to cope with the day-to-day stress in positive way. These are physical and mental exercises to reduce tension, diversion in various hobbies and activities to avoid negative thoughts, nutrition and healthy eating habits, lifestyle and congenial interpersonal relationship. The coping strategies usually employed by majority of people are distraction, situation redefinition, direct action, catharsis, acceptance, seeking social support, relaxation, and religion.

In cases where stress is severe and has consequently manifested in physical or psychological problems, help from the professionals should be taken. Stress inoculation training can help in coping with the stress.

Stress-Inoculation Training

Rajeev, a first-year college student, always breaks out in a cold sweat before taking an examination, is so tense and nervous that he forgets all the material and goes on to get a low grade on the test. Since Rajeev wants to do well at the university, he knows he will have to do something to overcome this debilitating test anxiety.

One thing Rajeev might do is to seek out a programme of stress-inoculation training. This approach uses techniques of behaviour modification to prevent stress in a variety of specific areas. These programmes educate individuals about their stressful reactions through an active give-and-take between leader and participants, give them a chance to rehearse ways to cope with the specific stressor being discussed, and then have them practice these coping skills on a variety of stressors, from mild to severe. In one programme geared to test anxiety, students are encouraged to learn new, helpful statements that they can say to themselves to replace the former anxiety-producing ones.

Stress-inoculation training has many other applications. It can help people overcome phobias, cope with pain, and control anger. One innovative way to use this same basic approach is to prevent stress before it occurs. Cognitive behavioural approaches have been used very successfully to manage problems arising from stress. Cognitive behavioural approaches are described in detail in Chapter 21.

Family Coping

The event that affects one human being—illness, a job promotion that requires a move out of town, the loss of a job, any major triumph or disappointment is likely to affect everyone in that person's family. Not only does the affected individual have to cope with the stress, the entire family must deal with it. Researchers who have studied family stress have found that families cope by the same basic means as individual's do by taking actions and changing their attitudes, both to solve the problems and to make themselves feel better.

Assessment of Stress and Coping

There are various methods to assess stress, these can be physiological measures or can be assessed on self-report, questionnaires, checklist and rating scales. One of the examples of rating scale developed for Indian population is given here. For children different scales are used as their stressors are different than those of adults (Table 10.1).

While psychological inventories and tests are also available that measure how the individual copes, clinical practice necessitates immediate empirical evaluation of the problem, the vulnerability level, and the coping strategies in use. The following list suggests guidelines of a generally useful approach to the assessment of patients, whether the predominant problem is ward-centred, and illness-related, or personality-related.

1. Do not use a set speech because each patient is different.
2. Introduce yourself, even to stuporous or confused patients.
3. Sit down and try to establish eye contact.
4. Avoid asking questions that can be answered 'yes' or 'no'.
5. Learn how to listen and observe.
6. Respond as seems appropriate, but make sure that the patient has the opportunity to talk, too.
7. Monitor your own thoughts because they may mirror those of the patient, or help explain your difficulties in getting across.
8. Modulate and measure your answers according to the needs of the patient.
9. Always ask yourself what the patient was like before becoming ill.
10. Clarification, control and cooling off are usually carried out simultaneously, just as perception, behaviour, and emotion are a unit.
11. Use the most timely, informative, and evocative questions, such as:
    a. What has bothered you most about this illness?
    b. How has it been a problem for you?
    c. What have you done (or are you doing) about the problem?
    d. What has been the most difficult thing you have had to face until now?
    e. What did you do then?
    f. Whom do you rely on most, or expect will be most helpful to you?
    g. In general, how do things usually turn out for you?
    h. Tell me what you think about this whole situation.

Clinical Applications

Effect of Stress on Health Coping is a problem-solving behaviour designed to bring about relief and equilibrium. The common denominator of coping is to have a problem. The common task of physicians and patients is to solve problems related to being sick, that is, the medical plight beyond mere physical changes and consequences. Coping, therefore, is an integral part of medical practice as well as illness. With the same disease at comparable stages, and with more or less equivalent treatment, patients may have different problems, and physicians may themselves respond with a wide variety of reactions, diagnoses and management.

Coping means that one has to overcome a threat or master a risky situation. How patients cope is a complicated mixture of cognitive appraisal and reappraisal, initial responses and corrected responses. Being sick is a problem in

Behavioural Sciences in Medical Practice

Table 10.1: Stress life events rating scale

S.No.	Events	Degrees of readjustment required
		Minimum ← 1 2 3 4 5 6 7 → Maximum

1. Death of husband/wife
2. Marital separation
3. Sent to jail
4. Death of a close family member, parent, sibling, child
5. Serious personal illness
6. Marriage of self
7. Losing job
8. Marital reconciliation
9. Retirement from job
10. Illness of a close family member
11. Difficulty in sexual relationship
12. Birth of a child
13. Significant increase in income unexpectedly
14. Significant decrease in income unexpectedly
15. Moving to another city
16. Death of a close friend
17. Argument/Fight with spouse
18. Borrowing money (Rs. 2,000 or more)
19. Promotion
20. Criminal or legal offense committed by close family
21. Demotion
22. Criminal/legal offense committed against a close family member
23. Son/daughter running away from house
24. Trouble with in-laws
25. Academic failure (in important examination)
26. Trouble with employer/boss, etc.
27. Moving to another house in the same city
28. Change of religion
29. Exit of close family member from household
30. Marriage of son
31. Marriage of daughter
32. Leaving home in search of spirituality
33. Partitioning of the joint family
34. A major theft in the house
35. Disappointment in love
36. Spouse unfaithful
37. Loss in business
38. Child marriage against parent's wishes

itself. But the fact of being sick sends waves into the far reaches of a patient's life, undoing psychosocial balance, and even initiating illness in significant others (family and friends).

Disease-related problem: Different diseases have their own special complications with which almost every victim must cope. A disfiguring scar, ataxia, a colostomy, a restrictive diet, and so forth require some form of primary rehabilitation and retraining that entails coping processes. Behavioural scientist in a general hospital deals with psychosocial problems. Some of these are complications of rehabilitative procedures. For example, it is not uncommon for an elderly person to prefer a wheelchair to a prosthesis after a leg amputation. The patient may be able to walk well with assistance in the hospital, but be reluctant to venture beyond his room when he returns home. The treating doctor can talk about the amputation with the patient, and then about the living arrangements, the emotional support received or not received from others, and fears about walking unaided or alone on a crowded street. Behavioural Scientist is now being asked more often to help patients suffering from "diseases of progress". Almost every advancement in medicine is followed by an unexpected complication. Treatments that save patients from one disease may expose them to several others. The secondary problems of immunosuppression are prominent examples that require psychosocial intervention.

Sickness-related problems: Illness have its interpersonal and intrapsychic qualities that may undo medical and surgical efforts. When the limits of medicine and surgery have been reached, psychosocial problems may just be gathering momentum. For example, a young father who develops carcinoma of the lung is not just physically sick. He worries about his job as well as about other psychosocial complications of illness and its treatment. He may complain about the physicians, argue with his wife, and even blame his children for his plight. All these objectionable results may conceal deep pessimism about survival and fear of abandoning people closest to him.

For some people, patienthood is easier than functioning in the outside world. A person who submits courageously to a series of operations may not be able to work when recovered and thereby becomes an even greater liability than before the surgery began. Every illness should be presumed to carry a balance of gains and losses for the individual. An unexpected improvement or recovery in a patient who has become accustomed to invalidism and the sick role may induce relative ego impairment if too many psychosocial responsibilities are thrust on the patient too quickly. Survival, support and self-esteem are only three important problems faced by chronically-ill patients, including those who are rescued from invalidism through newer medical and surgical treatments.

Vulnerability

Vulnerability refers to the emotional distress that is the most personal aspect of illness. It reflects impairment of competence, control and consciousness. Consequently, vulnerability not only signifies distress in the here-and-now, but a disposition to behave or conduct oneself at less than full efficiency. The ways in which the human being is vulnerable are both endless and unexpected.

Manifestation of poor coping: While dealing with other people you would meet people who are not good in coping with the daily hassles or stresses. Here are some behavioural patterns that can be observed in these individuals.

Vulnerability: Hopelessness -Patient believes that all is lost; effort is futile; there is no chance for recovery.

Turmoil/perturbation: Patient is tense, agitated, restless, indicating inner distress.

Frustration: Patient is angry about inability to resolve problems and get relief.

Despondent/depressed: Patient is dejected, withdrawn, tearful, and often inaccessible to interaction.

Helplessness/powerlessness: Patient feels unable to initiate positive action; complains of being too weak to struggle; surrenders and defaults decisions.

Anxiety/fears: Patient has specific fears or dreads; feelings of panic or impending doom.

Exhaustion/apathy: Patient feels depleted and worn out; expresses indifference to outcome.

Worthlessness/self-rebuke: Patient feels no good, defective; blames self for weakness, shortcomings, and failures.

Painful isolation/abandonment: Patient feels lonely, ignored, alienated from others who allegedly do not care.

Denial/avoidance: Patient speaks or acts as if unwilling to recognise threatening aspects of illness; minimises complaints or findings.

Truculence/annoyance: Patient is embittered, feeling victimised or mistreated by someone or something outside, beyond control.

Repudiation of significant others: Patient rejects, turns away from, or antagonises sources of potential help and support, usually a family member or friend.

Closed time perspective: Patient foresees a very limited future; day-to-day existence.

Vulnerability and the variations of coping have a somewhat reciprocal relationship, at least from the clinical viewpoint. Few patients use only one or two strategies to cope with very important problems, because in coping with important problems patients recall past experiences and apprehend future obstacles. Given a suitable combination or sequence of strategies, the patient who copes effectively will experience reduction of distress, relief, and perhaps even resolution of problems. Of the three principal parts of a patient's plight, coping is by far the most difficult to detect. The distress of vulnerability is usually far more obvious because high levels of vulnerability are what prompted consultation in the first place.

Good copers also have good doctor-patient relationships. They are optimistic and resourceful, can directly confront problems, and then can revise them in "cope-able" terms. Suppression and denial are only temporarily effective. Good copers are flexible in using all available options, just as they faced difficult situations in the past, even though the illness is the unique problem for every patient.

In contrast, patients who are poor copers tend to have higher emotional distress and do not clearly recognise pertinent psychosocial problems. The habits of avoiding, nullifying and disguising problems as well as the failure to be clear and communicative are diagnostic signs of poor coping. Blaming others or themselves is also an indication of poor coping potential. It is usually important to ask about time perspective and anticipated recovery, since these give a clue to how pessimistic or realistic the patient's view of the illness is. The doctor who works with patients needs experience in interview skills to deal with medical and surgical patients who are not primarily motivated to seek or use psychotherapeutic interventions.

SUMMARY

Stress is a stimulus event of sufficient severity to produce disequilibrium in the homeostatic physiological systems. The stimulus that evokes a stress response is called a stressor. A stimulus becomes a stressor either by the cognitive interpretation or meaning that the individual assigns to the stimulus or by the fact that the stimulus affects the individual by way of some sensory or metabolic process, which is stressful. In physiological terms stress is the body's response to any stressful demand. In psychological terms stress is an individual's cognitive judgement that his or her personal resources will be taxed or incapable of dealing with the demands posed by a particular event.

Stress comprises of stressor, stress response and the individual's coping resources like skills and social support systems. Stressor represents stimulus events requiring some form of adaptation or adjustment. Stressor can be internal stimuli like cognitions or thoughts or external stimuli like crowd, noise, and interpersonal difficulties.

Stresses are classified as positive or negative stresses.

An excessive number of 'life events' in a particular period of time can lead to increase ill health. The variety of illnesses that have been linked with life events range from heart disease, cancer and depression to the less life-threatening common cold or migraine.

Major stressful life events and daily hassles have been reported to have association with ill health. In children a significant association has been found between stressful life event and somatic complaints. The most frequent stressful life events were financial problems, moving house, death of a relative, chronic illness in the family and frequent change in job of parents.

Self-esteem has relevance to psychological distress and disorder. In many psychiatric problems self-esteem is one of the components for prevention and early intervention efforts in the service of mental health. Poor self-esteem is three times more in depressed patients.

Coping strategies in managing stress require change in yourself, others and the environment. Coping means the ways and means you adopt to keep stress at manageable levels. Coping has two components, the methods used and the focus of the coping response. Coping can be positive and negative. Some of the negative coping techniques are drinking alcohol, taking drugs, escaping from the stressful situation. There are certain ways to cope with the day-to-day stress in positive way.

There are various methods to assess stress, these can be physiological measures or can be assessed on self-report, questionnaires, checklist and rating scales. One of the examples of the common task of physicians and patients is to solve problems related to being sick. Coping is an integral part of medical practice as well as illness. Different diseases have their own special complications with which almost every victim must cope. A disfiguring scar, ataxia, a colostomy, a restrictive diet, require some form of primary rehabilitation and retraining that entails coping processes. Sickness-related problems have interpersonal and intrapsychic qualities that may undo medical and surgical efforts.

Vulnerability refers to the emotional distress that is the most personal aspect of illness. It reflects impairment of competence, control and consciousness. Consequently, vulnerability not only signifies distress in the here-and-now, but a disposition to behave or conduct oneself at less than full efficiency.

Personality

Sivati, 24 years old female, is pursuing a career in town planning. She is elder of two sisters in a nuclear family. She has had an outstanding academic record. She is very conscientious, overdutiful, perfectionist and rigid which is manifested in all forms of behaviour from handwriting to keeping clothes, things, dressing and other tasks. As she adheres to very high standards of performance, she expects similar standards of performance from others too. This expectation from others often causes anger outburst and creates problems in interpersonal relationship. She is always in a hurry to complete tasks, is not able to relax and often gets severe headache. This is an example of how personality determines behaviour of a person and its relationship in developing illness.

In our everyday lives we are accustomed to making some kind of assessment of other people. If we are asked to describe someone we know, we are likely to say something about his appearance and other aspects of behaviour, which characterise him as an individual who is different from others. There are always variations in individual's personality development, and functioning which results in a unique personality.

Definition

Personality is a stable, characteristic way a person feels and behaves in a variety of situations. Personality as a concept is difficult to define and psychologists also differ in their explanation of personality, some mention it in terms of qualities, some as characteristics of person's behaviour or may be both. RB Cattell, (1965) defines it, as that which determines behaviour in a defined situation and a defined mood. The assumption here is that the behaviour of the individual will depend not only on the situation in which he finds himself but also on his emotional state at that time. It is the stability during this period, which allows behaviour to be predictable within limits. Gorctn Allport, a pioneer in personality research has defined personality ' as a dynamic organisation within the individual, of psychological systems that determine his unique adjustments to his environment'. According to Mischel (1976) personality consists of distinctive patterns of behaviour that characterise each individual's adaptation to his life. Reference must also be made to two other terms used synonymously with personalities, character and temperament. Character is a word that tends to be used in a morally judgemental way; the individual is evaluated in terms of cultural norms against which he is seen 'good' or 'bad'. Temperament refers to the emotional responsiveness of a person, such as hot tempered-placid, fearful-unworried.

Determinants of Personality

Every child is born with certain potentialities. The development of these potentialities depends upon maturation and upon experiences encountered in growing up. The determinants that shape personality are viewed from different perspectives. The major distinction is drawn between biological influences, most likely to be genetically determined and environmental influences determined by family, school, peer group and culture.

Heredity

The relative contributions of heredity in the formation of adult personality have been studied by twin studies and statistical methods.

Eysenck studied personality dimensions in identical twins and nonidentical twins and found that the score on the dimensions of extra-version and neuroticism showed no significant correlation between the nonidentical twins but were closely related for the identical twins.

Physique: Further evidence of importance of biological factors in personality comes from individual differences to variation of physique. Kretschmer has given concept of personality types based on physique. The two types being schizothymic and cyclothymic personalities. These two types were correlated to major psychiatric disorders schizophrenia and manic-depressive psychosis respectively. The schizothymic is shy, inward looking with long and narrow body build. This type corresponds to Jung's introvert personality. This cyclothymic is sociable, outward looking, but liable to swings of mood have muscular or fat body build. This types corresponds to Jung's extrovert personality.

Sheldon identified three types of physique from a large number of photographs of male college students. According to him there are three personality types associated with functions of, the body organ and systems developed from the embryonic layers. The three types are: (i) the endomorphic, the viscerotonic personality is characterised by a love of comfort and of food, (ii) the mesomorphic, muscular build individuals with a somatotonic personality, are vigorous, active and assertive, (iii) the ectomorphic the cerebrotonic personality is dominated by the central nervous system with inhibition, restraint and little social contact. These physical body types and personality types represent the extreme dimensions rather than categories.

Environment

Personality characteristics are the result of interaction between the individual and the social and physical conditions of the situation. The environmental factors advocate that personality can be acquired. In the process of personality development psychosocial determinants play a crucial role.

Family: A family fulfils the basic physical and psychological needs of children as also seen in Chapter 16. During the early years of development the parents are the role models and through them various behaviours are learned, try to recall the time when you behaved just like your own mother or father. Family also transmits cultural values and norm, which influences your thinking process.

School and peer group: School environment is different in various schools; some emphasise competition, some high academic achievement, and some schools place greater importance to overall development and some devote more time on creativity. The differences in school environment contribute towards personality development of their students. Similarly the peer group influences are well known in the development of adaptive as well as maladaptive personality traits. If you are in the company of high achievers, you are also motivated to do well.

Culture: There has been a considerable amount of research on influence of culture on personality. Some cross-cultural studies have been conducted to study the effect of culture on various personality traits. McClelland found differences between ratings of achievement imagery in TAT stories of school boys in Japan, Germany, Brazil and India. Measures of field-dependence have also shown cross-cultural variations in many studies. The differences have been found in cognitive style and different child rearing practices. It has been found that a perceptual skill required for the performance on test of field-dependence depends upon past experience of similar task and which will vary from one culture to another. Cattell's 16 PF test has also been used to study cultural influences. If we apply cultural differences to study personality differences in our country, you would observe characteristic differences in individuals reared in urban or rural backgrounds. In some of the Indian studies conducted on disadvantaged children, it was found that learning of psychomotor skills was delayed in children with rural background. Similarly, cultural differences on personality can be seen in our context in individuals belonging to different communities like Punjabis, Bengalis, Biharis, Tamilians, etc.

Theories of Personality

Personality has been studied in a number of ways. The explanation of how people acquire and change the relative aspects of their behaviour comes from different theories of personality. Each personality theory has characteristic implications regarding the meaning of adjustment and deviance. However, two different approaches to study the concept are, the ideographic and the nomothetic—the former emphasises the uniqueness of the individual with intensive investigation of single cases and the latter with generalisation in the form of universal laws. Different theories may adopt any one of the approaches.

There are different schools of psychological thought about development of personality. There are number of different approaches to study personality. Cattell (1965) describes three historical phases in the understanding of personality. The oldest, though still continuing to the present day, is the prescientific or literary and philosophical phase. Many of the great poets, novelists and playwriters have, in their writings and especially in the characters have created and conveyed seemingly brilliant insights into the complexities of human nature. The second historical stage is called by Cattell the protoclinical, since it was based largely on observation of psychiatrically sick people by 'founding fathers' of psychiatry like Emil Kraepelin in Germany and Pierre Janet in France, but more especially Sigmund Freud and his early associates Carl Jung and Alfred Adler. Among the personality theories of psychodynamic approach, only the latter theorists would be discussed here. Two major limitations to this essentially descriptive historical phase in psychology are; first, the fact that it was derived from the study of psychological abnormality rather than the 'normal'; and second, the virtual absence of any attempt at measurement.

The characteristics of the third stage are evident from Cattell's description of it as quantitative and experimental. In other words, the scientific study of personality based on actual behavioural measurements. Four major theories of personality, psychodynamic, trait and type, social learning and humanistic theories are discussed in this section.

Psychodynamic Theories

The psychodynamic approach is ideographic, arising from observations made, during the course of treatment of psychologically disturbed patients. Psychodynamic approach has received considerable recognition on the basis of Freud's work. According to him, the structure of mind is seen as functionally differentiated into three parts; Id, ego and superego. The unconscious id energises primitive instincts or drives, which are satisfied, by wish-fulfilling fantasies. Id is governed by pleasure principles. The largely conscious ego, gradually develops in order to mediate between the demands of the id and the constraints of the outside world in accordance with the reality principle and guided by the third structure, the superego, which represents the values and controls of society and other controls of society through early identification with the parents and other figures of authority (Fig. 11.1).

The instinctual energy of the id, mainly in the form of libido is concerned with sex and self-preservation attached to different erogenous areas of the body—oral, anal and phallic—though as a result of excessive gratification or frustration it may become fixated at a particular stage. Later the libido becomes more outwardly directed as erotic feelings toward the parent of the opposite sex, with rivalry and fear of the parent of the same sex develops into an Oedipus or Electra conflict which should be successfully resolved by identification with the same-sexed parent and repression of the sexual drive during the latency period, until its reawakening at puberty in the final genital stage of development.

Another important aspect of psychodynamic theoryconcerns with the defense mechanisms used by the ego to reduce or avoid anxiety. The ego has several defense mechanisms at its disposal to protect itself from being traumatised by the stress arising from these conflicts. But the ego is not always aware of what the needs of the id and superego are, because many of these needs are unconscious. The occurrence of signal anxiety warns the ego that libidinal tensions have become so strong that it must either handle them or be disabled by stress.

All the defense mechanism has three characteristics in common: (i) they reduce stress and anxiety, (ii) they deny or distort reality, and (iii) they operate at unconscious level. Some of the common defense mechanisms are: repression, denial, rationalisation, displacement and sublimation, and identification.

Repression: It is the most important defense mechanism. It is the process by which the ego blocks off threatening thoughts or desires and thus keeps them from sweeping into the spotlight of consciousness. Most of these experiences have undischarged libidinal energy attached to them in some way. In repressing these experiences, the ego has to use up some of its own energy sources. And the more painful the memory, or the stronger the unacceptable urge, the more energy the ego must expend in order to keep the material repressed. Eventually the ego may run out of steam, and bits and pieces of the repressed material may leak though to consciousness as slips of the tongue, or as symbols in dreams.

Denial: As you would see during your clinical practice that many patients deny having an illness. Denial is a defense mechanism by which the ego shuts itself off from certain realities, especially which is painful facts.

Rationalisation: Again you would see patients who would give rationalisation for their non-compliance of treatment, e.g. a chronic alcoholic may rationalise for his drinking by saying that

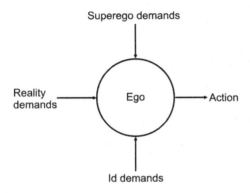

Fig. 11.1: Relation of Id, ego and superego

the drink provides him energy to earn money which is very important for bringing up of his children. Rationalisation is offering elaborate justifications for behaviours that are illogical or immature.

Displacement and sublimation: The child's ego gains the ability to displace the flow of libidinal energy from one object to another. But the ego may use this ability inappropriately, as a defense mechanism. If the child gets angry with its mother, it dares not hit her because it will be punished. Therefore, it displaces its anger towards a safe object—such as a doll—that cannot retaliate if the child strikes it.

Sublimation is a form of displacement and most mature of the defense mechanisms. In this the energy is channeled away from unacceptable to socially acceptable acts. For example, an unmarried female may sublimate her sexual drives in form of painting or art work.

Reaction formation: in reaction formation the ego changes unacceptable love into acceptable hate or *vice-versa*. If a mother hates a child—a feeling she must deny conscious awareness of—the mother may pat the child with affection. Or the mother's ego may indulge in projection by pretending that the child actually hates her. She thus projects her unacceptable emotions onto the child.

Identification: In the next Chapter 12 on Development—Infancy to Adolescence you will read about psychosexual development theory, which describes Oedipus complex and Electra complex. Many people resolve their Oedipus or Electra crisis by taking on the characteristics of their same-sex parent. The young girl identifies with her mother. In adolescence, the girl identifies with other women and strengthens the conscious portion of her superego. Ego-ideals help to reduce anxiety by allowing the person to release libidinal energy in socially approved ways.

Early splits with Freudian psychoanalysis resulted in Alfred Adler's school of individual psychology and Carl Jung's analytical psychology, Adler claimed that even in normal circumstances a child feels helpless and begins to develop a particular strategy or lifestyle, to compensate for feelings of inferiority and to reach the goal of superiority. Adler drew attention to the importance of the ego and nonsexual factors in the personality. Jung also reacted against Freud's emphasis on sex. The motivating force in Jung's view, although still called the libido, was nonsexual and more in the nature of a life force. Jung postulated not only a conscious mind and a personal unconscious, but in addition a much larger collective or racial unconscious containing the beliefs and myths of the individual's race and at a still deeper level, a universal unconscious shared with all humanity. Jung called the collective unconscious archetypes. Psychosocial developmental theory of Erik Erikson (see Chapter 12) who, with Erich Fromm, Karen Horney and Harry Stack Sullivan, comprised the sociologically oriented group known as the neo-Freudians that developed in USA during 1930s. Emphasis was placed on the interpersonal rather than the intrapsychic dimension and on the conflicts, which may arise in relationships between the individual and others as well as within himself. More recently object relations theory, describes 'object' in the sense of a psychologically significant person or part of a person, has stressed the relationship of the individual to such objects. The stages of development are then seen as different means of achieving such relationships (e.g. through feeding at the oral stage), and adult personality as being much influenced by the nature of these early relationships.

Trait and Type Theories

These theories focus on internal influences on personality. According to this viewpoint, personality is consistent from situation-to-situation not because of an emotional outlook coloured by early experience, nor because of universal needs. Rather these explanations focus on specific attributes peculiar to the individual, in some cases physical and in others psychological. Some of these theories divide individuals into distinct categories as being of one type or another. Jung's introverts and extroverts are types. Sheldon's classification according to the physique is also an example of personality types. Trait theories look at individuals not so much in terms of extremes of one type or another but as blends of many different characteristics that individuals have to a greater or lesser extent.

Allport differentiated between individual and common traits. A term trait was reserved for common traits and a new term personal disposition was introduced for individual trait. The implication is that a trait may be shared by a number of individuals. According to Allport, a specific act is always the product of many determinants not only of lasting sets, but also of momentary pressures on the person and in the situation. It is the repeated occurrence of acts that allow one to make necessary reference of traits and personal dispositions later on Allport distinguished traits and types in terms of the extent to which they are tailored to the individual. Allport maintained that each of us has a personal disposition made up of a cardinal, central and secondary traits. A cardinal trait is so dominant that it colours virtually every aspect of a person's behaviour and attributes. Central traits are handful of characteristic tendencies that we would ordinarily use to describe a person. The secondary traits are displayed by us from time-to-time, but are not strong enough to be regarded as integral parts of our personality.

Cattell assumes that there are natural elements of personality, which can be discovered using the technique of multivariate analysis. Cattell began his researches by taking trait names used in everyday language to describe human behaviour. He then rated individuals on the trait description and inspection of the ratings suggesting that about 40 basic dimensions are involved. The 16 first order or primary factors, which make up 16 PF questionnaires, have been most intensively considered by Cattell and his associates. These factors are called 'source traits'. We all have same traits but to different degrees and in this way, no two individuals are exactly alike.

Eysenck (1990) stated that each type is made up of a set of personality characteristics. Three major personality types or dimensions have been listed by Eysenck, namely extroversion, neuroticism and psychoticism. For example people who fit Eysenck's extroverted type are said to be characterised as sociable, lively and excitable. Each one of these characteristics can be broken into a habitual response, which can further be broken down to specific responses within specific situations. This progression from broad to specific responses made Eysenck's approach into a hierarchical theory.

The big Five: There are five basic dimensions, theorised to underlie the many traits used to described human behaviour, known as big five. Each of the dimensions is bipolar, one of the ends of the dimension describes the 'high' pole and the opposite end describes the 'low' pole. These five dimensions are—

- Openness to experience: creative intellectual and open minded *vs.* simple, shallow and unintelligent.
- Conscientiousness: organised responsible and cautious *vs.* careless frivolous, irresponsible.
- Extroversion: talkative, energetic and assertive *vs.* quite reserved and shy.
- Agreeableness: sympathetic, kind and affectionate *vs.* cold, quarrelsome and cruel.
- Neuroticism: emotionally stable, calm and contented *vs.* anxious, unstable and temperamental.

The big five theory is a comprehensive descriptive system. This approach accommodates many scientific approaches to personality. These five factors have been included in a personality assessment instrument, the NEO-pi (Caprara et al 1993). This inventory has been used to study personality characteristic in clinical and research studies (Costa and McCrae, 1992).

Social Learning Theories

The social learning approach to personality has derived its main impetus from the behavioural movement in psychology and partly from dissatisfaction with trait approaches. Behavioural psychologists take quite a different approach. Generally speaking, they see personality development as being a set of learned responses. Thus, according to BF Skinner, you became who you are primarily because that is what your social environment has conditioned you to be.

Skinner believes that behaviour is, above all else, lawful. By this he means that your actions (and hence your thoughts and emotional responses) are predictable because they are primarily under the control of external, measurable influences. You do not eat because you are "hungry", but rather because you have been conditioned to eat in the presence of certain environmental stimuli. Indeed, "hunger" has no meaning to Skinner because it refers to a subjective "inner state" rather than to an objective set of behaviours. Your "psychic energy" comes not from dynamic forces working deep within your unconscious mind, but from external inputs.

Skinner rejects not only all intrapsychic aspects of personality development, but most biological influences as well. Innate reflexes are always modified by experience. If you wish to study personality development, you should focus entirely on how a given society trains its children. For if you change the pattern of "parenting behaviours" in a culture, Skinner believes, you will completely alter the personalities of children reared in that culture. Social learning theories, especially that of Bandura and Walters postulated that all learning need not be direct (see Chapter 5). Imitation according to Bandura and Walters, plays a prominent role in learning. We try to imitate what we observe especially, when we identify with certain models in our environment. The selection of a model again depends on the age, sex, motives, etc. For example A child usually takes mother as a model. They have also pointed out how wrong models could set bad examples to the individual.

Situational determinants of behaviour have also been considered in social learning approach. Situations by themselves do not evoke any behaviour but it is given a meaning by the person. Different situations have their own meanings to people. Thus, situations influence one's behaviour in unique manner, on the basis of one's previous learning experience. To summarise, the social learning viewpoint places a great emphasis on the importance of learning and situations in personality. Human behaviour is only a resultant of person, situation variables and their interaction.

Humanistic Approach

A number of theorists have focussed on the concept of 'self' in personality. Self has two distinct sets of feelings. One set has to do with people's attitude about themselves, their self concept and second set relates to the processes by which the individual copes, remembers, thinks and plans. Self concept are central to humanistic theories. Carl Rogers and Abraham Maslow are two most influential humanistic theorists.

Rogers believes we are born with no self-concept, and no self—but we do have an innate urge to become fully functioning and actualised people. At birth, all we have is a confusing set of sensory impressions, physiological processes, and motor activities. Rogers calls this sum total of our experience the phenomenal field. As we mature, the outside world imposes a kind of order or logic onto this field. And, as we become aware of this logic, our self emerges and differentiates itself from the phenomenal field. The self is thus the conscious portion of experience.

Rogers believes you are most likely to run into developmental problems when society wants you to become something that conflicts with your own internal values or standards. If you yield to the demands of society too much, your psychological experience is distorted and your self-concept suffers accordingly. Most of your experiences are unconscious, i.e. below the threshold of awareness. But you can bring almost any experience above threshold if you merely give the experience a name or a label. That is, you make an unconscious experience conscious by developing word-symbols that allow you to describe (and hence think about) the experience. If a particular event threatens your self concept, then you may refuse to symbolise this even in words or thoughts. But if you cannot tolerate some of your own behaviours, you will have problems achieving full actualisation because you are continually hiding some of your own values or motivations from conscious expression.

When you can accept yourself completely, you become what Rogers's calls a fully functioning individual. You are open to all experience and you defend against nothing. You are aware of both your faults and your virtues, but you have a high positive regard for yourself. And, most of all, you maintain happy and humane relationships with others.

Abraham Maslow took his ideas about human behaviour from studying highly creative and psychologically healthy people. Maslow assumed these individuals had achieved a high degree of self-fulfillment or they would not have been so prominent and demonstrated such leadership. By determining the similarities among the members of this noted group, he arrived at the characteristics of a truly "self-actualised" person.

Most psychoanalytical theories focus on what can go wrong during the developmental years. That is, they emphasise the possibility of sickness, not the probability of success. Maslow's approach is different, for he looks primarily at the healthy side of human nature. As we noted in Chapter 8, Maslow has created a hierarchy of needs, of which self-actualisation is the highest. Maslow acknowledges the strength of our physiological instincts, but sees them as being "basic needs" easily satisfied in most civilised societies. Our drives for food and sex are part of a more impelling intrapsychic urge-an active "will toward health"—that drives us up the developmental ladder toward self-actualisation.

Humanistic theories emphasise the importance of people's subjective attitudes feelings and beliefs, especially with regard to self. Theories of this type are often criticised for their heavy reliance on subjective self report data but such data can provide one with respectable insights into people.

Personality Related to Illness

The idea that personality traits and psychological characteristics play a role in the aetiology of physical disease has its roots in medicine and philosophy before Descartes. Early physicians believed that intense emotions could produce imbalances in bodily function, culminating in various forms of physical pathology. In the first half of this century, the role of chronic emotional conflicts in the aetiology of physical disorders was emphasised. Based on observations of clinical groups, correlations between particular diseases and personality types were reported, and striking psychological similarities among patients suffering from the same organic disease were described. These similarities were formulated and linked to specific disorders such as coronary heart disease (CHD), peptic ulcer, and asthma. Later trait approaches suggested that certain dispositions, such as giving up, depression, and inability to express feelings were related to general susceptibility to illness. Recent studies suggest that epidemiological evidence for a link between Type A and CHD is no longer unequivocal. A number of studies have quantified the degree of coronary artery disease present in patient, undergoing coronary angiography and have correlated disease severity with measures of Type A behaviour. Patients with Type A personality were likely to have severe coronary artery disease in comparison to Type B patients. However, subsequent studies found that Type A was not associated with extensive coronary artery disease.

Behaviour Patterns and Coronary Heart Disease

Behaviour patterns and its relationship to health has been described in our ancient Indian system of medicine, Ayurveda. The fundamentals for prevention of disease and promotive health care were related to the following tenets:
- Achaar (conduct)
- Vichaar (thought)
- Vyavahaar (interpersonal dealings)
- Ahaar (nutrition).

These four tenets are components of personality and variations in these cause illness both physical and mental. While some of you would not agree that there seems to be an apparent relationship between physical health and our actions, but in all cultures it has been observed that the spiritual component energises and helps in coping with stress. A relaxed mind is certainly more productive than an agitated and tensed one. Tension and stress may lead to wrong decisions, thus to prevent and control stress relaxation exercises should be practiced (Wasir 1995).

Considerable attention has been devoted to the study of "coronary-prone" behaviour patterns, and two general patterns have been identified. The first consists of negative, disturbing emotions such as life dissatisfaction, anxiety and depression. Given generally fairly high correlations between these dysphonic characteristics seems reasonable to incorporate them into the broad rubric of "neuroticism". A second example of a "coronary prone behaviour" conceptualisation is the Type A behaviour pattern, which is the most extensively researched psychosocial risk factor of CHD. Individuals with the Type A behaviour pattern are characterised by action emotion complex, struggle to achieve more in short time, autonomous, status conscious, power hungry, inpatience, free-floating hostility. These individuals are intensely ambitious, competitive, short tempered and have time urgency. In contrast, type B individuals are relatively relaxed and easy-going.

Type A can be assessed by the structured interview in which individuals are asked to indicate how they usually respond in situations that is likely to elicit competitiveness, impatience and hostility in certain individuals. The evaluation of Type A is primarily based on speech stylistics, such as loudness and explosiveness, content of the answers. A number of questionnaires for assessing Type A exist; the Jenkins Activity Survey (JAS) (Jenkins, 1976) is the most commonly used. Studies that have correlated various Type A measures with other psychological scales. Self report measures correlate more highly with negative emotional states. In a classical study known as the Framingham Heart Study (Haynes, Feinleib and Kannel, 1980) an adhoc scale was used to measure Type A behaviour. Individuals who were classified as Type A were more likely to have developed CHD at the follow up eight years later than were Type B subjects. The framingham scale predicted the development of myocardial infarction alone, angina alone and myocardial infarction with angina.

Type A and Physiological Reactivity

Since associations between Type A and ischaemic heart disease cannot be explained solely by the standard coronary risk factors, research has attempted to determine physiologic mechanisms linking Type A to disease. Most explanations for this link suggest that behaviours exhibited by Type A individuals are accompanied by sympathetic neuroendocrine and cardiovascular responses, which might promote the development of coronary atherosclerosis or precipitate its clinical symptoms of ischaemic heart disease.

The results of this study suggest that there may be an underlying psychobiological or "constitutional" basis for Type A behaviour in cardiac patients. The impatience, hostility and speech patterns exhibited by Type A patients with manifest disease may, in part, reflect underlying sympathetic nervous system hyperactivity. This view is different from, but not necessarily contradictory with, the idea that Type A appraisals or behaviours produce elevated sympathetic responses. If Type A is a consequence of sympathetic hyperactivity, then Type A behaviour might be suppressed by treatment techniques that decreased sympathetic responsiveness. Beta-blockers such as propranolol are commonly used to treat cardiovascular disorders. These drugs antagonise certain sympathetic nervous system responses that would otherwise be activated by epinephrine. These responses occur primarily in organs such as the heart, and in smooth muscle of the blood vessels and lungs.

Clinical Applications

Personality has been of great clinical importance, as you would recall that no two patients even with a similar disease are same. The reactions to the illness have been found to be related to personality. An extrovert and an introvert may react differently to the restrictions imposed by illness. Someone with poor self-concept and self-esteem may feel further threatened by an illness as it produces feeling of failure to meet the demands of coping with illness. On the other hand, an individual habitual of using defense mechanism of projection may tend to blame others for his illness and find faults with the hospital system. The way a patient construes illness in general, and his own in particular, in relation to other aspects of life, will determine his response to it; an individual's strength of achievement motivation may be significant in relation to any disability threatening his career; that a sensation seeker would find any degree of sensory deprivation from illness particularly stressful; that those whose locus of control is internal may be vulnerable to the dependence on others often entailed by illness. Thus an understanding of patient's personality can help the physicians in providing specific treatment strategies. For example, when you realise that the patient X is taking secondary gains from her illness and thus is not showing any improvement, then providing attention to the healthy behaviour and ignoring illness behaviour would help the patient to recover soon.

From a more psychiatric standpoint, some knowledge of a person's 'normal' or 'previous' personality can be important in order to detect changes, which may have occurred as a consequence of disease either organic or psychological and also to assess the degree of recovery from such illness. An individual's personality will also 'colour' the clinical picture of any psychiatric disorder that he develops, so that it will never be identical with that of another patient. According to Eysenck the personality type determined the nature of illness for example, introverts are more prone to depression, anxiety, schizophrenia. The extroverts are more prone to disorders like somatoform and hypomania. Similarly personality has influence on the psychophysiological disorders. Studies have tried to correlate personality patterns of individuals with disorders such as irritable bowel symptoms, ulcerative colitis, headaches, etc.

There are some people whose personalities depart, in various ways, from the norm to such an extent that they experience difficulties themselves, resulting in anxiety or depression, or cause difficulties to others in their attempts to cope with the normal pressures and responsibilities of life; they may therefore be diagnosed as having a personality disorder.

Personality disorders themselves are classified into a number of types in a way that is generally quite different from that of the personality theories we have been considering. The definitions of the various personality disorders are essentially derived from clinical experience often being seen as personality 'equivalents' of particular psychiatric disorders (e.g. the 'schizoid' personality and schizophrenia, the 'hysterical' personality and hysteria).

Personality has been correlated with the studying skills. As a student you would be interested in knowing that certain personality characteristic predict greater academic success. Introverted boys and extroverted girls generally perform better in the academic performances. Since personality also influences which is interactional abilities hence in a working environment like hospitals where teamwork of multiple disciplines is required, understanding of personality is of greater relevance.

SUMMARY

Personality is a stable characteristic way a person feels and behaves in a whole variety of situations. Different psychologists view personality differently but many agree to the view that it is an interaction between the behaviour and a given situation. Character and temperament though different are terms used synonymous with personality.

Every child is born with certain potentialities. The determinants, which shape personality, are viewed from different perspectives. A distinction is drawn between biological influences, i.e. genetically determined and environmental influences determined by family, school, peer group and culture.

Personality has been studied in a number of ways by different theorists. These are psychodynamic theoretic by Freud, Jung, Adler and Erikson. According to Freud the interaction between the id, ego and superego results in personality development. Various defense mechanisms help to reduce stress and anxiety. The type and trait theories classify individuals according to types like introvert, extrovert and traits are personal dispositions. The traits can be cardinal, central and secondary. The big five factor theory includes five basic traits which broadly cover different traits given by all other theorists. The social learning theories emphasise role of learning and environmental situation in personality development. According to Humanistic theorists, self-concept, self-esteem and self-actualisation are related to success.

Early, physician believed that intense emotions could produce imbalances and bodily function, culminating in various forms of physical pathology. Specific disorders as coronary heart disease (CHD), peptic ulcer and asthma have been linked to personality. Epidemiological evidence is suggestive of link between Type A and CHD. Type A patients are more likely to have severe coronary artery disease in comparison to type B patients.

The study of personality has been of great clinical importance as one would recall that no two patients even with similar disease are same. An extrovert and an introvert may react differently to the instructions imposed by illness. People with poor self-concept, self-esteem and low motivation feel threatened by illness. Knowledge of a person's normal or previous personality can be important in order to detect changes, which occur as consequences of disease—organic or psychological, and also to assess the degree of recovery from such illness.

PART 3: Development of Behaviour

Development—Infancy to Adolescence

12

Sanjay, a 15 years old adolescent, has frequent temper outbursts, he does not get along with his parents, he has occasional fights with his parents and his younger sister. He frequently demands money from his parents, which the parents cannot afford. His parents feel that his academic performance is also going down, as he spends lot of time in looking at himself in the mirror, and is interested in talking to girls. Though he is a terror at home, but on the other hand, he is very popular amongst his friends. Sanjay is not suffering from any psychiatric problem, but is passing through an adolescent period. To understand normal deviations in behaviour, one should be aware of the normal developmental process.

The human life cycle influences health and illness at all its stages. Human development starts at the time of birth and continues till death. Development passes through important stages of life. These can be understood in terms of Infancy, Childhood, Adolescence, Adulthood and Old age. In this chapter, developmental process from infancy to adolescence shall be discussed, and in the next chapter, development process in adulthood and old age would be discussed.

INFANCY AND CHILDHOOD

The human infant has a number of adaptive reflexes, including the grasping and sucking reflexes. Infants are social creatures from the day they are born. Early social development, lays a foundation for later relationships with parents, siblings, friends and relatives. Self-awareness and social referencing (increased awareness of others) are two important elements of social development. Self-awareness is seen around 15 months of age. The core of social development lies in the emotional bonds that babies form with their caregivers. Infant attachment is reflected by separation anxiety, which appears around 8-12 months of age. Separation anxiety refers to the distress displayed by infants, when separated from their parents or caregivers.

Language proceeds from control of crying to loosing, to babbling, followed by use of single words and then to telegraphic speech. Pre-language communication between parents and child involves shared rhythms, nonverbal signals (in the form of touch, vocalising, gazing or smiling). Turn taking is the tendency of parent and child to alternate in the sending and receiving of signals and messages.

Stages of Development

Development occurs along multiple lines, it is overall physical development, cognitive, personality, social and neurological development. The personal experiences, organisational styles, coping strategies, feelings and thoughts, all contribute to create one's unique experience of life.

Development moves in a fixed, predictable manner, with minor variations in all individuals. Some of the important milestones of development are given in Table 12.1.

Table 12.1: Milestones of development

Age	Motor	Social
0-3 months	Lateral head movement Arms and legs thrust in play Eye coordination Head erect and steady	Fixes eyes and holds gaze Smiles at nodding head, high voice First social smile Discriminate between mother and others
3-6 months	Rolls over Head steady Elevates on arms Equilateral movements Turns from back to side Sits with support	Gives first laugh Expresses wariness Responds to mother differently
6-12 months	Pulls to sit Bangs in play Sits alone steadily Pulls to stand Stands alone Starts walking	Babbles Laughs at incongruity Fear of strangers Interacts socially Follow simple instructions

Cognitive Development

Jean Piaget (1896 to 1980) focussed on how children and adolescents think and acquire knowledge. His theory is referred to as genetic epistemology, which means to study of acquisition, modification and growth of abstract ideas and abilities on the basis of an inheritive or biological substrate.

The concept of schemata lies at the core of his theory. He defined it as a specific cognitive structure that has a behavioural pattern. As an individual grows, the schema becomes more and more complex. Later schemas are referred to as operations, which include imitation, abstraction and higher intelligence. Piaget spoke of two processes: (a) assimilation, and (b) accommodation. The former refers to taking in of new experience, through one's own system of knowledge. The latter implies modification of existing schemas to the demands of the environment. These two processes give rise to the—concept of adaptation, which is the individual's ability to adjust to the environment and interact with it.

Piaget gave four stages of cognitive development.

Sensory Motor Stage

It occurs in the first two years of life. It is characterised by learning that occurs through sensory observation. The child is concerned with learning to coordinate purposeful movements with the information from his senses. Object permanence is an important achievement that occurs during this period. It implies that object have an existence independent of child's involvement with them. The child is able to maintain a mental image of an object even though it is not visible.

Preoperational Stage

It occurs during the second and the seventh year. The child uses language and symbols extensively. Thinking and reasoning are at an intuitive level. The child lacks a sense of cause and effect. The characteristic feature of the stage is egocentric thinking that is, having a limited point of view and inability to take the role of other person. Animistic thinking, the tendency to endow physical events and objects with life like psychological attributes is also seen during this stage.

Concrete Operational Stage

It is the stage that occurs between the seventh and eleventh year. In this stage, the child operates and acts on concrete, real and perceivable world of objects and events. Operational thinking replaces egocentric thinking, which means that the child is able to attend and deal with a wide array of information and is able to take others perspective. In this stage, the child is able to form a logical conclusion from two premises and this is known as syllogistic reasoning. The child is able to reason and follow rules and regulations develop moral sense and a code of values. Children who become overly invested in views may show obsessive-compulsive behaviour, and children who resist a code of value often seem willful and inactive.

Conservation and reversibility are the other two characteristics of this stage. Conservation is the ability to recognise that the shape and form of objects may change but the mass remains the same. Reversibility is the capacity to understand the relations between things, to understand that one thing can turn into another and back again. For example, ice and water.

Stage of Formal Operations

This stage occurs from 11 years onwards through the end of adolescence. The adolescent is able to think abstractly, reason deductively, define concepts and deal with permutation and combination. Hypotheticodeductive thinking, which is the highest organisation of cognition, occurs during this time. The individual is able to make a hypothesis and test it against reality.

Psychosexual Development Freud was probably the first psychologist, to emphasise the developmental aspects of personality and in particular to stress the decisive role of the early years of infancy and childhood in laying down the basic character structure of the person. Freud felt that personality was well-formed by the end of the fifth year, and that the subsequent growth consisted for the most part of elaborating this basic structure.

Freud's notions about personality development came from many sources. But mostly his theory sprang from his observations of his own patients. Freud was fascinated by the fact that most of his patients seemed to have gone through very similar developmental crises as children. Freud believed that "the child is the father of the man". Eventually, he decided that one passes through various psychosexual stages of development, which correspond to the maturational stage of ones body at various times in the life. Each stage is associated with a unique crisis of some kind.

Oral Stage

Oral stage is the period which lasts from birth to about one year of age. The first crisis is that of birth, when one is thrust out into the world and becomes dependent on others to meet the needs. You had innate reflexes that help to survive by creating libidinal energy that had to be discharged; but the manner in which you release this energy changes as body matures. When you were newborn, the brain centres, which control mouth movements were physically, the most developed so libidinal energy released easily through such oral activities as sucking and swallowing.

Freud saw many child—like oral behaviour patterns in his patients, such as talking too much, over-eating, excessive smoking and so forth. He presumed that this "residue of their infantile experiences" remained locked away in their unconscious minds because of some traumatic experience they had while in the oral stage. These patients had problems because they were still trying to release libidinal energy through adult oral activities. Therapy for these patients would obviously involve some form of "catharsis" to allow the patients to discharge the libidinal energy that had been repressed while they were still in the oral stage.

Anal Stage

The second crisis occurs when parents begin making demands, which conflicted with instinctual need to obtain immediate gratification of all biological and psychological needs. The second crisis reaches a peak during toilet training, when parents insist that you learn to delay gratification. Freud assumed you resolved this crisis by creating an "ego" or conscious self that could respond to reality by gaining voluntary control over the release of libidinal energy through anal activities.

Some of Freud's patients were excessively neat, obstinate, and miserly. These three traits make up what Freud called the "anal character", and he saw all the three as attempts to punish the mother for the trauma of toilet training. The mother demanded that the child "be clean", so the patient became unreasonably tidy. The mother demanded the child to "produce", so the child rebelled by withholding its feces, and became fixated at the anal stage. As an adult, the patient still rebels by obstinately refusing to part with single paise. Again, catharsis and giving the patient insight into the roots of the problem-seemed to Freud to be the best therapy.

Phallic Stage

At stage three or so, sex organs began to mature, and did the centres in the brain associated with sexual activity. Thus, one acquires a new avenue for discharging instinctual energies. During this phallic period, boys build up a warm and loving relationship with their mothers, which Freud called the Oedipus complex. At the same age, girls experience an intense "emotional attachment" for their fathers, called the Electra complex. Freud stated that, during the phallic stage, boys experience incestual desires to possess their mothers and compete with (or even kill) their fathers, while girls like their fathers and fear or hate their mothers.

Latency Period

According to Freud, one enters the latency period at about age five or six. At this time, one starts to move out of the home more frequently, and friendships with peers taken on greater importance on one's emotional and intellectual development. Freud believed this was natural homosexual period during which boys found 'heroes' among older male friends and peers, and girls developed 'crushes' on other girls and older women.

Psychosocial Development (Erikson)

Erikson proposed a psychosocial theory of development. This means that the stages of a person's life from birth to death are formed by social influences, interacting with a physically and psychologically nurturing organism. In Erikson's words, there is a mutual fit of individual and environment that is, of the individual's capacity to relate to an over expanding life space of people and institutions, on the one hand, the readiness of these people and institutions to make him part of an enjoying cultural concern (Erikson, 1975).

Eight Developmental Stages: According to the Psychosocial theory, development proceeds in stages—eight in all; the first four stages occur during infancy and childhood, the fifth stage during adolescence and last three stages during the adult years including old age. Erikson has placed particular emphasis on the adolescent period because it is then that the transition between childhood and adulthood is made.

These consecutive stages are not laid out according to a strict chronological timetable, because Erikson feels that a given child has its own timetable, and therefore, it would be misleading to specify an exact duration for each stage. Moreover, each stage is not passed through and then left behind. Instead, each stage contributes to the formation of the total personality. Each of these stages is characterised by its own type of crisis, or conflict. Erikson saw these crises as being eight great tests of your character.

Trust Vs Mistrust

Erikson called the first developmental stage the "sensory stage", which corresponds to Freud's oral stage. To Erikson, the crisis at the sensory stage is that of learning basic trust or mistrust of other people. At this point in life, the infant is totally dependent on others for its needs. If his mother (or someone else) meets these needs, the infant learns to depend on others in later life. If for any reason, the mother is inconsistent in satisfying the infant's needs, the infant may carry suspicion and doubt through the rest of its years.

Autonomy vs Shame, Doubt

The second of Erikson's stage, similar to the anal stage, is that of muscular development. During toilet training the child learns to control its own muscles and begins to assert its individuality. The crisis here is that of autonomy, or the ability to control one's own bodily functions. The child either learns autonomy, or if it is unsuccessful, develops shame and doubt about its own abilities.

Initiative vs Guilt

The third stage, that of locomotors control, is similar to Freud's phallic stage. Now the child attempts to develop its own way of asserting its needs and gaining its rewards. Urged by its instincts to possess its opposite-sex parent (at least in fantasy) and to rival its same-sex parent, the child faces the crisis of inner desires versus society's demands. Erikson believed that if the child could channel its sexual needs into socially acceptable behaviours, the child acquired initiative. If not, the child might build up a strong sense of guilt that would haunt it the rest of its days.

Industry vs Inferiority

Both Freud and Erikson called the fourth developmental stage that of latency. During these (typically) school years, the crisis the child faces is that of competence or failure. If the child does well in school, he learns that he can succeed and thus becomes industrious. If he does poorly, it gains a sense of inferiority.

Identity vs Indentity Confusion

At puberty, Freud thought sexual interest returns and the individual must make the final adjustment, that of heterosexuality. Erikson saw the puberty crisis as that of either finding your identity, or of developing what he called role confusion. You must decide what the future will hold and who you will become. Although the social roles available may vary from one society to another, you must decide which of these roles to adopt. By discovering who and what you want to be, you are able to plan your life as a working, functioning adult.

Intimacy vs Isolation

Erikson postulated three final stages of maturation beyond the five that Freud spoke of. The first of these stages, which occurs in young adulthood, presents you with the crisis of intimacy versus isolation. If you have "found" yourself by now, you can then go on to the delightful task of "finding" someone else to share life's intimacies with. If you fail to resolve your identity crisis, however, you will remain isolated from the closest forms of psychological "sharing" with others.

Generativity vs Stagnation

Societies often pass through a period of rapid development, then settle into complacency when growth stops and stagnation sets in. Erikson believed that adults often experience the same "growth" crisis during their middle years. Human beings need more than intimacy. We must be productive and helpful to our fellow humans, and we must make a contribution to society. The crisis decision here then is, that between what Erikson called generativity and stagnation.

Integrity vs Despair

Erikson's final stage is that of maturity. If you live long enough, you have to face squarely the fact that you are mortal, and that some day you will die. By resolving your prior crises, you gain the strength to integrate even death into the pattern of your existence, You come to terms with yourself, content with the knowledge that you have done the best that you could under the circumstances. Knowing that your life has been successful, you can die as you lived, with integrity. But, if you fail to solve the earlier crises, you may see your life as having been useless, incomplete, and wasted. And thus, you may succumb to feelings of despair at the futility of existence.

Summary of these eight stages is given in Table 12.2.

Adolescence

Adolescence is a period (ranging from 11-19 years), during which a growing person makes a transition from childhood to adulthood. The biological, psychological, cognitive, emotional and social changes taking place in the years around puberty are greater than at any other age since the second year of life. Adolescence period has its importance in preparing a young individual to meet challenges of social and economic world. In the recent years, there have been tremendous changes in our Indian social environment and economic conditions, which has influenced the psychological development of an adolescent. Emotional and psychological development of an adolescent needs understanding and careful handling by adults as this period is the most sensitive period in an individual's life.

The late adolescent period is marked by selecting a career. Career development consists of four broad phases:

a. *Exploration phase* Possibilities are made an initial search for career.
b. *Establishment phase* The individual finds a job, enters a career, develops competence and gains status.
c. *Mid career phase* is a time of high productivity and acceptance by co-workers.
d. *Later career phase* The individual serves as a respected expert and a guide/role model for young workers.

Table 12.2: Stages of psychosocial development

Stage and Age	Psychosocial crisis	Major concern
Infancy 0-1 yr.	Trust *vs* mistrust	The infant develops a sense of trust/mistrust that basic needs like warmth, physical contact will/will not be fulfilled.
Early childhood 1-3 yrs.	Autonomy *vs* shame, doubt	Learn self-control as a means of being self-sufficient, e.g. toilet training, shame and doubt about the ability to be autonomous.
Play age 3-6 yrs.	Initiative *vs* guilt	Anxious to investigate adult activities, may have feelings of guilt about trying to be independent and daring.
School age 7-11 yrs.	Industry *vs* inferiority	Learns about imagination and curiosity, develops learning skills or feelings of inferiority if they fail to master task.
Adolescence 12-20 yrs.	Identity *vs* identity confusion	Try to figure out who they are, how they are unique, how they can establish, sexual ethnic and career identity. Confusion can arise over these decisions.
Young adulthood 20-30 yrs	Intimacy *vs* isolation	Seek companionship and intimacy with significant others or avoid relationship and become isolated.
Adulthood 32-65 yrs	Generativity *vs* stagnation	Need to be productive—create products/ideas/children or become stagnated.
Mature age 65 +	Integrity *vs* despair	Efforts to make sense of one's life. Reflecting on completed goals or despair about unreached goals and desires.

Emotions Experienced during Adolescence

To understand the adolescent, it is important to know what he does and thinks but it is even more important to know what he feels. During adolescence, emotion is involved in everything in which the adolescent is involved. Different emotions are expressed by an adolescent when his desires are fulfilled, or when he is blocked or thwarted, in his efforts, or when he is harmed or threatened with harm.

Adolescent Love

To achieve the tasks of loving, an adolescent needs to achieve emotional independence of parents. The need to love and to be loved is supremely important in their lives. Examples of love are also seen in devotion towards group by delinquents and impulse for doing idealistic things. With adolescence, one is faced with new demands, new situations, in which the task of love and sex must be faced. The capacity or ability to love serves function to fulfill and broaden the potential for enjoying one's life. A person who is unable to love, for psychological or social reasons starts comparing himself with other peers and feels depressed.

Sexuality

Adolescents engage in range of sexual behaviours. Experimentation with sex is becoming very common with adolescents due to the effect of media. At times, these involvements lead to unwanted teenage pregnancies, abortions and guilt feelings. If these guilt feelings are not handled appropriately, it can lead to negative repercussions for future sexual relationship. Some adolescents engage in homosexual activities, both as active and passive partners.

Anger

Adolescent's temper flares often and easily because he is overly sensitive, he tends to feel abused, and his self-esteem and confidence are shaky partly due to the occurrence of physical and hormonal changes.

It is through his anger that an adolescent most sharply asserts his demands and interests. The basic conditions that arouse anger remain much the same throughout life, but there are changes with age in the particular circumstances that provoke it. When we try to understand anger in the adolescent, it is easier to identify what it is that makes him angry than to tell why it makes him angry.

During adolescence, persons rather than things most often provoke anger. There are many unavoidable frictions in the give and take of everyday life. Many adolescents are annoyed, not only by specific parental practices but also by parental traits and habits. It is often observed that anger is frequently aroused by unjust criticism by parents, being treated like a child at home, clashes of opinion with parents, and troubles with brothers and sisters.

Anxiety

Many adolescents may experience a vague feeling of uneasiness, a feeling of being on edge, other feelings such as fear, anger, restlessness, irritability, or depression. The underlying conflict springs from a clash between incompatible impulses, desires, or values. Such a conflict prevails when a person is angry but is afraid of giving offense. Likewise, it exists when a person is eager to be popular but has strong scruples against doing what is necessary to become popular.

Anxiety-producing Stresses in Adolescence

Everything that an adolescent for the first time recognises about himself, every venture that he accepts or declines, every decision he makes, may threaten earlier ideas, perceptions, and attitudes he has acquired regarding himself.

The course of physical growth itself has many emotional repercussions in adolescence, such as the stresses connected with early or late maturing, adolescent obesity, concern about development of the genitals and secondary sex characteristics. In the sphere of sex, he has urges and faces temptations, choices, and hasards, which are more critical than his earlier experiences with sex. In his interpersonal relations, he faces problems of independence-dependence, conformity-nonconformity, and self-assertion-self-negation.

Anxiety and self-determination: Planning for career is the preoccupation of this period. Some adolescents work very hard to achieve their goals. But some, with high achievement drive face anxiety either in achieving their targets, which might have been set very high or due to hurdles and delay coming in the way of success. Currently, many adolescents have the urge to earn lots of money in no time; when they find that it is not an easy task, they feel frustrated and depressed.

Anxiety-producing stresses in adolescence: The need for intimacy normally first appears in pre-adolescence. Intimacy means emotional closeness and it involves mutuality. It may become anxiety provoking for an adolescent, if due to a slower rate of development, he has no need for intimacy when most of the other persons of his age have this need.

Relationship with parents and siblings: There is a general agreement that adolescence is a challenging and sometimes trying time for both the young and the parents. The rapid rate of social change, which we are currently undergoing means that the adolescents and the parents have grown up in markedly in different worlds. When the developmental experiences that shape our personalities and social changes that must be confronted are very different, a generational gap may be expected. The adolescents develop different cultural values and outlooks. Differences in their knowledge tend to magnify the conflict between parents and adolescents.

Parental support and guidance, in addition to meeting the basic needs of developing young people for nurturance, are especially crucial in the face of stressful nature of adolescent transition. The parent-child relationship affects the relative ease with which the young person adjusts to the changed role a new demands of adolescence.

Relationship with Peers

Peer group provides the adolescent with the arena for much of the learning and developing that occurs in all the life tasks. Peers play crucial role in the psychological and social development of most adolescents, especially in age segregated, technological societies like our own, where entrance into adult world of work and family responsibility is increasingly delayed. The peer group provides opportunities to learn how to interact with others, to control social behaviour, to develop age relevant scales and interest and to share similar problems and feelings. Role played by peers in adolescence is especially critical. Relationship between both same and opposite sex peers during the adolescent years come closer to serving as prototype for later adult relationship—in social relations, in work and in interaction with members of opposite sex. The young man or woman who has not learned how to get along with other of the same sex and to establish satisfactory heterosexual relationship, by the time he or she reaches adulthood is likely to face serious obstacle in the years ahead.

Adolescents are also dependent on peer relationships, simply because ties to parents become progressively looser, as the adolescent gains greater independence. In addition, relation with family members are likely to become charged with conflicting emotions in the early years of adolescents-dependent yearnings, exist along side independent striving, hostility is mixed with love and conflict occur over cultural values and social behaviour. Consequently, many areas of adolescent's inner life and outward behaviour become difficult to share with parents.

During this vulnerable stage of development relationship with peers may also be harmful. Adolescents may be pressurised by a group of their peers into suspending their own better judgement and engaging in behaviour they may later regret. These may range from relatively minor improprieties to more serious, sometimes tragic incidence.

Finally, the role of the peer group in helping an individual to define his or her own identity becomes particularly important, during adolescence because at no other stage of development is one's sense of identity so fluid.

Social isolation and alienation: The prevalence of reported loneliness, shyness and social anxiety among adolescents appears to be rather high. Research investigating correlates of adolescent loneliness and social isolation, has focussed on several factors that seem to contribute to these interaction difficulties. Occasional feeling of loneliness, isolation, and awkwardness are probably normal. Among more seriously adolescents, the investigations have identified deficits in certain social skills, social participation and cognitive behavioural characteristics and social outlook problems.

There are powerful forces in the culture that lead adolescents to disguise or repress their emotions. The most common example is repression of sexual feelings in traditional and conservative families.

Ego and Identity

The adolescent "search for identity" leads to increased conflict with parents. Increased identification with peer groups is commonly seen during this period.

An essential problem of adolescence is that of finding a workable answer to the question, "Who am I?" As you have seen, that Erikson has pointed out a strong sense of ego identity in the adolescent, so he sees himself or herself as a separate, distinctive individual. Indeed, the very word individual, as a synonym for person, implies a universal need to perceive oneself as somehow separate from others, no matter how much one may share motives, values, and interests with others.

The individual needs to have a sense of psychosocial reciprocity—a consistency "between that which he conceives himself to be and that which he perceives others to see in him and expect of him". Erikson's assertion that one's sense of identity is tied, at least partly, to social reality is important, it emphasises the fact that societal or individual rejection can seriously impair an adolescent's chances of establishing a strong, secure sense of personal identity. Any developmental influences that contribute to confident perceptions of oneself as separate and distinct from others, consistent and integrated, having a continuity over time, and similar to the way one is perceived by others, contributes to overall sense of ego identity. By the same token, influences that may impair any of these self-perceptions, fosters what Erikson calls "identity confusion".

Due to difficult transition from childhood to adulthood, and of sensitivity to social and historical changes, the adolescent during the stage of identity formation is likely to suffer more deeply that ever before or even again from a confusion of roles, or identity confusion. This stage can cause one to feel isolated, empty, anxious, and indecisive. Adolescents may feel that society is pushing them to take decisions, thus they become even more resistant. They are deeply concerned with how others view them, and are apt to display a lot of self-consciousness and embarrassment.

Adolescent might feel he is regressing rather than progressing. The term identity crisis refers to the necessity to resolve the transitory failure to form a stable identity, or a confusion of roles. Each successive stage in fact, "is a potential crisis because of radical change in perspective" (Erikson, 1968).

Negative identity is a sense of possessing a set of potentially bad or unworthy characteristics. The most common way of dealing with one's negative identity is to project the bad characteristics onto others. It can lead to a lot of social pathology, including prejudice and crime, but it is also an important part of the adolescent's readiness for ideological involvement.

Personality and Social Development

Change in self, or sense of self, is an important issue in adolescence. The sudden changes in their bodies bewilder young people and make them question who they have been and who they are becoming. "Am I the same person I used to be?" they wonder. "What will be like from now on?" As teenagers continue to question and puzzle over their greatest preoccupation, their life's work, they are in danger of becoming confused. This confusion can show itself by the individual's taking an excessively long time to settle on a career.

Inconsistency and impulsiveness in behaviour interferes temporarily in achieving unique personality. In some manner, the distinctive characteristic that differentiates one individual from others in the psychological and behavioural realms must be consistent over time so that the individual can psychologically and be "himself" to himself and others. During adolescence, with peer group identity one sees changes in value system, beliefs, attitudes and behaviour, which are an integral part of personality. Stability in family relationship and role modelling is equally important in the formation of personality at this stage.

Clinical Applications

Understanding of normal child development helps in identification, management of mental subnormality and specific developmental delays. As a part of normal growth and development, children commonly undergo the psychological problems. Problems like specific fears sleep disturbances, regression, sibling rivalry and rebellion. However, if these normal problems worsen or last for long periods, it may be a signal for more serious disturbances. The serious disturbances are in the form of toilet training (enuresis and encopresis), feeding disturbances (overeating, anorexia nervosa and pica), speech disturbances (delayed speech and stuttering), learning disabilities, attention-deficit hyperactivity disorder and autism.

Adolescent period is a very sensitive period hence maintaining positive mental health is very important. Many adjustment problems of minor nature and psychiatric problems of major/severe nature develop during this period. Psychiatric problems and substance abuse have been dealt in detail in other chapters of this book. Adjustment problems mainly occur due to lots of factors like unresolved conflicts, misunderstanding with parents, impulsiveness, anger outburst, aggressive behaviour and increased interest in sexuality. There has been an increase in awareness of adolescent problems so some adolescents seek psychological help, but still a large number of adolescents experience anxiety of growing within themselves.

Many adjustment problems occur due to lack of information on sex. As masturbation is a common experience for adolescent boys, but there are many misconception associated with that, dating behaviour is increasing in present generation adolescents, which is not acceptable to many of the parents, especially in case of girls. So conflict and interpersonal problems arise. For girls, the problems begin with demand for autonomy. For girls conflicts are generally related to type of dresses, they want to wear, visit to beauty parlors and attending late night parties. Environment has a key role in increasing mental health problems. To some extent, media is responsible for their increase. Violence, aggressiveness and sexual liberties shown on TV. Screens, movies and songs instigate adolescents to behave in similar ways. The changing values of our society are different. Pressures and challenges to the adolescents like show-off of wealth, smoking, drinking, driving recklessly, late night parties and free mixing of both sexes in some sections of societies becomes a reason of conflict for others due to peer group pressures.

During the last few years, adolescent medicine has started to deal with a number of social problems experienced by youths such as tobacco, alcohol and drug abuse. Inadequate resilience to stress and adversity, and sexually transmitted diseases. Indeed, alcohol is the most widely used psychoactive drug among adolescents (32) and initiation of the use of tobacco (at the age of >11) has increased rapidly, especially in girls. Almost half of adolescents have used an illicit drug before they finish high school, and 25 percent have consumed an illegal drug other than marijuana (30). Moreover, approximately half of fatal motor vehicle accidents and homicides, as well as substantial proportion of suicides among adolescents, are associated with the use of alcohol and other drugs (33). The high incidence of adolescents affected with sexually transmitted diseases also has been pointed out.

A fairly common medical subject such as adequate nutrition for proper growth and pubertal development has become an obsessive problem for many teenagers, whose greater awareness of their physical appearance causes dissatisfaction with their body weight and physical image. Excessive dieting and inappropriate weight loss in girls usually interfere with normal growth and menstrual cycles. Most of these adolescents are not excessively overweight. Many, are most concerned over the localisation of subcutaneous fat on their hips, thighs, waist and buttocks. Most young girls, with these concerns diet without medical supervision. They begin by skipping breakfast or lunch, and prolong fasting. They often take diuretics, laxatives and appetite suppressants and end up with unexpected secondary health problems. Inappropriate preoccupation over weight and poor diets may be predisposing factors to more serious eating disorders, such as anorexia nervosa and bulimia, with all the psychological, gynaecologic and metabolic sequelae associated with these conditions.

Medical doctors also have to deal with another fairly common eating disorder, i.e. some forms of obesity. Excessive overweight in pubertal boys and girls, not only causes important psychological problems, which affect social, educational and sport activities, but also is a predisposing factor for hypertension and elevated cholesterol with a greater risk of cardiovascular diseases later in adulthood. Excessive food intake, sedentary lifestyles, excessive television viewing habits, and poor physical activities are among the main causes of obesity in childhood and adolescence.

The relationship between overweight during adolescence and subsequent educational achievement, marital status, household income, and self-esteem on 370 obese patients aged 16 to 24 years, was studied by Gortmaker et al. These authors concluded in a seven year follow-up that this condition had important negative social and economic consequences, which were more adverse than those of many individuals with other chronic diseases. Practically all adolescents are over sensitive about body image, and fat teenagers are especially vulnerable to social discrimination. Medical doctors must see and talk to these adolescents without the presence of their parents, carrying out a private dialogue, even at ages of 10 or lower. Youngsters on their own usually become more friendly, open, receptive and cooperative than in the presence of their parents. Adequate counselling and properly balanced dieting, not fancy commercial diets, should be prescribed with a periodic weight check. No drugs for weight reduction should be administered. These patients should be counselled that while they are modifying their body to reach their final physical shape late in puberty, they are developing their personality; their self-assurance, and their self-control. Their efforts therefore, are not only directed to modifying their physical aspects but also to building up their personality.

Adolescent growth proceeds at an astonishing pace, the most rapid of any postnatal time (average weight increment during the adolescent growth spurt is 16 g/day for females and 19 g/day for males). It is also during adolescence and young adulthood that the skeletal mineral accretion is completed, the peak bone mass being critical for skeletal maintenance and prevention of osteoporosis. Lesions of arteriosclerosis also begin to accelerate at this age and peak incidence of anorexia and bulimia nervosa is in adolescence. Moreover, overweight and obese conditions occurring at this age show persistent health effects decades later. Furthermore, food habits which develop as the adolescent enjoys increasing independence and responsibility for his or her own dietary intake are believed to persist into adulthood, making this a critical time for preventive health interventions.

SUMMARY

The human infant has a number of adaptive reflexes, including the grasping and sucking reflexes. Early social development lays a foundation for later relationships with other people. Development occurs along multiple lines, it is overall physical development, cognitive, personality, social and neurological development. The motor development is mainly in the first few years of life. Cognitive development according to Piaget, occurs in four stages, sensory motor stage, preoperational stage, concrete operational stage, and stage of formal operations.

According to Freud, the personality development passes through various stages of psychosexual development. These stages are oral stage, anal stage, phallic stage and latency period. Erikson has proposed a psychosocial theory of personality development, which consists of eight stages. The first four stages occur during infancy and childhood, the fifth during adolescence and the last three stages during the adult years including old age.

Adolescents are a transition period in one's life from childhood to adulthood. Psychological and emotional development reaches its peak during this period. The changes occurring in an individual are varied and rapid which if not handled carefully can disturb the mental health of an individual.

Constitutional delay of the onset of puberty is a fairly common reason for adolescents (14 and 16 years of age) and for their parents to seek a clinical consultation. While the age of puberty onset varies, the delayed initiation of pubertal changes and of the growth spurt frequently worries a large number of adolescents, especially boys, because of the social dimension of perceived delays. Some who perceive that their development is abnormal, start having problems in school, stop participating in sports, are no longer willing to participate in social events, etc.

Most girls with delayed puberty accept the explanation offered, especially when one can give approximate dates when these processes will start taking place. Conversely, boys are more difficult to manage, because most of them are quite upset over their sexual infantilism and short stature. Boys usually seek clinical help because their growth velocity has not increased significantly, at a time when their peers are growing faster than they. Boys often show a considerable difference in height from one year to the next. Frequently, they do not mention their main concern, i.e. that they are shorter than their school friends and are often ridiculed by peers. Such patients should be assured that the present situation is transient. They should be provided with an approximate date for the onset of their growth spurt based on testicular volument and their bone age and an estimate of final adult height. Some boys with delayed puberty are also quite concerned over their sexual infantilism. This concern often leads them to abandon sports activities because they do not want to undress with their more sexually mature peers. Some respond by making efforts to obtain better physical development. They perform strenuous exercises at the gymnasium, two to three hours daily, using heavy weights to stimulate muscle development. Physicians should advise them that such efforts will have very limited results due to a transient lack of sufficient testosterone to stimulate muscle mass growth. A useful metaphor is to compare their efforts to a man who wishes to move a car by pushing it, without the car having gasoline; he will be able to move the car, but slowly; igniting the engine would be better but this is impossible without gasoline; in sense, testosterone is the gasoline needed by the muscle for it to develop when stimulated by exercise.

Adulthood to Ageing

A senior government executive, around 45 years old was referred for obsessive rumination. This problem was very severe and it interfered with his work, he felt insecure, so his wife, also an executive had to be with him always. Behavioural assessment revealed that besides his rumination about girl, he also was afraid to see gray hair, had intense anxiety as well as apprehension about his growing old. He had negative thoughts related to old age as nobody cares for, person becomes lonely and the life in old age is worthless. This case is not unique, as many of us can have problems of adjustment to age specific roles, illness, failing abilities and so on. On the other hand, we meet many people from various stages of life enjoying every bit of experience. This chapter shall help you to understand various developmental changes, which occur with the advancement of age so that you can identify the deviations and thus provide help.

According to the ancient Hindu literature, the development period was divided into four stages namely: Brahmacharya ashram, Grihasth ashram, Vanprasth ashram, and Sanyas ashram. The first two stages correspond to early period of childhood through adolescence and adulthood where the individual settles in job, gets married and has family responsibilities. The Vanprasth is equivalent to the middle age where the person after fulfilling some of the primary responsibilities of family, works for his self-actualisation joins religious organisations works for social cause; and finally, the sanyas being the old age where the individual retires and occupies himself with religious activities. Similar system of development has been adopted by the modern thinkers. Many of the developmental tasks described in ancient Hindu books are similar in nature with those described by modern thinkers.

Adulthood

The adulthood has been divided into three parts, namely, young adulthood (20 to 40-45 years); middle adulthood (40-45 to about 65 years); and old age (from 65 or 70 years onwards). This classification is only for the convenience of studying the developmental process in adult age, which is fairly a longer period than other stages like childhood or adolescence.

Stages in Adult Development

It is only recently that due attention has been given to the developmental process from early adulthood to middle adulthood. Thus, some longitudinal studies have been carried out to study this process. The findings of these studies are as follows:

The Early Adult Transition (17 to 22 years)

People feel halfway out of the family and sense a great need to get all the way out. They have a tenuous sense of their own autonomy and feel that real adult life is just around the corner.

Entering the Adult World (22 to 28 years)

People now feel like adults. They are established in a chosen lifestyle; independent of their parents, and pursuing immediate goals without questioning themselves about whether they are following the right course.

The Age 30 Transition (28 to 34 years)

People ask themselves, "What is this life all about now that I am doing what I am supposed to?" and "Is what I am, the only way for me to be?" They often reassess both work and family patterns. At this time, for example, career women think about having a baby, and homemakers begin to work outside the home.

Settling Down (33 to 43 years)

People make deeper commitments to work, family, and other important aspects of their lives, setting specific goals with set timetables. Towards the end of this period, is the state which Levinson calls "becoming one's own man", when men break away from the authorities in their lives and work at attaining senior status in their own right.

Midlife Transition (40 to 45 years)

People question virtually every aspect of their lives and values with an increasing awareness that time is limited. They may bridge the transition to the second half of life. They come to terms with the fact that the first part of adult life is over, and they will not be able to do all that they had planned before they grow old and die. The transition may be smoothly managed or it may assume crisis proportions, depending on their personalities and the specific situations they find themselves in.

While biology shapes much of what we do in childhood, culture and individual personality play a much larger role in adult life. The older we grow, the less our age tells about us. For example, two 45-year-old women may resemble each other physiologically, but the one who had two children in her twenties, remained at home would have a different outlook on life from that of her age-mate with a well-established career.

Traditionally, most adults have had strong feelings about the time in life, when certain activities are considered acceptable. People are keenly aware of their own timing and describe themselves as "early", "late", or "on time", regarding the time they got married, settled in a career, had children, or retired. This sense of timing seems to be shaped by environmental expectations, often affected by social class.

In recent years, however, as affluence has filtered down, as medical advances have kept people vigorous, and as the life span has lengthened, age-based expectations have become more flexible. We are more accepting of 40-year-old first time parents and 40-year-old grandparents, 50-year-old retirees and 75-year-old workers. As Bernice Neugarten and Gunhild Hagestad (1976) point out, we seem to be moving in the direction of what might be called an age-irrelevant society; and it can be argued that age, like race or sex, is diminishing in importance as a regulator of behaviour.

In adulthood, generally people are well-settled in their careers barring a few. We are much more flexible in dealing with the basic developmental tasks of adulthood. These are years of good health and energy, especially in our twenties and thirties, with very slight, gradual changes not becoming noticeable till about age 50. We are at the peak of our muscular strength and our manual dexterity at about 25 or 30. We see and hear most sharply in our early twenties, gradually there is a decline in these senses, as majority of the people become farsighted around forty years. Taste, smell, and sensitivity to pain, touch, and temperature remain stable until at least 45 or 50.

Certain relatively consistent events mark adulthood in our society. These range from escaping parental dominance in the late teens, to a noticeable acceptance of one's lot in life during the 50's. Research indicates that midlife affects many people in the 37-41 ranges, but this is not universal. Midlife crisis is characterised by feeling of instability and anxiety.

Biological ageing begins between 25 and 30 years, but peak performance in specific pursuits may come at various parts throughout life. Most of the health changes from young adulthood to middle age are relatively minor. The organ systems are not as efficient as they had been, tending to lose some of their reserve capacity. Men's sexual capacity declines, and high blood pressure becomes a problem. Metabolism changes, and both sexes tend to put on weight.

How do individuals cope with physical changes, and therefore, with the awareness of their ageing? Past health history, family attitudes, and individual personalities play a large part. Women tend to be more health conscious, both for themselves and their families. This may have something to do with the fact that pregnancy and childbirth have involved them more closely with medical care, as well as with their traditional role as guardian of the family's health. While men often turn to diets and exercise, they tend to ignore symptoms (Lewis and Lewis, 1977).

Middle Adulthood

Physical Changes

The ratio of the physical and the psychological changes in midlife vary, with the former affecting women universally and the latter becoming increasingly recognised syndrome among men.

Menopause: It is a biological event in every woman's life, when she stops menstruating and can no longer bear children. There are variations in the age at which it may come. It can occur any time between 38 and 60 years of age, with the average between 48 and 52 (Upjohn, 1983). At one time, a number of psychological problems, especially depression, were blamed on the menopause, but recent research shows no reason to attribute psychiatric illness to the physical changes in a woman's body. Such problems are more likely caused by environmental pressures against ageing, which remind a woman that menopause marks the end of her youth. In those cultures that value the older woman, few problems are associated with the menopause (Ballinger, 1961). A society's attitude toward ageing seems to influence a menopausal woman's well-being far more than the level of hormones in her body.

The male climacteric: Despite the fact that men continue to father children till quite late in life, there are some biological changes in middle-aged men. These include decreased fertility and frequency of orgasm, and an increase in impotency (Beard, 1975). Furthermore, men seem to have cyclic fluctuations in the production of hormones. About five per cent of middle-aged men are said to experience symptoms such as depression, fatigue, sexual inadequacy, and vaguely defined physical complaints. Since researchers have found no relationships between hormone levels and mood changes (Doering, Kraemer; Brodie and Hamburg), it is probable that most men's complaints are just as subject to environmental pressures as women's are. Some of the problems may be related to disturbing life events, such as illness of the man or his wife, business or job problems, his children leaving home, or the death of his parents.

Intelligence and Memory

For many years, it was believed that general intellectual activity peaked at about age 20 and then declined. We have strong evidence showing that certain types of intelligence continue to develop throughout life. We have discussed in Chapter 6 about two types of intelligence, fluid and crystallised. Verbal abilities, a type of crystallised intelligence, appear to increase throughout adulthood and old age. Performance in solving new problems such as spatial-relations tasks, an aspect of fluid intelligence, peaks in the late teens and then begins a slow, steady decline. Furthermore, the accumulated wisdom that comes with adulthood may offset any decline in fluid abilities. Wisdom, the ability to exercise good judgement about important but uncertain matters of life, also affects our relationships with other people.

Personality

Few of us hold the same outlook on life at 40 that we did at 20, showing the growth and development that takes place during adulthood. This growth comes about from many sources—the people we meet, the reading we do, the experiences we undergo, the challenges we face up to. Recent longitudinal studies of adults have dramatically illustrated the kinds of developmental tasks we deal with over the years.

Yet despite the changes that occur-in our lives and our thinking, we are still the same people. And we do tend to carry certain basic traits with us in all the twists and turns of life's pathways. The two threads of stability and change are intertwined throughout all our lives, with some of us showing more change and others more continuity.

One personality change, common in midlife is the tendency to express aspects of our personalities that we had repressed during our younger years. Sometimes, the repressed personality traits get a chance to manifest in middle age. With the recognition at this stage of life that some of our basic goals have already been achieved—the children reared, the career established, the identity in large measure achieved—both men and women feel freer to change from the stereotypical male or female role they had modelled themselves in younger age. They allow themselves to express long-buried aspects of their personalities, as many women become more assertive, competitive, and independent and many men allow themselves to be passive and dependent. You may find many men enjoying cooking in this age, which was never even dreamt in their young age. The significant aspect of such change is not of "contrasexual" nature but the fact that any trait that has been repressed for the first half of life may now flower, with the increased self-confidence and relaxation that often accompany middle age.

One other common personality change, which may help uncover such buried characteristics, is a tendency for people to become more introspective as they grow older. While younger people invest more of their energies in action rather than in thought, people at midlife and beyond tend to think about themselves more, analysing what they have done in their lives and why they have done it (Cytrynbaum).

Parenthood and Development

Parenthood can be a creative self-growth experience as parents go through its several stages: anticipating ahead of time what parenthood will be like, adjusting to new demands and learning how to meet them at every stage of their children's growth, and then disengaging from the active parental role as children mature. As children grow, parents get a second chance to relive their own childhood experiences and to work out issues they had not resolved with their own parents. In addition, their children, who bring their own unique personalities and demands to this intimate, intensely emotional relationship, influence them. This is the period when children settle in own professions, get married and leave home. The parents especially mothers may feel lonely in the house. This phenomenon has been called "empty nest syndrome". Persons with poor coping ability or with too much of dependency on children find difficult to adjust with the new circumstances.

Old Age or the Senescence

The interface between the body systems and the environment as it exists in senescence requires one to look at the older person in a special light. Most significantly, later life is marked by a number of progressive losses. For example, health, vocation, financial security, status, beauty, friendship, and even-eventually-life itself are all at risk for older people.

Abnormal development occurs when the elderly individual is unable to cope successfully with the large number of losses that he or she is apt to experience in the course of a life time. The symptoms that the elderly individual exhibits in the face of these stresses are likely to represent exacerbations of long-standing or well-established patterns of behaviour. Senescence leads to diverse physical and psychosocial changes that may affect the functioning of the older adult.

Developmental Tasks of Old Age

Gerontologists have proposed two theories of ageing. The disengagement theory holds that withdrawal from society is necessary and desirable in old age. The activity theory counters that optimal adjustment to ageing is tied to continuing activity and involvement. According to a report, well being in old age is characterised by self-acceptance, positive relations with others, autonomy, environmental mastery, a purpose in life and continued personal growth.

Those who do achieve a sense of wholeness and integrity may develop one of the hallmarks of successful ageing, wisdom. Our culture traditionally relies on selected elderly people for advice about complex life problems. One reason may be that older people who have been attentive to their life experience, often have a perspective on reality that is richer and more informed than the view most younger people take.

Health Changes

Physical functioning and health decline in old age. Although ageing does not affect the entire organism uniformly, we observe negative changes in nine body systems; they are musculoskeletal, cardiovascular, respiratory, nervous and special senses, gastrointestinal, urinary, integumentary, reproductive, and endocrine. Whether we look at the thinning of muscular fibres, loss of muscle tone in the bladder, or decreased basal metabolic rate, we discover a decline in the older person's vital functions. It is of special importance to the behavioural scientist, to recognise that all five senses suffer loss in even normal ageing, thereby skewing perception. For the most part, these conditions are more like chronic, debilitating illnesses, as opposed to acute episodes as seen earlier in life. The following pictures show physical changes that occur from adulthood to old age (Fig. 13.1).

Psychological Changes

Intelligence

Some intellectual abilities do not decline with age, while other abilities decline at different rates. In general, verbal abilities tend to be maintained while psychomotor speed and problem solving tend to decline. Studies using the Wechler Adult Intelligence Scale (WAIS), indicated the elderly do best on information, vocabulary, and comprehension subtests; less well on arithmetic and picture completion subtests; and worst on tests of object assembly, block design, and picture arrangement.

Learning and Memory

Because learning and memory are closely intertwined and both are crucial to intellectual

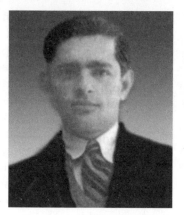 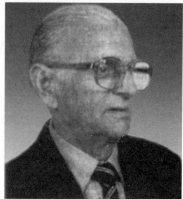

Fig. 13.1: Physical changes according to aging

functioning, it is important to find out how the two operate in old age. Many investigators have worked at this task, and some general trends are emerging from their work. First, though older adults can certainly learn via classical and instrumental conditioning.

Second, in verbal learning—learning lists of words, for example, adults over 60 generally do not perform as well as do young adults, but experts are now debating whether these performance differences reflect real differences in learning ability. Some attribute the inferior performance of older adults to pacing problems. It is on timed tasks that older people perform most poorly.

Third, overcaution and pacing problems may also contribute to some of the memory—performance deficits older people demonstrate. These deficits are not found in all aspects of their memory but are largely confined to processing of information.

Older people show deficits in the encoding and retrieval processes. They are less effective than are younger adults in coming up with good strategies for organising and rehearsing the memories they are encoding, and they often take longer than do younger adults to draw memories out of storage (Erber, 1982). Memories—be they words, pictures, or concepts—seem to be recognised about as effectively by older as by younger adults; it is recall, remembering from scratch or from partial cues, that tends to suffer with old age. As we have seen in Chapter on Memory that the memories are rarely lost, it just takes longer to find them in the file or takes longer to retrieve. The abilities may vary in the various components of memory—registration, storage and retrieval of information. Bellak (1976) reports that elderly individuals may remember better when information is personally meaningful, offered in small amounts, and presented in a way that is easy to code for storage.

Personality Changes

Adult development from early adulthood to middle adulthood and to later life has been a largely neglected area of study. Recently, some attention has been given to the study of personality in later years, by adopting a developmental approach. Thus, as during the formative childhood and adolescent years, the adult is viewed as passing through various life phases. During these phases, the individual's perspective on life and death, personal accomplishments, and interpersonal relationships are ever evolving. The many changes faced by the elderly quite often call for a team approach to deal with their problems. Mental health problems may be one of many issues confronting the older person.

Stressful Life Events

There is an increasing evidence that life events associated with older persons are higher due to death of the spouse, change in living conditions, at times rejection from children, lack of friends, restriction in financial condition and mobility. The physical disabilities like loss of hearing, poor visions, difficulty in walking, etc. may cause additional stress on the older person. These stressful events should be taken into consideration while understanding the problems of the aged, because the presence of stress can delay the recovery process of physical diseases (Chapter 10).

Indeed mental health conditions may be inextricably tied to other physical or social problems in the older person's life. An understanding of the role of body systems as well as needs for care and support are necessary, in order to be able to provide effective treatment to an older patient. Even the manner in which you communicate with the older patient is important in developing trust and good doctor-patient relationship. At times, it is good to integrate mental health treatment into the ovrall care plan for the older patient.

Social Changes

Social losses among the elderly are a major concern. Widowed elders lose the psychosocial role of being a spouse and are much more likely to experience isolation and loneliness. People who experience isolation and loneliness are documented as being at high risk for mental illness.

The economical problems in old age often result in the biopsychosocial crises experienced by the elderly. The elderly persons from lower or middle economic class may live on relatively fixed incomes. During illness, if expensive medication is prescribed, many of these elderly persons are not even able to buy them. Lack of mobility, limited public transportation, poor intergenerational relationships, loss of status due to retirement, society's prejudice can result in synergistic blend of conditions that lead to a high rate of psychopathology and need for services among the old.

Gerontologists have proposed two theories of ageing. The disengagement theory holds that withdrawal from society is necessary and desirable in old age. The activity theory counters that optimal adjustment to ageing is tied to continuing activity and involvement. According to Ryft (1989), well being in old age is characterised by self-acceptance, positive relations with others, autonomy, environmental mastery, a purpose in life and continued personal growth.

Clinical Applications

Ageing brings difficulties of adjustment and these may be of sufficient severity to lead to pathological states of anxiety or depression, which required treatment. Middle adulthood is a period of productivity, being on the highest scales of the career and thus more prone to stress. As we have seen earlier in the Chapter of Stress, that it can give rise to number of physical problems. Coping with these physical problems and fulfilling the aspirations and ambitions may get into conflict. Understanding the varying reactions to such situations can be used in the management of physical problems.

With the advancement in medicine, the life expectancy has increased. Thus, in any country the population of the elderly people is growing. With advancement of age, not only the physical problems increased but the psychological problems are also greater. Since memory problems are a frequent complaint of elderly people who are depressed, discriminating between memory problems that are organic versus functional in nature is of prime importance. Amongst the psychological problems, depression is the most common problem encountered in the aged population. The depressive feeling may be associated with loneliness, physical illness or simply due to the decline of abilities due to normal ageing. Understanding the family circumstances, social support system and coping resources of these people can enhance the efficacy of the treatment.

SUMMARY

The period of adulthood has primarily been divided into three periods, namely, early, middle and late adulthood. Depending upon the personality, attitude and lifestyle the differentiation between these three stages is not very clear-cut. Generally, there are not many physical or psychological changes in the early adulthood. The physical changes start showing up after the age of 50 years (middle age).

The middle age is the period, which can show some personality changes like the women becoming more assertive and the men taking the reverse role. The physical changes due to menopause can be associated with some psychological problems in some women. These being, who have negative attitude towards ageing or have not achieved what they wanted are more prone to depression at this age. The old age is generally considered around 65 years and above. In old age there are problems in learning new materials and deficits in memory primarily due to the difficulty in retrieval. There can be some personality changes as old age demands adjustment with retirement, limited resources and decline in functioning of the vital organs. Death of the spouse and children staying away can result in loneliness. Older people are at risk to develop mental health problems, especially depression.

Dealing with Death and Bereavement

A 3 years old child admitted in paediatric ICU, is in very critical condition. The patient is restless, crying with pain and has very little chance of survival. His parents are constantly enquiring about his condition. As a doctor attending upon the child, what should you do? Tell the parents about his critical condition or just do not talk to them. Often patients and family members have been ignored and not informed about the condition. Now more and more patients and family members wish to know all about the disease process, prognosis and treatment plans. In such cases, where the illness is fatal, the doctors' role in comforting the patient and family is very vital.

The care of the dying patient and the comfort of the bereaved are major responsibility of the doctor. It is as important as providing treatment. These areas have only in recent years been studied systematically. Death evokes fear and embarrassment among most people, as they have not experienced death till late in their lives. The medical professions also do not encounter death as frequent as it was in the past. With the improvement of life expectancy in this century, death has become less well known and therefore, perhaps, more frightening. Yet death is inevitable in many conditions and doctors have to be prepared to deal with such situations. They should be able to offer help in easing the process of dying. For doctors, it may also now evoke more of a sense of professional failure since the expectation is increasingly one of the cure from life-threatening diseases—a fact which colours the doctor's attitude to the death. It is of considerable value to understand and thereby help, both the dying and the bereaved.

The reactions of family members to death vary according to the nature of death. The ending of life may take a variety of forms—sometimes sudden and unexpected as with a fatal accident or heart attack, sometimes slow and expected following a period of 'terminal' illness. Many healthy elderly people die peacefully in their sleep without warning; death being simply due to 'old age'. Determinants of the psychological response to dying are associated with its cause (e.g. due to ageing or disease, and if so its nature), with the individual and with his environment. Fears of death are at times focussed less on the thought of death itself, and more on the process of dying. Sometimes, death is disturbing as it may result in extreme physical distress.

Many factors influence an individual's response to death. One of the common significant response is the presence of religious faith, since this often holds out the promise of eternal life. It has been observed in hospitalised patients, that those who had a firm religious faith have least anxiety. Consoling power of religion is seen in all types of patients, with different religious background. Sudden death due to accidents or cardiac arrest, are more difficult to accept than death due to chronic illness.

Another factor that influences responses to death is, age in the younger patient as the anxiety is further aroused by parenthood with apprehension concerning dependent children. Depression is also frequently seen among the dying. While this may by partly related to physical discomfort in some illnesses, it may also stem from feelings of isolation resulting from a tendency to avoidance or emotional withdrawal on the part of others when a person is known to be dying. At the same time, this disengagement may sometimes be a two-way process, with the dying person himself withdrawing, perhaps in anticipation of the final parting. Depression may additionally be explicable as part of a kind of anticipatory grief or mourning by the individual for the losses that he is experiencing or expecting by loss of life.

The patient (if conscious) and family members face a very difficult time as the death approaches. Many problems arise at this time due to lack of communication and doctors' ability to handle such situations. Often the doctors take death of the patient as a matter of fact and the patient may just be a bed no. 2 for them. This attitude and manner of communicating causes lots of harsh feeling in the family members. It is thus important for the doctors to understand different types of reactions and responses to death and thereby deal accordingly.

Methods to Deal with Dying Patients

Robert, a 43-year-old businessman, and his wife had two sons. Doctors had given him six months to live, but offered and even encouraged him to undergo chemotherapy which would give him a ten per cent chance of recovery. The chemotherapy had wrecked his body and made him physically much weaker. In spite of this, his family and his doctor desired him to continue. When he was asked as to what he wanted to do, that was the first time that he said that he wanted the treatment stopped and that he only wanted to spend the rest of the day of his life with his family and with as much peace as possible.

This incident supports the fact that the quality of time spent in the last days of life is most important for all concerned. The family members should be encouraged to support patient's attempts to remain as independent as possible. He can be involved in making decisions concerned with the family. In our culture there is a tendency to hide facts from the patient. When we do not talk about death with the patient, it does not mean that the patient is not aware of it. Rather, they conceal their anxieties and other thoughts to themselves, which might be more painful. If the patient is in a conscious state, talking about death, at least warning of impending death can help the patient to be prepared for it. Surely it is better to face death than to die suddenly. We need to be there willing to listen to the thoughts, feelings, fears and doubts about dying. Do not brush aside the topic, so as not to cause any unnecessary upsets or avoid the subject because you cannot cope up with the patients, and family's reaction. In some situations, the patient may not want to talk about the pending death. In those situations we should not push this subject. Chapter 23 gives details of communicating with dying patients.

There are two areas of decision making that concern the dying patient. One has to do with the treatment and the other has to do with practical needs and plans for the immediate future such as organising finances, making will for legal matters, seeking spiritual readiness and rekindling relationships. Lack of information is one of the primary causes of anxiety among the terminally ill. We should therefore take all things into consideration before deciding to withhold any information about the patient. It would be tragic if one were to die without fulfilling or expressing one's wishes regarding areas of one's wishes.

If the family members are well-informed about the pending death, they can either fulfill their certain religious rituals or mend their relationship with the dying person, if it was disturbed.

By not warning the family members, we often generate guilt feelings in them. I have encountered a situation, where the wife when informed about her husband's death said that if she was informed earlier, at least she could have offered some prayers to improve her husband's next life (a Hindu belief).

There are many practical and thoughtful things that we can do to help the patients in their final days. Life is precious, even when death is near. We should do all that can make them comfortable.

Bereavement

The effect of death on those who are still alive has also received systematic investigation in recent years. A fairly consistent pattern of mourning has been identified (Parkes, 1965). Typical or uncomplicated grief is usually seen following the death of a parent, child, sibling or first-degree relative with whom there has been at least a moderate amount of social contact within the preceding year.

Stages of Bereavement

Bereavement involves several stages. The first response to an unexpected death is one of shock and disbelief—a period of denial, which may last from a few hours to a fortnight. A 42 years old woman lost her husband while he was undergoing angioplasty. When the news was conveyed to her by the relative, she became absolutely shocked, did not cry, and kept saying that 'Deepak is feeling better, he has sent me home to look after children. Tomorrow he will be discharged from the hospital.' She was not able to give any reasons why the other relatives were crying. She came out of this state after half an hour. During this period, bereaved person feels numbed but is able to carry on with the usual routine, as well as coping with arrangements for the funeral.

Gradually however, this protective denial begins to give way to a full realisation of the loss and is associated with feelings of despair. Attacks of yearning may be accompanied by great distress, with reminders of the deceased (such symptoms may include feelings of tightness, etc.). Between these waves of distress, there is a general state of depression, apathy and sense of futility. Sleep is disturbed and appetite poor. There is a preoccupation with thoughts of the deceased and often a characteristic restlessness which may appear aimless but probably represents a searching for the dead—sometimes acknowledged by the bereaved person, who consciously looks in places previously frequented by the dead person. Irritability and anger are as responsible for the death. Often in the hospital, sometimes the medical staff is blamed, and at times the relatives become very aggressive and abusive towards the doctors. On the other hand, there may be feelings of guilt and self-blame for past behaviour towards the deceased, whose memory tends to be idealised. In the earlier part of this stage, however, there is a tendency to think of the dead person as still alive to feel his presence or to actually see or hear him but gradually this is replaced by full realisation of the loss. Another frequent characteristic is the appearance of traits of the deceased in the behaviour of the bereaved including often the symptoms of the last illness. Finally, the intensity of this stage begins to decline after a few weeks and is generally minimal by about six months, with full acceptance of the death. For several years thereafter, however, there may be occasional brief periods of depression and yearning, usually precipitated by reminders of the loss and especially by anniversaries.

A great deal of mental activity is involved in the process of grieving. Freud (1917) described his mental activity as grief work and Lindemann (1944) subdivided this into three components: (1) emancipation from bondage to the deceased (2) readjustment to the environment from which the deceased in missing, and (3) formation of new relationships. The first of these tasks is the most crucial and depends upon the bereaved person remembering, often repeatedly, the many shared experiences that formed the basis of the relationship with the deceased. This process is initially extremely distressing but becomes progressively less, so with passage of time such recollections do not bring pain but pleasure. Table 14.1 summarises the stages of bereavement.

Table 14.1: Stages of bereavement

- Shock and disbelief
- Protective denial
- Preoccupation with thoughts (Feeling of guilt and self-blame)
- Tendency to think of dead people alive
- Appearance of traits (of the deceased person in the bereaved)
- Depression
- Full acceptance

A person's mourning does not of course take place in isolation, but within a sociocultural context, which includes the particular beliefs and rituals of his culture Anthropological studies have shown that these vary widely between different societies, each of which seems to have developed its own beliefs about the meaning of death together with a set of rituals concerning the disposal of the bereaved. Now, the ritual associated with bereavement has declined, and Gorer (1965) claims that this loss of recognition and support for the expression of the grief is responsible for increased psychological disturbance among bereaved people today. In this respect, the Orthodox way of ritual mourning appears to provide a more favourable environment. In our culture, there is also a tendency to encourage the strict control of feelings on the part of the mourner.

Religious beliefs are also important in bereavement. Just as belief in an 'after-life' can colour the attitudes of the dying to their condition, so too it affects those who are left behind. The idea of ultimate reunion can be a great comfort to the bereaved, though it sometimes leads to suicide in order to hasten the process.

Children also have problems in accepting death of their dear ones. Children develop the concept of death around seven years of age. Due to the incomplete understanding, very young children often cannot accept the absence of the person due to death. As children do not openly express their fears regarding death, they often develop emotional problems, which are manifested in a sudden drop in their academic performance, sleep disturbances, development of fears, depression and insecurity. Children should be helped to talk out their fears and anxieties.

Clinical Applications

The care of the dying is also one of the responsibilities of the doctor. A great deal can be done to provide relief from physical discomfort, and especially pain; but care of the whole person includes consideration of his psychological welfare, and this is a matter which has received more systematic attention in recent years.

One of the most frequently discussed problems, is how much information should be given to dying patients, in particular, whether and if so when, they should be made aware of the fact that their illness is fatal. This question is often put in relation to cancer—should the patient be told? the implication being that this is like pronouncing a death sentence. In fact, the matter is nowhere near as simple at this. By no means all patients diagnosed as having cancer will have their lives shortened by the disease, while there are obviously many of other diseases that can threaten life. Nor in the presence of a fatal disease, is the doctor usually able to predict with any degree of accuracy when death will occur. For their part, patients often suspect and sometimes are sure that they are dying before being told so. Doctors vary in their attitudes to telling patients the truth about fatal illness, ranging from those who consider it never right to do so, to those who believe in always providing such information. Most, probably take a position somewhere between these two extremes and try to judge what is best for each individual patient.

Most dying patients ultimately come to an awareness of the truth, whether or not they ask for and are given it. Greater stress should be given on listening to what patients have to say and ask than on what should be said to them. If they are given the opportunity to talk about their situation, to voice their concerns and to express their wishes, it is usually possible to judge the best response to any question about prognosis. Some indicate quite openly that they do not want to know if their illness is fatal, and this wish should be respected. Others, ask the question in such a way that it indicates the need for reassurance, or at least hope ('It's not cancer, is it doctor?'). In this event, rather than giving an immediate denial and perhaps untruthful reply, which will be of more lasting value to the patient than a consoling but false picture of the future; by allowing him to talk freely and repeatedly in this way, and by giving simple explanations of his disease, the patient's awareness of dying may gradually grow in an atmosphere of sympathetic understanding.

Attitude towards death, namely, the sense of failure felt by medical and other staff in the face of a fatal illness. This may sometimes lead to a tendency to withdraw from contact with the dying, which may be sensed by the patient. Many patients are sensitive to this difficulty on the part of some doctors and feel unable to talk openly to them about their illness, for fear of causing embarrassment. However, that a shift may be occurring within the medical profession towards greater frankness, and this is associated with an increasing emphasis on the care of the dying in medical education.

An awareness of the normal sequence of events in typical grief, together with an understanding of the psychological processes involved, should be of assistance to those who are concerned with advising and helping the bereaved, and indeed it has become recognised that bereavement counselling requires more than common sense if it is to be effective.

During the early stage of numbness, the bereaved person needs a certain amount of assistance with simple decisions and practical matters to do with the registration of the death, funeral arrangements, etc. Once the initial phase of shock has passed, sharing of the feelings of grief may be most helpful, while advice to 'stop thinking about it' can be positively harmful. Expression of emotions should be allowed but not forced by insensitive probing. Individuals will vary in the degree to which they actually express their grief—what is important is that they should be able to feel it. This means rejecting the customary social attitude, which seems to imply that grief can be avoided by not talking about it, and by restricting conversation to trivialities instead. The bereaved person needs sympathetic understanding but not pity, and at this time, social support system provided by relatives and friends in our culture is very helpful in coping with the loss. Bereavement sometimes leads to abnormal reactions, which may be of clinical importance, both physically and psychologically. There is evidence for an increased incidence of both morbidity and mortality from organic disease, following bereavement. Bereavement may also result in a psychiatric illness such a neurotic illness, depression, schizophrenia, or mania, for example. In this case, the actual nature of the psychological disturbance is probably not determined by the bereavement, which simply acts as a nonspecific precipitating stress.

Sometimes you may encounter abnormal grief reactions, which may be seen as variants of the normal process, and are thus 'stress-specific', i.e. they only occur following a loss. Parkes (1965) describes three types of abnormal grief. Chronic grief represents an intensification and prolongation of the typical form, and is frequently associated with recurrent ideas of guilt and self-blame, and with physical symptoms, similar to those of the final illness of the deceased. Inhibited grief tends to occur in the very young or the very old, and is characterised by the prolonged inhibition of a large part of the total picture of typical grief, with substitution of other symptoms instead. Delayed grief is typical or chronic grief occurring after a delay of months or years.

Parkes reviewed the evidence, mostly from studies of bereaved women, concerning the determinants of severe grief reactions, and concluded that the high-risk case would have the following characteristics; a young widow with children and no close relatives nearby; a timid, dependent personality, history of depressive illness; a relationship with her husband which was closely dependent or ambivalent with no preparedness for his unexpected death; and finally, a family and cultural tradition which inhibits the expression of grief.

SUMMARY

The care of dying patient and comfort of the bereaved are major responsibility of doctor and as important as providing treatment. Determinants of psychological response to dying are associated with its cause (e.g. due to aging or disease), and with the individual and his environment. Fears of death are at times focussed less on the thought of death itself, and more on the process of dying. Sometimes, death is disturbing and may result in extreme physical distress. Some measures can be taken by the clinician in consultation with the family members, to make the dying person more comfortable by talking to them, listening to their wish and reducing their apprehensions and anxiety.

The effect of death on those who are still alive has also received systematic investigation in the recent years. A fairly consistent pattern of mourning has been identified. Typical or uncomplicated grief is usually following death of a parent, child, sibling, or first-degree relative, with whom there has been at least moderate degree of social contact within preceding year. Bereavement involves several stages, including the shock following the death within few hours to six months, till the individual has a full acceptance of death. Children also have problems in accepting death of their dear ones. As children do not openly express their fears regarding death, they often develop emotional problems, which are manifested in sudden drop in their academic performance, sleep disturbances, development of fears, depression and insecurity.

Attitude towards death, on part of medical staff and how the matter is conveyed is of utmost importance. On awareness of the normal sequence of events, in typical grief together with an understanding of the psychological processes involved, should be of assistance to those who are concerned with advising and helping the bereaved, and indeed it has become recognised that bereavement counselling requires more common sense, if it is to be effective.

PART 4: Social Behaviour

15. Attitudes

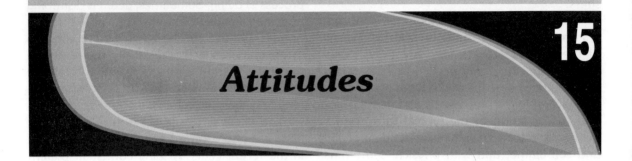

Dr Krishan Kant, is taking history of a patient, admitted in surgery ward. The patient has past history of abusing illicit drugs, he is not employed, and his appearance is not good. Presently the patient is having fever and has an infected wound on his right thigh. When this case history is presented, the consultant is surprised that in spite of being a good resident doctor, Dr Kant has neglected to elicit some common details, which were important to diagnose this patient. This incomplete case history was not due to lack of competence, but due to negative attitudes towards patients with substance abuse.

There is an increasing awareness of the importance of the role that attitudes and ability to communicate play, in the delivery of effective clinical services. It is extremely important for a doctor to be a congenial person who has the sincerity and tact to strike a good relationship with the health care team, his patients and their families. Attitudes related to patient care, taking responsibility and working in a team develop during the training of the medical students. Hence, it is necessary to assess attitudes of students from time-to-time.

Nature of Attitudes

An attitude is a tendency to behave in a preferential manner. It denotes certain constant traits in an individual's ways of feeling and thinking, and his predispositions towards action with regard to another person such as, a patient Attitudes are our expressions of likes and dislikes towards the people and objects. They determine and guide our behaviour in different social situations. One may have noticed that a doctor's behaviour is different while treating an elderly person as compared to an adolescent, or if treating a critically-ill patient. These differences in behaviour are because of his attitudes towards old people and adolescents. Our attitude towards a critical, terminally-ill patient determines how we interact with him or his family members. An attitude has three components:

- *Cognitive* what a person knows and his belief about the attitude object.
- *Affective* how he feels about the attitude object.
- *Conative* behavioural tendency towards the object, both verbal and nonverbal (Fig. 15.1).

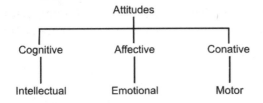

Fig. 15.1: Components of attitudes

Let us take an example to illustrate these three components of an attitude. Consider the views of an imaginary person named Dr Arvind Verma on the issues of drug addiction. Dr Verma has some beliefs about persons taking illegal drugs, the conditions under which they are taken and the problems these persons can create. All of these beliefs constitute cognitions about drug addiction. Dr Verma also has some feelings about drug addiction. Whenever he comes across such a person, he feels sorry and has sympathy for the family members of the addicted person. What does Dr Verma do to help these persons reflects his behavioural tendencies towards drug addicts. Thus attitudes are more than the mere knowledge of the subject matter. There is feeling associated with it and this determines the action that the person would take in that particular situation.

Attitudes are predisposed 'tendencies to respond in a particular way and not a fixed response. These are not innate. The whole personality structure of an individual and his behaviour are constituted by a complex of interlinked attitudes. Attitudes are influenced by a number of factors. Attitudes are preferences towards a wide variety of attitudinal items such as likes or dislikes, anti or pro, positive or negative. Anything that arouses evaluative feelings can be called an object of attitude, e.g. an attitude towards assessment of teachers. A distinction is commonly made between attitude and opinion. An opinion is a belief that one holds about some object in his environment. It differs from attitude, being relatively free of emotion. It lacks the affective component central to attitude.

Role of Attitudes in Nursing

In medical, students' attitudes vary according to patient's characteristics, quality of teaching and attitudes of teachers. A significant relationship has been reported between attitudes and the learning material. The choice towards a 'particular medical speciality' plays significant role in determining the ultimate career choice. Attitudes influence the behavioural responses of the individuals. The professional attitude of the doctor is not only concerned with his feelings, beliefs and behaviour towards the patients, but also towards other elements of professional functioning like health care delivery, scientific interest and collaboration with other professionals. Importance of the assessment of attitudes for doctors can be related to the following factors:

Patient care: Any negative attitude towards race, community or disease results in a prejudicial behaviour that affects the patients.

Formation of attitudes of peers or juniors: Senior doctors has a significant impact on the students for the formation of opinions concerning health-related issues.

Acceptance of new technology: In the present times, many new innovations in techniques, equipment and methods of health care delivery are taking place. Our attitudes can bias acceptance of new technology and high profile specialities.

Interpersonal skills: Studies have shown that during training of undergraduate students there is a gradual decline in their interpersonal skills. This affects skills of history taking and elicitation of information from the patient.

Curriculum planning: While planning a new curriculum or revising the existing curriculum in educational courses, one needs to identify the attitudes of the students and teachers.

Effects of attitudes on meaningful learning and retention: Attitudinal bias has a differential effect on the learning of controversial things. With a favourable attitude, one is highly motivated to learn, puts greater effort and concentrates better. Negative attitude leads to close-minded view to analyse new material and hence, learning is impaired. Attitude structure exerts an additional facilitating influence on retention that is independent of cognition and motivation.

Effect of attitudinal bias on training/learning: Attitudinal bias often causes loss of objectivity in a clinical setting. This is encountered in situations where either a relative patient is being examined or a patient revealing a history resembling the student's own life. Class or racial differences also impair a student's ability to relate effectively.

Marcotte and Held (1978) have suggested a set of responses that reveal attitudinal bias while examining the patients. These are:

1. *Premature closure and dogmatic response*—an early referral is made prior to taking a complete history, a simplistic solution may be provided in the initial contact.
2. *Evasion*—student misses the patient's history and directs the conversation under his control.
3. *Premature reassurance*—here the student negates the concerns of the patient and reassures the patient without having substantial evidence.
4. *Rejection*—student may avoid conflict areas and reject patient's concerns by neglect.
5. *Condescension*—Value-laden language is used so as to shame, embarrass or humiliate the patient.
6. *Too many technical jargons* are used by the student that confuses the patient.

Developments of Attitudes

Attitudes can develop through different modes. Heredity may play only a very small part through differences in the physical characteristics and intelligence. It is mainly the environmental factors that are responsible for development of attitudes. These are through family, peers, conditioning in sociocultural environment (Fig. 15.2).

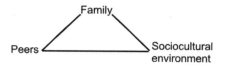

Fig. 15.2: Development of attitudes

Family

Family is the first place for formation of attitudes. Parents begin the information flow that forms beliefs and attitudes about things. Categories are formed in our head on the basis of early information.

Sullivan has observed that the information provided by the parents in the earliest stages of life is very difficult to undo. Erroneous and nonadaptive attitudes moulded from parental feedback have tremendous implications for further personality development.

As we grow, we tend to be influenced by other sources such as friends and group members. They serve as reference group in the development of attitudes. One identifies oneself with friends and moulds one's attitudes in relation to the prevailing norms of the group concerned.

Peers

Just as we learn from family in the early childhood, later our peer group has a tremendous influence on the development of attitudes. One may form very different or opposing attitudes in the company of friends, e.g. attitudes towards patients with AIDS or addictions, etc.

Conditioning in Sociocultural Environment

There are ample examples in our sociocultural environment, which are responsible for conditioning our attitudes. One such example is words, which have acquired effective meaning.

They can create positive or negative attitudes. Many attitudes developed on the basis of classical conditioning are found to be irrational, as they have been paired with an emotion producing unconditioned stimulus either accidentally or in a quite extraneous situation. Similarly the appropriate attitudes can be developed through classical conditioning.

An attitudinal response can be learnt through instrumental conditioning by reinforcing a response that occurred in the presence of a discriminated stimulus. Any responses, which have a reinforcing consequence, are learnt more readily than those without reinforcement. Inter-racial and intercaste attitudes are prevalent in our culture, so if your interaction with persons from other caste is satisfactory, you tend to develop positive attitudes towards persons of that caste.

How to Facilitate Development of Attitudes?

The problems of ensuring teaching as well as the development of attitudes may be ideally resolved by selection of medical students who will pay attention to humanistic concerns and by recruiting faculty members who can serve as role models for the younger students. However, a more realistic approach would be to build learning opportunities, and to ensure periodical assessment of the same. One needs to organise educational methods that cut across disciplines and provide the right setting for developing attitudes besides imparting knowledge.

Teachers motivate and facilitate the development of attitudes in students. Attitudes of senior students and peers also help in shaping those of future students. Though there are no guaranteed methods of teaching attitudes, yet teachers must be aware of all learning experiences that facilitate the development of worthwhile attitudes.

Providing Information

Information can bring changes in attitudes. For example, information about smoking as a cause for cancer and heart diseases is likely to bring about changes in attitudes towards smoking. It may not work in all cases, but it is generally found to be helpful. Information about attitudes may be imparted through lectures, or audiovisual aids, especially, video and films. The attitude of even health professionals towards AIDS patients can be changed dramatically, by effective utilisation of video films and other audiovisual media.

Providing Examples or Models

Most advertising is designed to change attitudes. A common technique is to show an ideal person using a certain product. The advertiser aims to provide a model or an example, which will be followed by the reader. Many students consider their teachers as a role model and often emulate their teacher's behaviour. If the teachers are rude to patients, then their students will tend to do likewise. It is therefore, essential to set good examples for the students.

Providing Experience

Medical training provides a number of experiences, which shape the attitudes of the students. They may see patients with sores that have not been treated and that have become septic and possibly disabling. This direct experience of seeing the patient's suffering will have far more impact on shaping students attitudes than a whole lot of theoretical information about the need for early treatment of sores and superficial wounds.

Discussions

Discussions in small groups are generally thought to be helpful in shaping student's attitudes.

Discussion also helps to make the previous three methods more effective. For example, it is helpful for students to describe and discuss the experiences that they have had with their patients. During the discussion, they can share their experiences with other members of the group. Discussions also help to change students' attitudes by the process in which a student gives his opinion and sees the reactions of other students. Discussions are more effective in small groups.

Role-play

Role-playing is an exercise in which the students play roles of suffering patients, doctors, paramedicals, etc. and begin to experience different kind of behavioural attributes. In a role-play, the participants exaggerate a situation or an incidence so that the audience can better appreciate the gravity of the situation. Not only the participants benefit from the role-play, but also the audience who can empathies with the characters of the role-play. The job of the teacher is just to play a theme for the role-play and brief the participants on the theme. A group discussion can be conducted at the end of the role-play to analyse the theme and to identify the 'take home message'.

Attitudes to be Developed by Undergraduate Medical Students

It has been felt that medical students need to develop more humanistic attitudes towards patients and their relatives. It is difficult to list all the attitudes that one would like students to have. Some of the essential and primary attitudes expected from the medical student are given below.
1. Eliciting psychosocial aspects of the illness.
2. Giving due respect to the patient's age; communicating patiently with older patients.
3. Examination of female patients in privacy.
4. Informing the relative about the patient's condition.
5. Breaking the news of death to the relatives.
6. To elicit history concerning very personal aspects of patient's life, like sexual history.
7. Informing the patient before giving an injection or doing a procedure.
8. Understanding individual differences and reactions to illness.

Methods to Change Attitudes

During the development stage if a student has developed certain negative attitudes, which later interfere with his professional competence, then it is desirable for the student to modify the negative attitudes. It is not an easy task to change attitudes, as they are consistent ways of reacting towards object. Attitudes can be changed under different conditions. It is necessary to modify unhealthy or irrational attitudes for learning new things.

Attitude change is influenced by both factors that are external as well as internal to the person. One should pay attention/consider the communicator, communication and the audience to bring about a change in attitude (Fig. 15.3).
a. Source or the communicator should be very effective and highly credible. He should be trustworthy and an expert to produce the change. Communicators, if they are similar to the target audience, their message is well taken, that means the communicator should is be someone from your profession, speciality and should be considered as a role model by you.
b. Content of communication has also been subjected to research. The findings are that communications, which discuss both the pros and cons to the point, are more effective in situations where there is initial resistance to accept. Communications associated with pleasant emotions can also enhance effectiveness.
c. Personality characteristics of the audience have been linked with attitude change. However, self-esteem and intelligence do not

play a very important role in changing attitudes. Increased discrepancy between the audience's attitudes from the target's position can help in change of attitudes. Committing the audience to take challenges or do something has proven to be an effective technique for attitude change. General susceptibility or suggestibility of an individual will also determine their tendency to accept/reject new information.

Similarly role playing, bringing change through smaller steps, distracting the audience are some other methods which have been used to change attitudes.

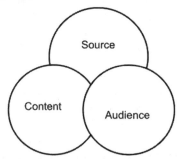

Fig. 15.3: Methods to change attitudes

ASSESSMENT OF ATTITUDES

In the studies conducted by the consortium (Verma et al 1993), it has been revealed that some departments discussed attitudes at times while imparting the news of illness to the patients and their families, but no one assessed them. Medical educators assess the acquisition of student's skills but not attitudes. Assessment of attitudes seems to be ignored because of the following reasons:
1. Attitudes are often vague and ill-defined entities.
2. The teachers frequently differ on what attitudes are really desirable.
3. Our instruments for measuring attitudes are not really good. Hence many teachers consider it inappropriate to use these instruments of poor reliability and validity for the purposes of grading certification.

Measuring an attitude is a difficult task, as it has to be measured in an indirect way. One cannot see the attitude directly; it must be measured from what the individual says or does. Even when one talks about the behavioural component of an attitude, the predisposition to act in a particular way is concerned with the preparation to act rather than with the act itself. Attitudes do refer to internal aspects of behaviour but there are also external manifestations of attitudes, as they are often expressed in actions. What a person does, and the manner in which he or she does it, most directly expresses a person's behavioural tendency. Actions may also express beliefs or feelings, though not so directly as they do the behavioural component. Occasionally, physiological indicators may be used, but even these are only indirect by-products of the internal arousal associated with an attitude.

The most common approach in attitude measurement is to find out how favourable or unfavourable is the individual to an idea. There are different methods of measuring attitudes. Some of these are very simple while others are complex. Broadly, attitudes can be measured by self-report methods, attitude scales and involuntary behaviour methods. Attitude scales are more often used because of their reliability. The commonly used scales are the Likert scale and the Osgood's semantic differential scale.

The various instruments in current use for assessment of attitudes are:

Rating Scales

A series of statements concerning attitudes being measured are made, and the answer is expected on a 3-7 point scale. The most commonly used scales are Likert scale which ask the rater to rate the attribute on a five point scale *viz.* strongly agree/agree/undecided/disagree/strongly disagree. Osgood's semantic differential scale is another commonly used scale.

Likert scale: In Likert scale, an attitudinal object is assessed on a five point scale ranging from extremely positive to extremely negative. It forms a continuum extending between two extremes of a scale. Each pole of the scale is represented by the attitude intended to be assessed. The scores are given from 5 to 1. Some of the examples of this type of scale are given below:

Behavioural science is of minimum relevance in UG medical curriculum   A B C D E

Knowledge of behavioural sciences helps in understanding psychosocial aspects of illness   A B C D E

Each patient needs an different way of communication to explain his problems.   A B C D E

(A: strongly agree, B: agree, C: cannot decide, D: disagree, E: strongly disagree).

Monchy et al (1988) had developed a scale to measure professional attitudes of students on doctor-patient relationship. Some of its items are as follows:

The emotions of the doctor should agree ideally never play a role in his dealings with patients.	Strongly agree	Agree	Neutral	Disagree	Strongly disagree
Only a small number of patients are able to understand complex health problems.	Strongly agree	Agree	Neutral	Disagree	Strongly disagree

Osgood scale: In Osgood's scale, two opposite adjectives are given with gradations. Following are some examples of this scale:

Behavioural Sciences course in medical curriculum is:
Useful -------------------------- Not useful.
Informative -------------------- Not informative.
Interesting ---------------------- Uninteresting.
Relevant ----------------------- Irrelevant.

Observational Rating Scales

In clinical settings, the students' attitudes can often be assessed through observational rating scales. This requires repeated and standardised direct observation of student's behaviour (activity) over a long period and in natural professional situations such as in the ward with older patients, outpatient clinic or in primary health centre. Attitudes are assessed on a standardised rating scale. If the rating is not done carefully it can lead to various errors in the measurement. One example of this type is as follows.

If a student is being observed when he is examining a patient, and an evaluation is needed of how he gains the patient's confidence, the following rating scale may be used:

The student has:
Taken all the necessary precautions, and the patient appears completely relaxed   5
Taken the necessary precautions and has reassured the patient several times   4
Made an effort, and has followed it up   3
Made an effort, without following it up   2
Seems to be quite unaware of the problem   1

Though assessment of attitudes is a difficult task it is worth taking the trouble, as it would ensure positive development of attitudes in medical students. This can be integrated with assessment of skills and knowledge.

Indirect Methods

One of the methods is based on the principle that people remember better the things that they consider to be important. A group of student might be shown a filmed interview with a patient followed by a series of multiple choice questions, some of them relating to biomedical aspects and others to the social aspects of the case. The answers to questions relating to social aspects would indicate the attitudes of the candidate.

Construction of an attitude scale: One often faces difficulties in deciding what aspect of an attitude is to be measured. We cannot measure

everything at one time, so we must choose precisely what we wish to measure or examine. Often attitude scale needs to be constructed for a particular aspect that one wishes to measure. Following are the steps in construction of an attitude scale:
1. Specify attitude variable that is to be measured.
2. Collect wide variety of statements.
3. Edit the statements.
4. Sort out the statements into (an imaginary) scale.
5. Calculate the scale value.

Writing of the statements is difficult yet most important aspect of constructing an attitude scale. Some of the guidelines for writing the statements are given in the box.

Reliability and validity: Since most of the time, attitude scales are constructed for the specific aspect of behaviour, one should do item validation of the statements and estimate reliability and content and construct validity of the scale using standard procedures, such as test retest method, split half method, etc.
1. The statements should be brief.
2. Each statement should convey one complete thought.
3. The statement should belong to the attitude variable that is to be measured.
4. Care should be taken on language:
   - use simple sentences
   - avoid double negatives
   - avoid "all, always, none or never"
   - use with care "only, just, merely"
   - avoid words with more than one meaning.
5. The statements should cover the entire range of the effective scale of interest.
6. Statements should be such that they can be endorsed or rejected (agreed/disagreed).
7. Acceptance and rejection should indicate something about the attitude measured.

SUMMARY

An attitude is a tendency to behave in a preferential manner. It denotes certain traits in an individual's ways of feeling and thinking, and his predispositions towards action with regard to another person such as a patient. Attitudes are our expressions of like and dislikes towards the people and objects. They determine and guide our behaviour in different social situations.

An attitude has three components, Cognitive—What a person knows and his belief about the attitude object, Affective—How he feels about the attitude object and Conative—Behavioural tendency towards the object, both verbal and nonverbal.

Attitude development in itself is a long process. The formation occurs on three different modes. The family, peers and the conditioning processes both operant and instrumental provide explanation for formation of rational and irrational attitudes. Balance theory tries to explain how attitudes change to create a balanced structure. However, if a imbalance exists, there is a tendency to move towards this balance.

Once we understand our attitudes we work in the direction of change especially modifying irrational and unhealthy attitudes. Attitude change is influenced by both internal and external factors. It involves a communicator, the quality of communication, the content of the message and the receiver's personality. For facilitation of development of new attitudes in such clinical settings we need to provide more information, a model, have more discussions, look into experiences of medical students and exact patient-doctor role plays. A list of essential and primary attitudes expected from medical students has been given at the end of the chapter. Thereby correct attitudes would bring in satisfaction of needs bringing in satisfaction of work.

Family

Ms S, 16 years old, weighing 25 kg, five feet tall, was diagnosed as having an eating disorder —anorexia nervosa. She presented with complaints of loss of weight, poor appetite, irritability, acting out aggressively, both at home and at school. On detail history taking, it was noted that her family consisted of her grandmother, parents and four siblings. Out of the four siblings, she was the eldest girl with the youngest child a brother. There was marital disharmony between her parents. The mother perceived her husband as extremely harsh and communicated more with the patient. Though the family was very well off, yet the mother often borrowed money from her parents to fulfill the needs of the children. Grandmother was punitive and abusive to children, and they often had verbal fights in the family. This caused anxiety in the patient. Her problems reflected instability, erratic, unpredictable environment in the house. The mother was afraid to face uncontrollable temper-tantrums of the patient and gave in easily to fulfill, even irrational demands by her. As a result, the homeostasis of family as a system was disturbed, with poor understanding of the needs of the family members.

This is an example of how family can predispose, precipitate and reinforce the illness. In this chapter, you will learn the importance of studying family, their relationships, communications and developments of psychopathology, and role of these factors in therapy.

Structure of Family

The family is a system of social relationships, which trains its young in different dealings in the society. A family cares, protects and educates its young, not only in the ways of its culture but also in ways that helps to establish identity, self-concept and functioning of its children. The family is the most powerful force for the promotion of health, as well as for the production of disturbance in members. Ackerman (1966) has described the disturbed family as one, in which the members sacrifice one of their own members in order that their needs are gratified. Assessment of presenting quality of family interaction are essential components in its understanding.

The family structure may be nuclear, extended or joint. As shown in Figure 16.1, the nuclear family consists of a married couple and their children; extended family has parents, their son and his wife and children. The joint family is a kin group, which may contain 3 or more generations within one household. It may have parents, all their children with their families, and in some households it may extend further, i.e. children of the third generation may also live in the same house. All the family members share a common kitchen. The joint family system was very prevalent in our culture, but now this system is breaking for extended and nuclear family system. The nuclear family is a product of modern culture and values. In other words, the nuclear family is more of a new generation concept and it views the child to be more independent and engage in self-actualisation.

In accordance with the present day demands, the nuclear family may experience disturbances due to the confusion and conflict arising from past and present changing values.

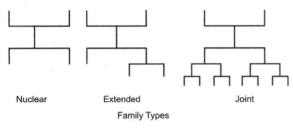

Fig. 16.1: Structure of family

Functions of family are normally centred around satisfaction of basic needs as food and shelter, the provision of love and security and the promotion of psychosocial development. The family also fulfills the sexual needs and reproduction. Just as the individual undergoes sequences of development throughout, so does the family pass through succession of developmental changes during its life cycle? At the start of the family life, the couple's main task is to establish their own relationship or the arrival of the children, one needs to adapt to the parental roles and also make children adapt with demands of the external roles; later on families promote the independence of adolescent children, with maturational tasks of career setting and adult sexual role; then as grandparents. In our Indian society, varying roles are taken up according to the needs of a particular family. For example, in some families where the young couple is working, grandparents may look after the household and bring up the grandchildren.

Every human group has devised prescriptions to ensure that the family accomplishes not only the biological and developmental missions essential for survival and growth, but also in most cultures, that it attends to enculturating tasks in the service of society. In this way, the family is the link between generations that ensures the continuity of the culture, but is also an element in cultural change.

Role of Family in Health and Illness

Individual's behaviour and its interaction with the environment provide important information for the understanding of health and disease. Health can be defined as that state in which an organism's internal components function harmoniously, and are interacting harmoniously with the environment. Knowledge of the patients, and of the human and inanimate factors in the environment that surround them—factors that shaped and continue to shape individual development is as essential to diagnosis and treatment, as is laboratory data of body fluids or electrical tracings. As William Osler stated, "It is more important to know what kind of patient has the disease than what kind of disease the patient has."

"What kind of patient", is determined critically by the earliest social environment involved in shaping that person; it will be adoptive parents, who take over at the earliest possible time. Usually however, one family provides the offsprings with the biological, psychosocial, and cultural heritages, that ensure the infant's survival and humanisation.

A family has major importance in the dissemination of disease. It is the base unit, which is involved in the transmission of genes and culture from one generation to the next. Like the transmission of genetic disorders, it also transmits major psychiatric disorders and minor psychological problems through the psychological environment. Each family is unique in terms of its environment, some being healthy which promote positive mental health and some being maladaptive, thereby promoting negative mental health. As you have read in other chapters of this book (learning, emotion, motivation, illness behaviour and pain), that family also plays a crucial role in teaching adaptation to physical illness. It also provides the immediate environment for the sharing of genes, diet, toxins, infections, stress, emotions and social attachments that may interact to affect expression of underlying physical and behavioural traits, and also to cause various mental disorders and to influence the outcome of these disorders.

This is specially true for children's behavioural disorders, which are related not only to genetic factors (inherited from parents and shared with other family members) but also to family environmental factors as the family forms the earliest, immediate and most persistent socio-psychological environment for the infant and small child and shapes its behaviour and attitudes. Even when child comes out of the family, its subsequent experiences are perceived, understood and emotionally reacted according to the foundations established within the family. The role of family in causation and outcome of various mental illnesses has been proved by various studies showing positive or negative association between specific behavioural disorders on one side and certain types of family psychopathology on the other side. We are more concerned with the psychological dysfunctions, so we shall limit our discussion on family dysfunctions rather than positive aspects of the family.

There have been various studies in which illness has been correlated with the family. Family can transmit illness through heredity, both in physical and psychiatric disorders, for example, diabetes, coronary disorders, blindness, and mood disorders. A family can also transmit illness through its psychological environment for example, inconsistency in disciplining, marital discords, broken homes, financial problems, chronic illness and so on. Perception and experience of pain (see in Chapter 25) is also influenced by the family members. Family environment is very important in the causation of childhood psychiatric disorders. Some of the studies conducted have shown that abdominal complaints in the immediate family members of the children with recurrent abdominal pain (RAP) was six times higher than the matched controls. Out of this, mothers accounted for 2/5th of the family members affected by RAP.

Psychological problems in family members have been reported by several authors. Friedman (1972) noted that children with RAP experience stressors such as psychological illness in one on both parents, parental discord, parental absence and unsatisfactory parent-child relationships. Hodges et al (1985) emphasised that both parents of a child with RAP demonstrated significant anxiety levels, with mothers out numbering fathers - 25 to 40 percent of the mothers had mild depression also.

Families represent more than mere collection of individuals. There are patterned regularities in transactions among individual family members, and between the family and the larger community, that may have important implications for their health and well-being. Family theorists have sometimes underestimated the large areas of autonomy in the lives of family members, and their ability to transcend the limits of the family's influence. Nonetheless, they have alerted us to the need to observe how involvement in a family regulates and constrains or facilitates the coping of the individuals.

It should be made clear, that no argument is made that only the family transactions cause the psychosomatic problems occurring in a given family member. Instead in some families, symptoms may foster the development of problematic family organisation.

Weakland (1977) has coined the term 'family somatic', to indicate the family's involvement in health and illness. He argues that it is important to describe concretely how both illness, and the maintenance of health pose problems for a given individual and other members of the family, and how they cope with it.

Affective Involvement

Optimally the family meets emotional needs of all members and provides cohesion, security and sense of being valued that contribute to the development of trust, self-esteem and independence.

The degree of affective involvement varies in the families, with some having more intense and involving family relationships. The quality of involvement determines, whether the relationship is nurturing and supportive or destructive and self-serving (Epstein and Bishop, 1981). In the uninvolved family, both the degree and the quality of involvement are low. Such families encourage premature emotional separation, often resulting in pseudoindependence that markedly impairs the capacity to tolerate true intimacy. Families whose intensity and quality of involvement are only slightly greater than those of unemotional family, may be described as showing interest which is devoid of feelings. Some families still show a still higher intensity of affective involvement, but withdraw their acceptance as soon as any member fails to satisfy the others' needs. Such parental narcissistic involvements are destructive in quality and usually excessive in degree.

Intense but destructive involvement occurs when two or more members are enmeshed (Minuchin, 1974). The concept of enmeshment is identical to those of symbiotic relationships (Solnit, 1978). It has pseudomutuality, undifferentiated family ego, and too richly cross-jointed system. Enmeshments are always reciprocal. They are destructive as they are incompatible with the development of autonomy and usually involve tolerance, and reinforcement by other family members. Those involved are overly sensitive and react with panic or rage to any attempt by the other partner at withdrawing.

Control Styles

Family members influence each other to ensure the accomplishment of the instrumental tasks and role requirements of daily life. Families vary in predictability and constructiveness, and each family has its own prototypical control styles. Generally control styles have been classified into four types: (i) rigid, (ii) flexible, (iii) laissez-faire and (iv) chaotic.

Rigid families are quite successful at maintenance control, but their rigidity interferes with successful adaptation and assumption of personal responsibility.

A flexible control style combines moderate predictability with high constructiveness. In a flexible style, task accomplishment is relatively easy to achieve because its supportive and educational tone encourages family members to participate and to identity with the rules of the family.

In laissez-faire style, members do as they please so long as to avoid bothering others and as little responsibility is assumed or expected. Because of their constant disorganisation, role integration is rarely achieved, task accomplishment is haphasard and communication is frequently insufficient, unclear and indirect.

A chaotic style is extremely low, both in predictability and constructiveness. Changes depend more on the mood of the dominant members in the family than situational demands. Instability and inconsistency typify these families and the overall effect is destructive.

Values and Norms

Every aspect of the family functioning, directly or indirectly reflects 'the family's values and norms'. The way in which roles are defined, the forms of communication considered acceptable, the predominant patterns of affective involvement and the control style are all shaped by values derived partly from the references of the parent's families of origin, to partly from the culture and subgroups to which a family belongs.

Family Temperament

As any clinician is aware, families vary dramatically in the character and flavour of their internal environments. Family temperament measures the underlying regulatory principle in families. Family temperament, is a product of three properties of family personality—family's energy level, preferred interaction distance, and characteristic behaviour change.

The family sets various guidelines and limits for it's functioning. The family's energy level establishes guidelines about behavioural activity, the family's preferred interactional distance establishes guidelines, regarding boundary permeability and their behaviour range establishes guidelines about the degree of variability, that the family manifests in its patterns of interactional behaviour.

Pathology and Communication in Families

Disturbances in the communication pattern are characteristic of the 'emotionally disturbed' families. Family psychopathology generally revolves around two concepts, which are central in understanding of psychopathology and used in therapy; these being the double-bind and the family homeostasis.

The double-bind form of communication has been labelled by Bateson et al (1968). The double-bind messages are peculiar to families, in which one of the members is schizophrenic. This type of communication may also be found in other families and may be induced in many common interpersonal situations.

The family as the social system is seen as maintaining a cooperative balance or homeostasis. In a disturbed family, the members interact with one another in ways that are exploitative or disturbing: "The emotional give and take" of family relationships is crucial in the development of mental health. The family determines the emotional fate of the child; it affects the emotional development of the adolescent and adult members as well (Ackerman, 1966).

The goal of communication amongst the family members is towards the achievement of a mutual understanding, which is possible only when the messages sent are clear, direct, and sufficient and the receivers are psychologically available.

In content, communication can be an affective (i.e. expression of feeling) instrument, which is either related to the ongoing tasks of everyday life or neutral (neither instrumental nor affective). At the same time, communication can be clear or masked (vague), disguised or ambiguous. The more masked is the message, the more likely it is to arouse confusion, anxiety and subsequent distortion in the receiver. The directedness and the indirectedness of the message depend on whether the message was received appropriately by the receiver, especially in indirect communication. The components of communication are presented in Table 16.1.

In disturbed families there may be paradoxical communication, which moves in two opposite and internally inconsistent directions at the same time.

Research on family interaction represents one aspect of the broader field of inquiry, referred to as Family Studies of psychopathology. The theoretical and methodological perspective, which we refer to as family interaction embodies two major commitments: (a) to identify family patterns and processes that are precursors, concomitants and consequences of disordered behaviour, (b) to the integration of this knowledge into the broader family studies literature, concerned with the independent and interdependent effects of genetic, sociocultural and personality factors on the development of perpetuation of psychopathology. These

Table 16.1: Components of communication

Essential Processes	
Exchanging information	mutual understanding
verbal	verbal
nonverbal	nonverbal
Critical aspects	
Sender	Receiver
clarity	availability
Directedness	openness
sufficiency	
Contents	
Instrumental	regarding the mechanics of day-to-day life.
Affective	regarding the emotional aspects of family life
	Consider: range and intensity of affect timing and duration of affect
Neutral	neither instrumental nor affective

interactions in greater depth with respect to the level of emotions is reviewed in the following section.

Systems Theory

Systems theory is a general theory to explain the interactions and relationships between the individual components comprising a larger structure. This theory provides a framework to understand the behaviour of the individual subsystems of the family such as the children or the parents, as well as their relationships to the outside world. This theory has gained popularity as it not only explains how families work and function, but also provides a method of analysing faults and flaws in the daily activities of family life. For instance, poor delineation of the boundaries between the parental and child subsystems can be responsible for problems of control and discipline with the children. The four other concepts in the general system theory that have influenced mainstream thinking about the family include:

Wholeness

It states that the system cannot be understood by dissection and study of its individual parts. We study the system as a whole. If one member in the system changes, then all the members of that system will change because of that one member's behaviour in terms of response to that change.

Equifinality

The concept of equifinality implies that there are many paths to the same destination. Applied to the family system, it means that the particular path a family takes as it evolves, its form is less significant than the final form itself. This is because there are more than a set of events leading to a certain end state and therefore, studying the events will not produce much useful information as studying the end state.

Feedback

Feedback refers to how individual units in the system communicate with each other. Feedback is circular rather than linear. In a systems theory, we understand the network in terms of a circular feedback loop, i.e. a change in A may produce a change in B and subsequently A again. Each person's behaviour becomes a reinforcing feedback for the behaviour of the other.

Homeostasis

Feedback either reflects change (positive feedback) or reinstates stability (negative feedback). The tendency of a system to seek stability and equilibrium is referred to as homeostasis. The homeostatic balance may be achieved by reducing deviations in process. This concept has been enormously helpful for family therapists in understanding a family's reluctance to change.

The system theory is different from traditional psychoanalytic theory, where the intrapsychic disturbances in the individual disrupt family functioning. The key differences in the two theories are highlighted below:

Past vs Present

Psychoanalytic therapists use their knowledge of the past to help the patient better understand what is going on in the present. Systemic therapists, view behaviour within the current interactions in the family.

Content vs Process

When family members come to therapy they focus on the content. Parents may say that their child does not come home on time. A couple may describe about their relationship being 'empty'. Although the therapist listens to what family members say about each other (concept), he is chiefly interested in how family members interact with each other (process). Different emphasis is given to the process of family therapy in various approaches.

Intrapsychic vs Interpersonal Context

The psychoanalyst focusses on the individuals past to encourage insight (intrapsychic), whereas systemic approaches focus on the current interactions (interpersonal) to alleviate symptomatic behaviour. Most of the systemic approaches deal with other significant contexts also. Transgenerational therapists include extended family members (grandparents) to change interactions in the nuclear family.

Model of Individual Psychopathology and Family Dysfunction

The fundamental tenet of a systems theory perspective is that traditional problems in and other psychiatric disorders as schizophrenia, depression, drug abuse and anxiety are best understood as manifestations of disturbances in the family (Haley, 1976; Minuchin, 1974; Stanton, 1981; Watzlawick, Weakland and Fish, 1974). The family member with "symptom" is little more than a messenger or family scapegoat; his/her symptoms serve to cover up the generalised family disturbance. In this sense, the symptoms of the identified "patient" are viewed as serving a function for the family as a whole, despite the overt distress that may occur as a consequence of these symptoms, e.g. a disruptive or delinquent child may consume an inordinate amount of attention from other family members, and thereby prevent parents from attending to the emptiness and lack of intimacy in their own marital relationship. As long as the child continues to engage in delinquent acts; the parents are protected from having to focus on their marriage. The functional value of the child's symptoms is usually beyond the awareness of all family members.

The notion that symptoms are functional reflects a view of families as complex interpersonal systems. The family system is relatively stable and organised according to implicit rules governing the behaviour of all family members in their inter-relationships with one another. The roles and the functions of family members behaviour are associated through a series of interconnected feedback loops that defy simple linear causal explanation. These behaviour patterns are repetitive and tend to occur in particular sequences. We can consider the following example:

Spouse A is driving and spouse B is in a hurry to get to their destination (also conveys this before starting). A accelerates and moves fast with a jerk, B holds on to the glass and criticises A, B protests more loudly, A shouts back and the child C starts to cry. At this point, the argument stops while B attends to C and A slows down.

This sequence exemplifies one form of a repetitive dysfunctional family process, where the child behaves in such a way that attention is withdrawn from the conflict between the spouses and refocussed onto the child. Thereby, when we discuss homeostasis in families the behaviour of the identified patient must be understood as being a part of that system. Despite the expressed concern with the patients' symptoms on the part of all family members, the family is inherently motivated to maintain homeostasis and will thereby resist any effort on the part of the therapist to modify the symptomatic behaviour of the identified patient. This makes the task of the family therapist exceedingly difficult.

Many of the prominent family theorists have identified triangles (e.g. mother, father, son) as the basic unit of family transactions. A third person is brought into diffuse to eliminate tension between the other two. According to Haley (1976), most behaviour problems in children are brought about by a cross-generational alliance between the child and over involved parent (usually the mother). The third party in the triangle is the absent parent (usually the father). It is a safe assumption that symptomatic behaviour on the part of the child is maintained by both parents, with the child serving as a buffer between the parents and saving them from a more direct relationship.

Family Therapy

If symptoms serve to stabilise the family and maintain homeostasis, it follows that the individual cannot be expected to change unless fundamental changes occur in the family system. This notion that family members will persist the therapists change attempts, has led to the development of this strategic therapy called family therapy. The model also implies that changes in individuals will effectively come about only when the structure of the family undergoes a change. Therefore, whether the therapist is treating one client or the entire family, the target of change is the family system.

Family Counselling

Family counselling is widely used in medical practice. You come across a family with Down's syndrome, and the family wants to have another child. You have to provide genetic counselling to this family. Similarly, role of family counselling in patients with AIDS, addictions, child psychiatric problems, development delays, patient undergoing painful procedures, all require family counselling. More details of counselling process are given in Chapter 19.

Clinical Application

The importance of understanding family in relation to medicine is best understood when you are working in community medicine and you make family visits. In all the hospitals, a concept of family medicine is emerging and has led to creation of separate departments of family medicine. The significance of the family in relation to health and illness lies in the fact that almost every patient or potential patient, is a member of a family and the interaction within the family is a two way process. The family may be considered from two points of view, one as possible causative or modifying agent in the patient's illness, and on the other hand as more immediate social environment within which the illness occurs—including the reaction of the other family members to it. Family provides social support, which has been considered very important in the recovery of the patient. In patients where there is no social support, the physicians have to work out in providing social support through nonvoluntary organisations. Family pathology, or sickness of the family itself may lead to codependence; this means that in chronic illness, the spouse may also develop similar symptoms. In some cases, chronic illness can lead to family breakdown, separation or divorce. This is especially true in patients having addictions or chronic mental illness. The separation or divorce between parents, due to the social changes prevalent in the present time is also giving rise to psychological problems in children. In patients with AIDS, the relevance of understanding family and providing counselling cannot be understated. The difficulties extended to the family members in looking after the sick patient also often calls for family counselling, to provide support and help to the entire family in the crisis situation.

Cultural factors may also be important in immigrant families, where conflict arises between the first and the second generations owing to the influence of different values. At times, social mobility causes conflict in children related to the values.

SUMMARY

The family is a social system, which cares, protects and educates its members to establish identity, self-concept and adapt to various stressful situations. The family is the most powerful force for the promotion of health as well as for the production of disturbance in members.

A family has major importance in the dissemination of disease. It transmits genes and culture from one generation to the next. Family is responsible in transmitting genetic disorders; it also transmits major psychiatric disorders and minor psychological problems through the psychological environment. Each family is unique in terms of its environment, some being healthy which promote positive mental health and some being maladaptive, thereby promoting negative mental health.

There are four types of controlling methods adopted by the families, these are—rigid, flexible, laissez-faire and choatic. The values and norms are also learned through family. Emotionally disturbed families have double-bind communication, in which no clear messages are given. Family psychopathology evolves around the concept of homeostasis, which reinforces illness in some member of the family to maintain its homeostasis. Systems theory has provided the framework to understand the relationships within the family and has also provided a model for family therapy.

Family counselling is the need of the present day medicine. Family members want to be informed about the illness and are being involved in the management, especially where child is the patient. To prevent certain diseases which have high genetic loading is a prime field for family counselling.

Understanding of family behaviour is of great relevance to medicine, as a result of this family medicine is emerging as a specialised field of medicine.

Compliance with Health Care

You are examining patients in endocrinology OPD. You come across an eighteen years old female, 5.1 feet tall, weighing 84 kg. All her investigations have been reported to be normal. The consultant seeing this patient advises diet restriction and vigorous activity. After one month's follow up, the patient reports no loss of weight. Why this girl has not lost any weight? Is her diagnosis wrong or she has not complied with the consultant's advice. Most likely her cause of not losing weight is noncompliance of the advice.

One of the significant problems in health care is patient's noncompliance or lack of adherence to medical treatment. Interest in adherence to health regimen has proliferated in recent years and has been directed to medication taking, where reports indicate that 33-80 per cent of patients do not follow or err in following their regimens (Garb et al, 1974). More recent reports suggest that other health regimens fare as poorly. Dropout rate in weight loss programmes reach as high as 70 per cent within two years and dietary compliance is about 50 per cent (Dunbar and Stunkard, 1997). Patients with postmyocardial infarction dropout of exercise programmes. The increasing professional interest in the area of compliance can probably be accounted for by an influence of several factors.

Thus, a substantial portion of individuals fail to receive maximum benefit from health regimens. The problem is further compounded, when one realises that good adherence is necessary and that knowledge of the degree of patient adherence is required to monitor treatment efficacy, safety and side effects. This is not only crucial to the evaluation of treatment for the individual patient, but also to the interpretation of clinical research involving self-administered regimen.

From a biomedical perspective, noncompliance in a patient means that they are ignorant, lazy or willfully neglectful. For example, you may have a patient with diabetes who does not comply with diet restriction. Similarly, in a number of other medical conditions, compliance is required not only related to drug in-take but also related to restrictions in diet, activities, smoking, drinking and change in lifestyle. The health care provider may not be aware of the antecedent environmental conditions for a patient's symptoms, his/her decision to seek treatment and also the failure to comply with treatment. At times, it may become difficult for the doctor to decide whether the treatment prescribed is not effective or the patient does not show improvement because of noncompliance.

The role a patient plays in his own therapy has subtly changed from a largely passive one to a largely active one. The life-threatening diseases have moved from those of infectious diseases to those of chronic diseases or diseases in which the person's lifestyle is implicated. This has resulted in the need for a long and continuous adherence to medical regimens and changes in patterns of living. Under these conditions, the person assumes more responsibility for the health outcome because of the very nature of the health problem and the long duration of the therapy. Patients need to continue the therapy, even if long periods of time intervene between their contacts with physicians.

Another reason that patients assume a more active role in therapy is because chronic diseases have a direct and potent effect on their health status. Recommendations for the maintenance of health extend beyond those of taking drugs, to those of changing habits such as modifying smoking or eating patterns. Since there are a large number of examples in which health outcome is not determined by the doctor's actions alone, but rather that of the doctor's and patient actions jointly, the health provider might at first feel less responsible for the outcome. There may, for example, be some professional resistance accepting this different kind of responsibility, which includes gaining the patient's cooperation. Doctors and their coworkers are assuming greater responsibility to protect health hence the interest in helping the patients to comply has increased. When one remembers that recommendations to nonhospitalised people constitute to be the bulk of the practice of medicine, one realises that concern about patient compliance is unavoidable. It is quite reasonable to believe that future doctors will assume that their responsibility encompasses minimising those factors such as patient's educational level and understanding those which influence compliance.

The problem of compliance focusses on the environmental conditions promoting adherence to a structured treatment programme. For example, in case of evaluating adherence to weight reduction programme for obese individuals, the questions to be addressed would include frequency, quantity and type of food eaten, stimuli preceding eating, nature of eating—fast or slow, the consequences of eating. The research is being focussed on changing behaviour of the patient for long-term adherence of treatment. Behavioural scientist have developed strategies to resolve long-term adherence by understanding patient's behaviour and using behavioural strategies to bring change in patient's lifestyle.

Most of the doctors feel confident that they can identify noncompliers; but in reality, it is a difficult task. Several studies have been conducted on the degree of accuracy with which health care providers can identify noncompliant patients—usually with respect to medication. Since the physician's subjective assessment of a person's compliance seems to be inadequate, one begins to consider other ways of measuring compliance as well as to look more closely at what is meant by the term compliance.

The compliance or recommendations for health ranges from advice about periodic health examinations, to making radical changes in daily habits such as abstinence from alcohol. With a little reflection, one would certainly expect compliance with some recommendations to be higher than with others, and this proved to be true in several studies. For example: (1) the greater the change in the person's long-standing personal habits, the less likely he is to comply; (2) the more complex the drug regimen, the less compliance is obtained; and (3) the longer the duration of therapy, the lesser is the compliance.

Types of Compliance

Compliance varies according to the type of health recommendation: (1) making a contact with a health provider, (2) adhering to a drug regimen, or (3) making lifestyle changes (Fig. 17.1).

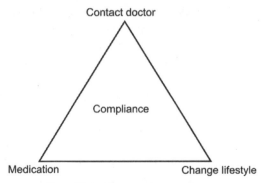

Fig. 17.1: Types of compliance

Contact with Health Provider

Perhaps the most pervasive type of behaviour involving compliance, is that in which the patient is asked to either initiates or continue contact with a health provider. This request involves the simplest form of compliance. It is a truism that nothing can be done if the patient does not present himself for help. Still the serious consequences of such a non compliance is often seen when a person does not seek help at all or waits until his disease has crossed beyond the point of intervention. There have been many attempts to find the reasons for such delay.

The factors found to be related to delay in or failure to seek health care are—fear, ignorance, level of education, cultural beliefs, financial status, and convenience of location. Almost half of all missed appointments are related to ineffective communication. Differences in the effectiveness of communication may account for some of the variation in rates of missed appointments that have been reported.

To sum up, there is a substantial amount of evidence that suggests that very simple efforts will increase compliance with all types of appointments.

Medication Compliance

The patient himself, his support system, his relationship with the clinician, and his experience with the clinic itself, all contribute to his ability and willingness to follow a medical regimen. But perhaps the single most important determinant of compliance is the regimen itself.

It has been found that on an average, there is about 50 per cent compliance with medication recommendations. Compliance to medication is related to the degree of complexity. There is a poor compliance if the medication regimen is complex and a large number of medicines are to be taken in a single day. It has also been observed that if the medication does not have any benefit, the patients on their own stop taking it.

Medication compliance is an issue in any health problem and has been found in such widely varying cases as—prescribed for pregnant women with anaemia, to antihypertensive medication for those with elevated blood pressure. There is some suggestion that older patients have more trouble than younger ones in complying. It has been suggested that it is possible to increase drug adherence by assisting patients with the establishment of the required routine. Education of hospitalised patients to take their medication when they are discharged should be used more extensively.

Lifestyle Changes

The most difficult compliance to achieve is related to changing personal habits such as eating patterns, exercise, or alcohol intake. Although these types of behaviours are known to relate to health status, patients have proved to be refractory when doctors have tried to change them. This type of health behaviour change seems to be particularly resistant to mere advice, which is left to be implemented by the patient on his own. Perhaps, part of the lack of success is that health providers themselves are somewhat hesitant to give advice about personal habits.

The physician might well be most effective in initiating health advice and reinforcing successful health habit change—that his efforts can be strengthened by working with other personnel who see patients more often. This seems to be the most effective method in helping patients with health recommendations, which involve making changes in lifestyle.

Factors Related to Compliance

Studies on the identification of factors that predict compliance behaviour have focussed on psychological characteristics of the person such as attitudes and perception of illness and health behaviour; environmental factors such as family instability, living alone, the therapeutic regimen itself and finally the doctor-patient interaction. Davidson (1982) reported that there was no relationship between therapeutic compliance and factors like education, socioeconomic status, family interaction, and distance to the clinic or hospital or the diagnosis. Research examining attitude and perception of the patient is related to health belief system, which the person learns from his sociocultural environment.

There are three general categories of factors that have been studied (Gillum and Barsky, 1974), which determine relation to the compliance behaviour of patients: the personnel characteristics of patients, the personal characteristics of providers and the structural characteristics of the health care setting.

Patient Characteristics

Considerable effort has been expended to assemble information about the types of individuals, who are noncompliant. Unfortunately, there are large numbers of studies, which taken as a whole, have reported contradictory information about the sociodemographic variables of sex, age, and economic status. The most ambitious attempt to synthesise knowledge in this area has been by Sackett and his colleagues. What emerges from this and similar attempts is that it is difficult to identify noncompliers on the basis of knowing their sociodemographic characteristics. One physician, who studied noncompliance in considerable detail concluded that each person should be considered a potential noncomplier. Noncompliance should be assumed, especially when no evidence of benefit from the recommendation is seen. This should not be interpreted as recommending an adversary relationship; quite the reverse is necessary.

Despite the lack of an easy method of identifying noncompliers, there are certain personal characteristics, including attitude, towards therapy and disease, which should alert the physician that the patient may be at a greater risk of noncompliance, for example, those who live alone. This is consistent with the finding that noncompliance increases, depending on whether the individual is an inpatient, day patient, or ambulatory patient. In other words, lesser the support the patient has or the more he is on his own, the greater is the likelihood of noncompliance.

Persons who understand the therapeutic benefit of the recommendation and who have immediate negative feedback if they fail to comply are more likely to have better compliance.

There are some persons, for example, who deny their illness and are therefore unable to comply with the health recommendations, since denial and compliance are incompatible. Usually, the denial stems from being unable to deal with a "weakness" or with the fear that accompanies being told of the illness. There are other patients who, because of a lack of trust, do not accept the validity and truth of the illness or the prescribed treatment. These are persons, who for a variety of reasons, are convinced they are not ill, and therefore there is no rationale for compliance with any treatment.

On the other hand, there are those who accept the fact that they are ill but are noncompliant because they are motivated to remain ill. They, for instance, get either attention or tolerance because of their illness or are given special dispensation from work or other demands.

Provider Characteristics

There have not been as many studies to identify personal characteristics of the provider related to compliance, as there have been to identify patient's characteristics. This may, however, be misleading, for the provider-patient encounter is an interaction in which both persons' characteristic contribute to the process, and to separate these characteristics is in some ways arbitrary.

There have been a few studies of the relation between the quality of the doctor-patient relationship and patient compliance. Several studies have shown acceptance and satisfaction with practitioners and paramedical assistants, which seems to be related to the ability of these providers to establish rapport and continuity of contact with the patient as with physicians.

There are other studies that show that improved compliance is related to a long-time relationship with the physician (Charney, 1967) and that private physicians are better able to obtain compliance than clinic physicians. It is not possible, of course, to study these characteristics without considering the patients' characteristics. Nevertheless, studies do suggest that a good patient-physician relationship, which is maintained over a fairly long time, increases the chances of compliance. It has been found that the physician's attitudes toward treatment and medication are important in determining the patient's compliance behaviour. The physician's degree of conviction in the treatment is also related to the patient's cooperation. If the prescribing physician believes in the efficacy of the treatment, he is much more apt to obtain patient compliance than is his counterpart, who is unconvinced about the benefits. Seemingly, this conviction is, intentionally or unintentionally, communicated to the patient. Several authors attribute all noncompliance problems to failure in communication between the provider and the patient. Those physicians or providers, who spend time establishing the patient's understanding of the reason for the required regimen, do get better compliance.

Assessment of Compliance

Compliance can be measured by number of methods, for example, interviews, pill count, clinician rating, biochemical indicators and self-report. Since each of these methods has their own limitations, thus a combination of two or more forms of assessment should be used. Biochemical procedures provide a direct measure, whether or not the treatment has been carried out, but provides no knowledge of the degree of compliance. The pill count offers information on the degree of compliance over time, but does not offer any information on the problems encountered or side effects. The self-report can be insufficient due to the memory lapses. Self-monitoring can provide a continuous record on compliance, as well as patterns and problems specific to regimen. It is not suggested to use physiological outcomes as measure of compliance, as there is individual variability in response to treatment that allows some patients to achieve a therapeutic goal with poor compliance rates.

Clinical Application

Recently some approaches and techniques have been developed to facilitate compliance. These include patient education, accommodation, modification of environmental and social factors, change in therapeutics regimen, and enhancement of doctor-patient interaction.

1. *Education*—Patient education can have a greater impact, if education about the illness

is provided in an active way, for example, making the patient read the information himself through handouts or self-help books.
2. *Accommodation*—The personality characteristics, which interfere with compliance, are understood and the treatment is planned out in terms of negotiations. This makes the person an active participant in the treatment. This type of treatment negotiations, have been found to be very useful, especially in de-addiction of drugs and substance abuse.
3. *Modification of environmental and social factors*—The family members and friends can be included in the treatment and they can be oriented to reinforce compliant behaviours. Any interpersonal problems at home interfering with the treatment can also be resolved with the family members.
4. *Change in therapeutic regimen*—The regimen can be made as simple as possible, and the patient should be involved in the planning. Compliance can be shaped by: first, giving simple components of the treatment regiment and reinforcing success, and gradually adding the other components of the regimen.
5. *Enhancement of doctor-patient relationship*—Good communication between the doctor and patient can resolve some of the problems of noncompliance. By understanding patient's expectation, his viewpoint and problems encountered in adhering to the treatment regimen, the doctor and the patient can work out schedule for treatment.

SUMMARY

One of the significant problems in health care is patient's noncompliance or lack of adherence to medical treatment. A substantial portion of individuals fails to receive maximum benefit from health regimens. The problem is further compounded, when one realises that good adherence is necessary and that knowledge of the degree of patient adherence is required to monitor treatment efficacy, safety and side effects.

From a biomedical perspective, noncompliance in a patient means that they are ignorant, lazy or willfully neglectful. For example, you may have a patient with diabetes who does not comply with diet restriction. Compliance is required not only for the intake of medication but also for compliance with restrictions in diet, activity or lifestyle.

The average person in our country has a larger number of contacts with the health care system than ever before. He has found that there are more and more ways in which such contacts can give him relief in times of illness or even prevent its occurrence. As knowledge has continued to be accumulated, curative medicine has become possible for an increasing number of diseases; knowledge about the pathogenesis of disease has resulted in the prevention or control of some diseases at an early stage.

Compliance is of three types: first, making a contact with health provider; second, adhering to the medication regimen; and third, making lifestyle changes. There are various factors related to compliance, these are primarily related to patient characteristic and characteristic of the provider.

In the present day medical context, when more of psychosocial factors are playing role in the aetiology of illness, compliance to treatment has become one of the important aspects of total health care system. Motivating the patients to comply specially in disorders, like substance abuse, AIDS, coronary heart diseases, diabetes has become important for the physicians. Behavioural therapy techniques are used to intervene with noncompliance patients.

PART 5: Assessment and Management

Assessment in Behavioural Sciences

18

Assessment methods used in behaviour sciences are very comprehensive and have a variety of instruments. Both qualitative and quantitative methods are used in the assessment. These methods are being employed not only in psychiatry but in all clinical disciplines, especially to understand the role of psychosocial factors, e.g. to rule out depression in patient with low back pain, or to rule out possibility of secondary gains in the same patient with low back pain.

Assessment refers to the procedures and processes employed in collecting information about or evidence of human behaviour Assessment, a broader term, refers to the entire process involved in collecting information about persons and using it to make important predictions and inferences.

Goals of Assessment

The goal of assessment is to identify and understand the individual's symptoms within the context of his or her overall level of functioning and environment. This includes determining the nature and severity of any maladaptive behaviour and understanding the conditions that may have caused and/or be maintaining it. To do this, the clinician must gather, weigh, and synthesise as much information as possible about the patient, usually within a brief period of time and often with limited information. The individual may manifest a perplexing array of psychological problems, and his or her medical and social history may be unknown. In addition, there may be seemingly unsolvable problems in the individual's life situation. Equally important to evaluate are the individual's strengths and resources, including such personal factors as motivation for treatment capacity for change, ability to participate in the treatment, programme, and available support from family and others. With all this information in hand, the clinician must then arrive at a working formulation concerning what can be done to promote the individual's well being. It is an awesome but necessary task.

The assessment provides a basis for making decisions concerning the best treatment programme, be it hospitalisation, the use of medication or psychotherapy, the modification of family patterns, or some other approach. The initial assessment also provides a baseline for comparison, later with other measures obtained during and following treatment. This is important but sometimes forgotten aspect of assessment. It makes it possible to check on the effectiveness of an ongoing treatment programme, to see if modifications may be needed; it also allows for comparison of the relative effectiveness among different therapeutic and preventive approaches. This is important not only in treating the individual, but also in conducting the research that can advance our understanding of the disorders themselves, as well as the development of new and more effective assessment and treatment techniques. All of which ultimately, will enhance the prognosis for individuals suffering from psychological disorders. Furthermore, the importance of assessment has increased dramatically as the demand for accountability in therapy has grown. Assessment is not necessarily a onetime venture, it is an ongoing process.

The foremost goal of assessment is to identify the problem. Is it a situational problem, produced by an environmental stressor, or is it a more pervasive and long-term disorder? How is the individual dealing with the problem?

For many clinical purposes, a formal diagnostic classification is much less important than having a basic understanding of the individual's history, intellectual functioning, personality characteristics, and environmental pressures and resources.

It is also important to understand the person and his problems in the social context in which the individual operates. What kinds of environmental demands are typically placed on the individual, and what supports or special stressors exist in the individual's life situation?

Assessment helps to understand why the person is behaving in maladaptive ways. The diverse and often conflicting bits of information about the individual's personality traits, behaviour patterns, environmental demands, must then be integrated into a consistent and meaningful picture. The formulation should allow the clinician to develop hypotheses about the patient's future behaviour as well, e.g. what is the likelihood of improvement or deterioration if the individual's problems are left untreated? Which behaviours should be the focus of change and what treatment methods are most likely to be successful? How much change might reasonably be expected from a particular type of treatment?

Sources of Assessment

Since a wide range of factors can play important roles in causing and maintaining maladaptive behaviour, assessment may involve the various assessment procedures like physical, psychological, and environmental assessment procedures.

Physical Evaluation

In some situations or with certain psychological problems, a medical examination is necessary to rule out physical abnormalities or to determine the extent to which physical problems are involved. The medical evaluation may include both general physical and special neurological examinations. A common example of this is recurrent abdominal pain, headache, or panic attacks.

Psychosocial Assessment

Psychosocial assessment attempts to provide a realistic picture of the individual in interaction with the environment. This picture includes relevant information concerning the individual's personality makeup and present level of functioning, as well as information about the stressors and resources in his or her life situation. For example, early in the process, clinicians may act like puzzle solvers, absorbing as much information about the client as possible—present feelings, attitudes, memories, demographic facts, and so on—and trying to fit the pieces together into a meaningful pattern. They typically formulate hypotheses and discard or confirm them as they proceed. Starting usually with a global technique, such as the clinical interview, clinicians may later select more specific assessment tasks or tests. The following are some of the psychosocial procedures that may be used.

Assessment Interviews

The assessment interview usually involves a face-to-face conversation conducted in such a way that the clinician obtains information about various aspects of the patient's situation, behaviour, and personality makeup. The interview may vary from a simple set of questions to a more formal format.

In order to minimise sources of error, an assessment interview is often carefully structured in terms of goals, content to be explored, and the type of relationship the interviewer attempts to establish with the subject. Here, the use of rating scales may help focus and score the interview data. For example, the subject may be rated on a three-point scale with respect to self-esteem, anxiety, and various other characteristics. Such a structured interview is particularly effective in giving an overall impression of the subject and his or her life situation and in revealing specific problems or crises—such as marital difficulties, drug dependence, or suicidal fantasies that may require immediate therapeutic intervention.

In recent years, several researchers have attempted to improve further the reliability of the clinical interview by eliminating the human factor and using computers instead to actually conduct the interview. Highly sophisticated computer programmes have been written to "tailor-make" a diagnostic interview for the patient. One of the examples is Computerised Diagnostic Interview for Children that can conduct a standard psychiatric interview. Several more specific clinical assessment tasks have been adopted for computer administration.

Self-Assessment

A type of assessment that is related to the interview is the self-report. This approach recognises that individuals are an excellent source of information about themselves. Assuming that the right questions are asked and that people are willing to disclose information about themselves, the results can be quite valuable. One of the most efficient instruments for obtaining specific information about an individual's problem area is the self-report schedule or problem checklist. Such checklists may include items that measure fears, problems, moods, and conditions that may be operating as reinforcers in the person's life. Thus they can provide useful information for structuring a behavioural treatment plan. Quality of life is also assessed on self-reports.

Clinical Observation

Direct observation of the individual's characteristic behaviour has always been an important method of psychosocial assessment. The main purpose of direct observation is to find out more about the person's psychological makeup and level of functioning; though such observations would ideally occur within the individual's natural environment, or they are typically confined to hospital settings. For example, a brief description is usually made of the patient's behaviour at the time of admission in the hospital and more detailed observations are made periodically in the ward. These descriptions include relevant information about the subject's personal hygiene, emotional behaviour, delusions or hallucinations, anxiety, sexual behaviour, aggressive or suicidal tendencies, and so on.

Psychological Tests

Interviews and behavioural observations are direct attempts to determine the individual's beliefs, attitudes, and problems. Psychological tests, on the other hand, are a more indirect means of assessing psychological characteristics. A psychological test is essentially an objective and standardised measure of a sample of behaviour. Psychological tests are like tests in any other science, as observations are made on a small but carefully chosen sample of an individual's behaviour. In this respect, the psychologist proceeds in much the same way as the biochemist that tests a patient's blood. The diagnostic or predictive value of psychological tests depends on the degree to which it serves as an indicator of a relatively broad and significant area of behaviour. The psychological test is a standardised measure that implies uniformity of procedure in administering and scoring the test. The testing conditions are also controlled for scientific observation. The tests are evaluated for their reliability and validity. Many times, a battery of psychological tests is administered to assess wide range of behaviours.

Objectives of Psychological Tests

Psychological testing is done primarily with four objectives.

Screening of certain traits or behaviour: Certain personality traits like psychopathy, extroversion, neuroticism, poor coping resourses, emotionally labile individuals, are more prone to acquire behavioural or emotional disorders. Psychological tests are used for screening individuals who are at high risk to develop these disorders. The screening is often required when a research is to be carried out or for early identification of 'at risk' population.

To assess psychopathology and to help in making diagnosis: Patients often have comorbid conditions such as schizophrenia, depression, anxiety, personality disorder or organic brain syndrome. The clinical presentation of these comorbid conditions often are not presented in the clear cut manner and thus cause problems in making the diagnosis. In these situations psychological test finding can help by providing evidence for psychopathology, thought disorder, signs of organicity or personality profile.

To elicit factors that are causative as well as maintaining maladaptive behaviours: There is a complex interaction of psychosocial and biological factors in the aetiology of many psychiatric disorders as in any other medical disorder. At present there is shift of focus on understanding and treating the underlying causes, and factors that could maintain the maladaptive behaviour like addiction. Often the underlying aetiological factors are psychosocial factors operating at an individual level or in the family dynamics, or in the job situation. These factors are often not reported by the patient, as they do not recognise an association between psychosocial problems and addiction. Moreover, the conflicts may not be operating at the conscious level. Psychological tests help in digging out this information from both conscious as well as subconscious level systematically. After determining and assessing the impact of these factors on the addictive behaviour of the patient, they can be the foundation for planning treatment. If the underlying factors are treated then the relapse rate can also be reduced considerably.

In planning of rehabilitation assessment of cognitive ability and aptitude: Planning of rehabilitation for patients with psychiatric illness or neurological disorders, handicaps, head injury patients, is as important as the treatment. If rehabilitation plans are not made and executed then chances of relapse or developing psychiatric problems are higher. At present in most of the medical centres more attention is being focussed in helping patients to rehabilitate. This requires an understanding of patient's level of cognitive functioning, i.e. attention, memory, intelligence, aptitude, interest and adaptability. The psychological testing can provide valuable information on all of these aspects, which can be used in planning the rehabilitation.

Types of Psychological Assessment

Psychological assessment generally is classified as neuropsychological tests, personality tests and tests for assessment of psychopathology. The tests are selected according to the aim of assessment, e.g. diagnosis, rehabilitation or research.

In a clinical setting these tests are given on an individual basis. Observation of behaviour during testing is as important as the test performance, as the nonverbal clues indicate useful information like motivation, persistence, concentration and manipulativeness.

Neuropsychological Assessment: Neuropsychological assessment comprises of cognitive functions, namely, attention, concentration, perception, memory and intelligence. Some of the examples of these tests are as follows:

Attention and concentration: All cognitive functions are dependent on attention span and ability to sustain attention. Clinically attention can be assessed through observation during history taking and in interview sessions. Formally it can be assessed by asking the patient to repeat digits forward and backward. Forward digits are started from 3 and continued till 8-9 digits. The test is stopped after two consecutive failures. Backward digits are given from 2 to 8. The digits should not be presented either very fast or very slow. The ideal rate of presentation should be one digit per second. These can also be assessed on the subtest of Wechsler's Adult Intelligence Scale namely Digit Span and Digit Symbol test.

The other methods used for formal and objective tests include letter cancellation, colour cancellation, counting 20 to 1 backwards and serial subtraction 40-3.

Perception: Bender Visual Motor Gestalt test (Fig. 18.1) is a simple and short method of

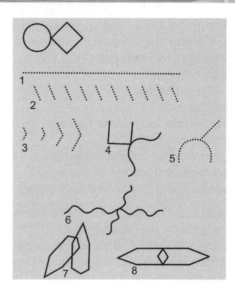

Fig. 18.1: Bender visual-motor Gestalt test

assessing organicity and visuomotor coordination, useful for both children and adults. This test consists of simple 9 designs printed against a white background on a separate card, which are to be copied by the patient on unlined paper. Objective scoring system is available. Evaluation of the protocol depends both in the form of the reproduced figures and on their relationship to each other. Probably the most frequent clinical use for the test with adults is as a screening device for detecting signs of organicity.

Memory assessment: Memory tests help to assess degree of impairment in memory functions. They also provide a baseline on which treatment programme can be planned specifically to enhance memory. An ideal test of memory should estimate deficits in all types of memory processes and should suggest anatomical localisation as well as the aetiological nature of the pathology. There are no biological tests that indicate memory deficits. The currently available neuropsychological tests are also far from meeting this ideal goal.

Most of the tests used at present may be grouped under the following categories:
1. Single tests of memory
   a. Verbal tests.
   b. Nonverbal tests.
2. Test batteries for memory.
3. Neuropsychological test batteries including tests for memory.
4. Questionnaires to assess memory.
5. Clinical examinations of memory.
6. Specific rating scales and inventories.

Digit span tests: The Wechsler's Adult Intelligence Scale includes a digit span subtest in which an increasing number of digits are presented for immediate verbal recall. The digits are recalled both in a forward and a reverse order. The rate of presentation for all digits is 1/sec.

In the Number Span technique, the patient is given increasingly longer number of sequences. However, each succeeding sequence differs from the one before it in its last number, e.g. 6-2, 6-2-4, 6-2-4-8, and so forth. It is reported that young adults could recall an average of 9.06 numbers, whereas older persons (> 65 years) could retain only 5.87 numbers.

Letter span tests: These tests are similar to the digit span tests except that letters are substituted for digits. The norms for letter span are 6.7 letters for people in their 20s and 6.5 letters for people in their 50s.

Memory for sentences: An average adult can correctly recall sentences of 24 or 25 syllables in length. The Stanford-Binet Scales include a sentence memory test at several age levels, beginning with 12 syllable sentences for 4-year-old, 16 to 19-syllable sentences for 11-year-old, and 20-syllable sentences for 13-year-old. The syntax and vocabulary become more complex at higher age levels.

Memory for paragraph and stories: It is generally not possible to memorise a paragraph or a story word by word. However, most people can recall the ideas presented in the paragraph using some of their own words and some from the actual presentations, omissions, additions, elaborations, and shifts in the story's sequence. Several methods of scoring have been suggested. Rapaport et al (1968) developed a system in which they scored all segments of the story as correct in which "the change does not alter the general meaning of the story or its details". They also included a four-point "distortion score" that reflects the extent of minor alterations as accurate "meaningful memories".

Several of the paragraphs and stories that have been standardised for testing immediate and delayed recall include stories in the Stanford-Binet Test, the Wechsler Memory Scale, the Babcock Story Recall Test, and the Cowboy story.

Test batteries for memory Wechsler memory scale is a rapid, simple and practical memory examination. This test is used all over the world. It consists of the following seven subtests.
1. *Personal and current information*—The subject is asked for age, date of birth, and identification of current and recent public officials.
2. *Orientation* is assessed by questions about the time and place.
3. *Mental control*—This subcategory is designed to test automatism such as repeating the alphabet and simple conceptual tracking as in counting by fours from 1 to 53.
4. *Logical memory*—This subtest includes immediate recall of verbal ideas from two paragraphs. The examiner first reads the two paragraphs but stops after each paragraph to get the subject's immediate recall. Paragraph A contains 24 memory units or ideas and paragraph B contains 33. The subject is given one point of credit for each correct idea recalled. The total score is the average recalled and extends upto 23.
5. *Digit span*—This subtest differs from the Digit Span Subtest of the Wechsler's Adult Intelligence Scale by omitting the three-digit trial of digit forward and the two-digit trial of digit backward and not giving score credits for performance of nine or eight backward.

6. *Visual reproduction*—Each of the three cards with a printed design is shown for 5 sec. following each exposure, the patient draws what he remembers of the design. This is an immediate recall test but some examiners also recommend a delayed trial.
7. *Associate learning test*—This subtest consists of ten words, of which six are called "easy" as they have common associations such as "baby-cries" and the other four pairs are uncommon or "hard" associations such as "cabbage-pen". The list of the word pairs is read three times. The subject tries to recall as many pair associates as he can remember after each reading. The total score is on half the sum of all correct associations to the easy pairs plus the sum of all correct associations to the hard pairs. The highest possible score is 21.

PGI memory scale: This scale has been standardised by Pershad for Indian population. It is used on both literate and illiterate adults and older persons. It has ten subtests, namely remote memory, recent memory, mental balance, attention and concentration, delayed recall, immediate recall, verbal retention for similar pairs, verbal retention for dissimilar pairs, visual retention, and recognition. Figure 18.2 is the stimulus card for recognition test. The testee has to identify these objects from the larger object table (Fig. 18.3). This test has objective scoring, and norms according to age and sex have been developed.

Memory questionnaires: For assessment of working memory simple questionnaires can also be used. The content of these questionnaires is related to historical facts, salient life events, and memory of specific situations on the basis of repeated experience with every day memory tasks. Generally immediate recent and remote memory is assessed. These terms also are referred to as short-term and long-term memory.

Clinical examination of memory: Most neuro-psychiatric examinations includes a mental status examination to determine the patient's neurological and psychiatric status. Memory assessment is an important part of a comprehensive mental status examination. However, in order to reach some conclusion about memory deficits, it is necessary to assess other mental functions such as the patient's level of awareness, verbal functions, attention and concentration, emotional status, and intellectual potential. A deficit in any one of these areas is likely to affect functions in other areas as well as memory. In fact, most mental functions overlap with each other and a separation of such functions is artificial.

Brief cognitive rating scale (BCRS) (Reisberg et al, 1983): Patients with Alzheimer's disease show a fairly uniform decline on BCRS, which utilises seven, rating categories for each of the five axis. Several other diagnostic categories such as mania and acute anxiety will cause some deficits on the concentration axis. The five axes include the following: concentration and calculating ability, recent memory, past memory, orientation, functioning and self-care. Items in each axis are scored from information obtained during a clinical interview with the patient in the presence of spouse or the caretaker.

Global deterioration scale (GDS) (Reisberg et al, 1982): The Global Deterioration Scale is a clinical scale that describes clinical characteristics of Alzheimer's disease in seven stages that correspond to seven clinical phases as follows:

GDS stages	Clinical phases
1. No cognitive decline	Normal
2. Very mild cognitive decline	Forgetfulness
3. Mild cognitive decline	Early confusion
4. Moderate cognitive decline	Late confusion
5. Moderately severe decline	Early dementia
6. Severe cognitive decline	Middle dementia
7. Very severe cognitive decline	Late dementia

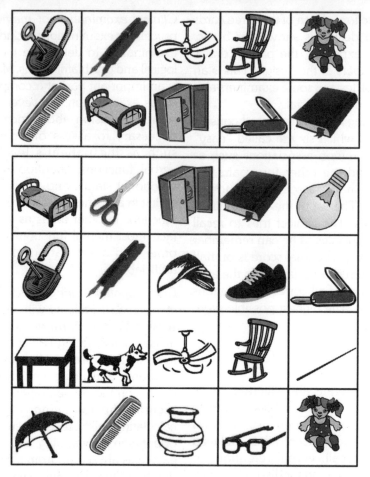

Figs 18.2 and 18.3: Recognition tests in PGI memory scale

Intelligence: Assessment of intelligence is the most common referral received by the psychologist. Intelligence tests are divided into verbal tests and performance tests.

1. *Wechsler's adult intelligence scale (WAIS)*— is the most widely used intelligence scale. It consists of verbal performance scales of which are further subdivided into subscales. The details of these subscales are as following:

Verbal	Performance
Information	Block design
Comprehension	Picture completion
Arithmetic	Picture arrangement
Similarities	Object assembly
Digit Span	Digit symbol
Vocabulary	

Indian Adaptation of both of these verbal (Pershad and Verma) and performance (Ramalingaswamy) scales are available. Figure 18.4 is an example of picture completion test, and Figure 18.5 is example of object assembly test.

2. *Bhatia's battery of performance test of intelligence*—The test was devised by Dr CM Bhatia in India. This test measures performance intelligence. The test consists of five subtests that are loaded with the general factor (G) and a specific factor (S). These are:
   a. Kohs block design test consisting of 10 designs. The time limit for the first 5 designs is 2 minutes and for the next 5, it is 3 minutes. The test is the measure of perceptual motor coordination, mental coordination and ability for analysis and synthesis.
   b. Alexander's Passalong test, which consists of 8 designs. The time limit for the first four designs is 2 minutes and for the next four is 3 minutes. It provides with the measure of spacial, perceptual and motor coordination.
   c. Pattern drawing test consists of 8 items starting from a simple square (Fig. 18.6). The subject should draw each pattern without lifting the pencil and without retracing. It measures motor coordination, perceptual motor ability, imagery and spacial component.
   d. Immediate memory subtest has 2 subparts, in part 1 the subject is to recall the digits as provided to him whereas in the second the subject is to recall them backwards.
   e. Picture construction test consists of 5 items. It measures the ability to apprehend relations, mental imagery and conceptualise part of the whole.

3. *Standard progressive matrices (SPM)*—this test was developed by Raven and has three forms. Besides standard progressive matrices (Fig. 18.7), the other two are Coloured progressive matrices and advance matrices. SPM has five sets of matrices, with 12 patterns in each set. The age range on which the test can be administered is ≥ 12 years. This test is considered a culturally fair test, as familiarity with any specific language is not required. This has an objective scoring and

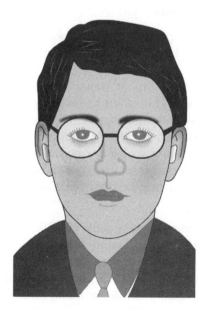

Fig. 18.4: Picture completion test item

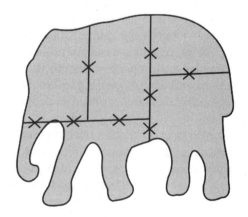

Fig. 18.5: Object assembly test

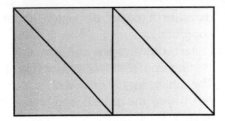

Fig. 18.6: Pattern drawing test

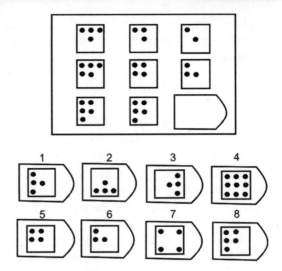

Fig. 18.7: Standard progressive matrices

intelligence is expressed in terms of percentile ranks. The task is to choose the missing insert from the given alternatives. The easier items require accuracy of discrimination, the more difficult items involve analogies, permutations and alternations of pattern and other logical relations.

Personality Tests

Clinical assessment of personality and psychopathology is a complex task, and it is one of the most critical aspects of working with emotionally disturbed individuals. Personality testing is done for many reasons. Its aim is to assess what the person is usually like in thoughts, feelings and behaviour patterns. Personality tests tap individual differences of reacting to certain situations.

The thoroughness and accuracy of assessment can determine the extent to which an individual's problems are understood and how well his or her needs are met through therapy. In recent years, objective assessment has grown more popular and important due to its varied applications and advantages, e.g. quantification in improvement, research, consumer protection, etc.

Personality test most often refers to measures of emotional states, personality type and traits, e.g. introversion-extroversion, interpersonal relations, interests, motivation and attitudes. Personality tests are in form of: (a) rating scales, (b) questionnaires, (c) semiprojective tests, and (d) projective tests. All these tests have their own advantages as well as disadvantages. Generally a test is selected according to the aim of the assessment. Some of the commonly used personality tests are as following:

Rating Scales

To measure psychopathology objectively rating scales can be used. Rating scales enable the observer to indicate not only the presence or absence of a trait or behaviour, but also its prominence. The rating scales are generally of two types—self-rating scales and observer rating scales. Beck's depression rating scale and Hamilton rating scales are commonly used to measure depression. Anxiety can be measured on state and trait anxiety scale and hamilton anxiety scale.

Brief psychiatric rating scale (BPRS): This is the most widely used rating scale for recording observations in clinical practice and in psychiatric research. The BPRS provides a structured and quantifiable format for rating clinical symptoms such as somatic concern, anxiety, emotional withdrawal, guilt feelings, hostility, suspiciousness, and unusual thought patterns. It contains 18 scales that are scored from ratings made by the clinician following an interview with the patient. The distinct patterns of behaviour reflected in the BPRS rating, enable clinicians to make a standardised comparison of their patients' symptoms with the behaviour of other psychiatric patients. The BPRS has been found to be an extremely useful instrument in clinical research, especially for the purpose of assigning patients to treatment groups on the basis of similarity in symptoms.

Questionnaires

1. *The Minnesota Multiphasic Personality Inventory (MMPI)*—is certainly among the most widely used psychodiagnostic instruments. The test consists of 550 unique items whose content ranges from psychiatric symptoms to political and social attitudes. As such, many researchers have felt that the MMPI can be a particularly useful diagnostic measure in instances where there is a denial of problems. The ten basic clinical scales of MMPI include—HS: Hypochondriasis, D: Depression, HY: Hysteria, Pd. Psychopathic deviate, Mf. Masculinity-femininity, pa: Paranoia, Pt. Psychasthenia, Sc: Schizophrenia, Ma: Hypomania, Si. Social Introversion scale.
2. *Eysenck's Personality Questionnaire*—Compared to MMPI, Eysenck's Personality Questionnaire measures only three dimensions of personality namely, introversion-extroversion, neuroticism, psychoticism and lie score. This questionnaire consists of 86 items and has been commonly used in research studies in India.

Semiprojective Test

Sentence Completion Test (SCT): Responses on this test are often most helpful in establishing level of confidence regarding predictions of overt behaviour. The SCT is designed to tap the patient's, conscious associations to areas like self-relationship with father, mother, opposite sex and superiors. It is composed of series of sentence stems, such as, "I like..." "Sometimes I wish....:" which patients are asked to complete in their own words. The SCT usually elicits information that the patient is quite willing to give, the level of inference is usually less than in the Rorschach Test or TAT interpretations.

Projective tests: These test are based on the projective hypnothesis derived from Freud's psychoanalytic theory. The basic idea is that the test taker responds to a relatively unstructured stimuli and much of meaning to the responses comes from within the person. Thereby, revealing the hidden aspects of the personality. It is a prolonged, intensive and extensive assessment of that individual's personality. It is from these responses that deductions are made about the personality dynamics including underlying conflicts and ego defenses.

a. The Rorschach inkblot technique was developed by Herman Rorschach (1921 / 1941). He produced a set of 10 inkblots. The blots, 5 are black and white (Fig. 18.8), 2 grey and red and 3 multicoloured and appear on separate cards. Subjects are presented with one card at a time and asked question as 'what might this be?' or 'what does this remind you of?' After writing down the first response the tester goes back through each response asking for more details. The first phase of the test is called the free-association phase, and the second is called the inquiry. Scoring combines objective and subjective procedures looking into the area of the stimulus, and other properties of the blot as form, content, etc.

b. *Thematic apperception test* Another projective approach was taken by Christina Morgan and Henry Murray (1938) in developing TAT. It is based on Murray's theory of needs, which come-up in the stories given by the patient.

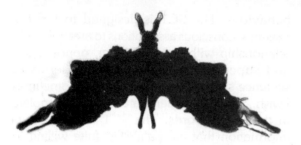

Fig. 18.8: Rorschach inkblot test

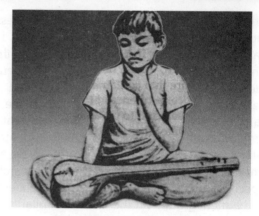

Fig. 18.9: TAT stimulus card

The Indian adaptation of this test is available. A set of 10 cards is selected (Fig. 18.9). To guide story production, tester instructs while giving a picture, that based on the picture a story has to be made by incorporating who all are in the picture, what had happened before, what is going to happen and what are the people involved thinking and feeling. Trained psychologists pick up themes coming out from each story and thereby make personality inferences.

Assessment of Alcoholism and Substance Abuse

CAGE questionnaire: The CAGE questionnaire has become one of the most widely used screening devices for alcoholism. It derives its name as an acronym, for the following four questions that are asked of patients:
1. Have you ever felt you ought to CUT DOWN on your drinking?
2. Have people ANNOYED you by criticising your drinking?
3. Have you ever felt bad or GUILTY about your drinking?
4. Have you ever had a drink first thing in the morning to steady your nerves or get rid of a hangover (EYE OPENER)?

Michigan Alcoholism Screening Test (MAST): The Michigan alcoholism screening test, or MAST (Selzer 1971), is a widely used 25-items, true/false questionnaire that contains questions about alcohol consumption and consequences of alcohol use. The test can be administered either as a self-report questionnaire or as a structured interview. The items are differentially weighted, resulting in a summary score that ranges from 0 to 50. Although different cut-off scores for identifying alcoholism have been recommended, these scores generally range between 5 (the original cut-off) and 7, with higher scores reflecting greater impairment and a higher likelihood of significant alcoholism.

Drug Abuse Screening Test (DAST): The drug abuse screening test, or DAST (Skinner 1982), is a 28-item, true/false self-administered questionnaire that contains questions about the extent and consequences of substance use. The items were selected to parallel items from the MAST. Unlike the standard scoring of the MAST, each DAST item is equally weighted so that summary scores ranges from 0 to 28. Skinner (1982) emphasised that the DAST score is best conceptualised as a quantitative index of substance abuse problems.

Alcohol Dependence Scale (ADS): The ADS (Skinner and Horn, 1984; Skinner and Allen, 1982) was designed to provide a brief measure of the extent to which alcohol use has progressed from psychological involvement to the point of impaired control over drinking. The scale is patterned after the concept of the alcohol dependence syndrome described in a World Health Organisation (WHO) Task Force Report, which portrays alcohol dependence as existing in degrees rather than as an all-or-none phenomenon.

The ADS consists of 25 multiple choice items, pertaining directly to alcohol use and its consequences; scores on the scale range between 0 and 47.

Assessment Motivation: Readiness to Change

Outcome of any intervention is primarily dependent on motivation of the patient and his willingness to change. Often it is difficult to obtain the correct information about the patient's, motivation on direct interview due to response bias and manipulative behaviour of the patient. Indirect assessment of motivation to seek treatment and to bring positive change in behaviour can be assessed through projective tests like Thematic Aperception test and Sentence Completion Tests.

The use of Psychological Tests in Personnel Screening

Many people who experience personal problems or extreme psychological distress are not able to function well enough in their job. In some organisations, where the job demands are high, the employers get the psychological screening done through experts handing psychological tests. The high stress producing jobs like army personnel, police officers and firefighters, air traffic controllers, and nuclear power plant workers, require a consistently higher level of psychological performance or greater emotional stability than others and allow for less personal variations in the performance of the job. Emotional problems in some employees can be extremely dangerous to the employees and to society as a whole. For example, an individual who holds a key position in a nuclear power plant control room and who is experiencing symptoms of severe depression can have his or her ability to function significantly impaired, possibly resulting in a failure to recognise critical problems. In India, various organisations have psychological screening as a regular feature. For example, members going to Antarctica for winter time for sixteen months are also psychologically examined.

Psychological Assessment of Children

Childhood disturbances are rarely as clear-cut as adult psychiatric disorders, and there are often too many explanations for child's problem behaviours in current family interactions, or in child's school experiences. Modern day psychological assessment is likely to contribute to build a plan of management. There may be a need for assessing the cognitive functioning and academic achievements. It may be important to study the personality characteristics and the way the child is perceived by others. Or it may be valuable to get a family account of present symptoms and the problem within. Keeping the above in view we may use one or a combination of tests depending on the problem as mentioned below.

Intellectual Assessment: In infant's developmental schedules are used to assess intelligence. Adaptive behaviour is considered very important in young children.

Vineland Social Maturity Scale: This test was developed to assess the individual's developmental level. It is most often used on mentally retarded children, extending within an age range from birth to 25 years. The test gives a pattern analysis on eight different areas, such as self-help in eating, dressing, socialisation, etc. This test is also useful in screening and in assessment for uncooperative children. This scale has been standardised for our population.

Wechsler Intelligence Scale for Children-R (WISC-R): This test is similar in its format to WIAS, and its Indian standardised version is known as Malin's intelligence scale for Indian school children. The subtests are classified into verbal and performance scales yielding verbal, performance and full scale IQs. There is another test for children in the age range of two and half years to six years, Wechsler Preschool and Primary Scale of Intelligence (WPPSI).

Coloured Progressive Matrices (CPM): This test is used for younger children within an age range of 5½ to 11½ years. It is a nonverbal test with percentile norms by half years and supplementary norms for mentally retarded children. It is a culture fair test with simple, easy to comprehend instructions. It consists of 36 items divided over 3 subtests reflecting on abstract and reasoning abilities.

Assessment of Specific Learning Disability (SLD): A battery of tests have been developed at NIMHANS, to assess children having specific learning disability. This consists of the following subtests:
1. Test of general abilities
2. Attention
3. Perceptual motor abilities
4. Visual discrimination
5. Auditory discrimination
6. Memory
7. Language skills
8. Arithmetic skills.

Personality Tests

Projective tests are commonly used with children to assess their needs, conflicts and general personality. Some of the commonly used tests are:

Children, apperception test (CAT): This test is designed for children in the age range of 3 to 10 years. The CAT cards have pictures of animals, more like in human situations relating to problems of feeding, sibling rivalry, parent-child relations, aggression, toilet-training and other childhood experiences (Fig. 18.10). The Indian version of CAT is also available. CAT supplementary cards depict different situations like classroom, interaction in the playground, and reactions to illness.

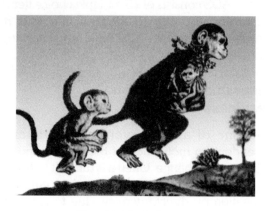

Fig. 18.10: CAT card

Ravens Controlled Projection Test (RCPT): This projective test can be administered in the age range of 6½ and 12½ years. The child is asked to draw whatever he wishes to and construct a story for which a set of questions are asked by the examiner. The child's concerns over lies, worries, dreams, friendships, etc. are elicited, which provides a better understanding of the child.

Draw-A-person Test: This test (Good enough) assesses both intelligence and the personality characteristics. The child is given two sheets of paper, and asked to draw a child followed by a figure of opposite sex to the one drawn. A set inquiry is carried out by putting up questions on ambition, family, friends, attitude toward sex and marriage, etc. bringing out hidden meanings followed by psychoanalytic interpretation.

House-Tree-Person Test: This test is used for children of 5 years age and older. The child is required to draw a house, a tree and a person in a sequence. The examiner takes notes on the spontaneous comments and the behaviour during the drawing, followed by a planned interview, eliciting details, clarification and material with symbolic significance. This is very simple but provides lots of information about the child and his interaction with his parents. Figure 18.11 illustrates a drawing by a child undergoing play therapy for emotional problems.

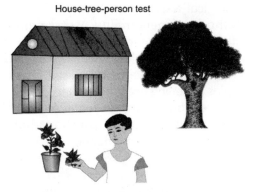

Fig. 18.11: Drawing by a child: house, tree and person

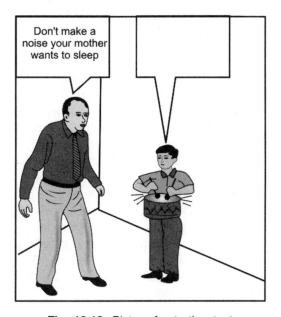

Fig. 18.12: Picture frustration test

Picture Frustration Test: This test elicits child's reactions to frustrating situations. The Indian test developed by Udai Pareek (Fig. 18.12), has 24 pictures and the child has to write his response to the situation in the box. Frustrations could be directed inwardly or to the external world.

Innovative Approaches to Assessment

Computer softwares are being developed to make scoring of psychological testing easy and less time consuming. Computers are used primarily in three ways :
i. to gather information
ii. to put together all of the information gathered
iii. to stimulate and predict the functioning of social systems.

Computers can also be used to compare a patient's adjustment in the community prior to and after treatment, and to show whether the outcome of treatment was better or worse than the expected level.

Ethical Aspects of Psychometric Testing: To use psychological tests, a professional has to follow some standards, which require that test administrators should be familiar with a test's research basis, use tests only in contexts in which they have been shown to be reliable and valid, and not go beyond their expertise or the test's empirically demonstrated applicability.

Problems in Assessment

Confidentiality

Psychological tests and other assessment procedures often elicit very personal information. Under some circumstances, professional mental health personnel are obliged to reveal this information to the legal authorities. So they may be abridged.

Issue of Cultural Bias

Most tests have been designed and have been standardised on middle or upper socioeconomic groups. Persons from other backgrounds might be handicapped in taking such tests and their scores would not be a fair measure of their potential. A great deal of effort has gone into attempts to develop tests of intelligence and other abilities that are "culture fair".

Criticism of Psychological Test Theory: An even more basic challenge has stemmed from the questioning of the assumption that maladjustive behaviour can best be understood by looking within the individual, at his traits and characteristics. The development of tests to assess these continuing inner characteristics was a logical extension of this concept. However, much of the behaviour observed does not fit anywhere in the established classification scheme, and the result is a further disenchantment with classification and labelling in general.

What can be done is to improve the existing procedures of psychological testing and erect safeguards to prevent the misuse of such assessment data.

SUMMARY

As assessment is the primary step in any treatment, thus there have been attempts to refine assessment instruments. The technologies that have been developed in the course of studies include structured interviews, observational rating scales, and self-report inventories. These methods have a place in daily clinical practice.

The large repertoire of instruments gives clinicians greater flexibility. They can select the particular method or instrument that suits their particular assessment needs. However, such a large quantity of tests can only leave the naive clinician feeling overwhelmed and uncertain about what should be used in any given clinical situation. An introduction to the general principles of how to use research instruments in clinical settings is necessary, along with some examples of how they may be used, and a historical review of the changes in psychiatry that have permitted this development.

Psychological tests are standardised measures of behaviour. The most common psychological tests are those, which assess intelligence or personality. Intelligence is commonly assessed on Wechsler Adult Intelligence scale.

Rating scales, questionnaires and protective tests, such as Rorschach Inkblot test, and TAT, can assess personality. There are different psychological tests for children.

Methods of personality assessment are essentially similar to those used previously like: Interview, Rating Scales, Questionnaires and Protective tests. Of late Standardised Interview Schedules are being used more often. There has been tremendous growth in rating scales especially for measurement of psychopathology. Similarly, as newer diagnostic classification systems are introduced, application of personality types is being applied to various medical conditions, and many new questionnaires are developed.

As in the case of interviews, the use of rating scales in clinical observation helps not only to organise information but also to encourage reliability and objectivity. That is, the formal structure of the scale is likely to keep unwarranted observer inferences to a minimum. The test findings provide valuable information about patient's current psychological functioning and his premorbid level of functioning. It provides the baseline on which intervention programmes can be evaluated and outcome can be objectively measured. The test finding can also help in deciding type of intervention useful to a given patient, e.g. patient having psychosocial problems, poor social skills, poor decision making, would benefit more from psychological intervention. Testing is time consuming thus a judicious and focussed assessment should be done for cost effectiveness.

Counselling

Counselling has wider applications in health care, and is not only restricted to the mental health problems. You are probably aware about career counselling, marriage counselling; and in health care, genetic counselling, family counselling and parent counselling are often practiced. The scope of counselling is becoming wider, as physical diseases with psychosocial aetiological factors, e.g. AIDS, substance abuse, are on increase. This chapter deals with the counselling process and skills that must be developed by any clinician.

Definition

Counselling is a process involving an interaction between a counsellor and a client, with the aim of helping the client change his behaviour. Counselling helps by explaining how the behaviour is learnt and how personality changes occur. Counselling can be explained as:
1. It influences change in voluntary behaviour of the client.
2. The purpose is to provide conditions, which facilitate a behaviour change of the clients.
3. As in all relationships, limits are imposed upon clients.
4. Conditions facilitating behaviour change are provided through interviews.
5. Listening is an important component.
6. Counsellor understands the client.
7. Counselling is conducted in privacy and discussion is confidential.

Activities Appearing Different but Similar to Counselling

To understand the characteristics of counselling, we should examine some of the controversies, relationships and helping activities that resemble counselling. There are also some activities that may appear different from counselling but have the same intentions. These range from friendly advice giving to more sharper differences between counselling and psychotherapy.

Advising and Influencing

Counselling has historically been associated with advice giving in every day life. Advice can be conveyed in strong terms as 'my advice to you is to get a job immediately', or 'I would advise you to consider my options before you act'. An advice can be acted upon or ignored. There are occasions when we all need instructions or advice. For example, we may ask about a travel route to somebody who is more familiar with that. But the final route X or Y is chosen by us. If one encounters a bad experience in that route we may blame the adviser. Daily life may be filled with more examples like asking for advice as what to wear, what to eat or buy.

Counselling is then not advice giving, but is telling clients what they should do, facilitating their efforts to arrive at their own decisions with personal and psychological issues. Generally our patients want the clinician to decide for them, or provide solutions to their problems.

Friendship

Friendship implies an acceptance, safety and loyalty. A real friend will come to your aid, if you need him. A real friend will not talk about you behind your back. He will understand you and your problems. But your counsellor is not your friend. Counsellors make clear boundaries between the counselling relationship and any other kind of relationship. Traditionally, counsellors and psychotherapists do not offer their services to close personal friends, but today the blurring of boundaries between friendship and counselling would lead to a compromise or damage both kinds of relationship. Some counsellors do not consider counselling distinct from relationships like friendship at all. We all help our friends by listening and responding helpfully to their problems. Though friendship cannot be disciplined the way counselling is, yet the importance of social support and listening by a friend cannot be undermined. In the developed western countries, patients with HIV and AIDS are assigned to a supportive friend on a long-term basis. Another example of this is Alcoholic Anonymous groups. There are fellow recovering alcoholics who offer committed support.

Friendship probably may help people more with their problems than formal counselling. But sometimes people do not want to be burden on their friends or they may feel their friends do not want to listen about their depression, one may have few or real geographically accessible friends or relatives. Some people may not be able to make good friends. Then the counsellors may functionally replace close friends teaching them how to seek secure friendships.

Teaching

Counselling is not teaching. It is rarely a didactic teaching, but counselling helps individuals to understand their values, and coping resources. Counsellors working with certain models often explicitly teach their clients new ways of looking at matters in the form of psychological concepts. Transactional Analysis, Cognitive Analytic Therapy, Rational Emotive Therapy, Cognitive Behavioural Therapy, all teach skills to modify maladaptive behaviour and effective functioning. Familiarity with the basic parent-adult-child model of transactional analysis, progressive relaxation techniques, social skills, assertiveness training are taught to the clients.

Distinctions Between Counselling and Psychotherapy (Table 19.1)

Psychotherapy and counselling are the two terms you often use while referring to psychological forms of treatment. These two are not the same, though both forms of therapy share many features in common. Psychotherapy is a psychological approach to treatment of emotional disorders as opposed to pharmacological or physical (ECT) approaches. This form of treatment involves an interaction between two people or more individuals.

Table 19.1: Difference between counselling and psychotherapy

Counselling	Psychotherapy
1. Education, career, health related	1. Supportive, reconstructive
2. Situational	2. Depth rooted
3. Problem-solving	3. Analytical
4. Focusses on present	4. Focusses on past
5. Deals with normal age—appropriate developmental tasks	5. Deals with severe emotional problem
6. Short-term	6. Long-term
7. Emphasis on preventive mental health	7. Emphasis on present mental health problems

The distinction between these two forms of therapy is not always clear-cut. Instead of viewing them as distinct forms of therapy, these should be viewed on a continuum with regard to various elements like goals, clients, setting, practitioner and method. In therapy, it is customary to designate the person, receiving help as "patient" and in counselling as "client" although this distinction is only superficial. In this chapter, patient refers to the person having physical illness, and client refers to persons having a problem rather than an illness. In comparing the goals of counselling to the goals of therapy, it seems apparent that a frequent goal of counselling is to help individual deal with the developmental tasks appropriate to their age. Counselling is more concerned with preventive mental health and therapy with remediation. Counsellor's deal with individuals who are not necessarily ill, but who have encountered problems, which may well be temporarily generating unhappiness.

Goals of Counselling

There are five major goals of counselling, namely:
1. Facilitating behaviour change
2. Enhancing coping skills
3. Promoting decision making
4. Improving relationships
5. Facilitating client potential.

These goals are not mutually exclusive, nor are they equally appropriate for every client. A more appropriate classification of counselling goals has been given by Byrne (1963). These are:
a. *Ultimate:* Goals which appear to be ideals and we could achieve the desired outcome from counselling.
b. *Intermediate:* These relate to reasons for seeking counselling and usually require several sessions to achieve this. The first four counselling goals mentioned above are intermediate goals i.e. they are outcomes, which can reasonably be achieved.
c. *Immediate:* These goals are moment by moment intentions of counseling, e.g. encourage a client to verbalize an unexpressed feeling.

Skills of Counselling

Most people probably agree that the kinds of skills, which form the basis of practical counselling training are not entirely distinguishable from the kinds of interpersonal and communication skills used in everyday settings. While imparting training in counselling skills, it is necessary that the clinicians should also be trained in communication skills (see Chapter 23) and should be motivated, as counselling requires time and patience. The counselling skills are:
1. Listening
2. Attending
3. Perceiving
4. Responding
5. Initiating
6. Summarising.

Passive Listening

Possibly the most basic of all skills is listening within the counselling interview. Patients need opportunities to explore their feelings, attitudes, values and behaviours; initially they need someone to listen, even passively, to what they wish to share. New counsellors are typically uncomfortable with time lapses during the interview, but if the counsellor can become sensitive to the various meanings of silence and skillful at handling these pauses, these silences can prove very useful. First, silence lets patients know that the responsibility for the interview lies on their shoulders. Too often counsellors rush into fill up the space, thus assuming inappropriate responsibility for the session. Second, silence allows patients to delve further into thoughts and feelings and to ponder the implications of what has transpired during the session, patients need this time to reflect and process without feeling pressured to verbalise every thought and feeling.

Listening is the process of tuning in carefully to the client's messages and responding accurately to the meaning behind the message. This type of listening is crucial in moving social conversation to different levels of communication, and it is the core of effective counselling. Listening at its simplest level calls on the counsellor to reframe the content and feelings that the patient has expressed.

Listening is a synthesis of the skills of restatement of content and reflection of feeling. It promotes within the patient, the feeling of being understood. It must be emphasised, that listening, though has an important role in the counselling process, is not sufficient to produce the desired growth and change in the patient.

Attending

Attending refers to the physical behaviours you use while listening to the patient. Posture, eye contact, facial expression, tone of voice, and gestures, all communicate without the use of words. Attending makes it easier to listen and remember, it enhances self-respect of the patient, it also helps to build good doctor-patient relationship. On the other hand, poor attending behaviour distracts from the relationship.

Perceiving

Perceiving as a skill differs from listening and attending, as in this listening and attending involve collecting all the cues the patient provides: words, meaning, tones, expressions and gestures. Perceiving is bringing all the cues to personal awareness in an attempt to comprehend the patient's compliance.

It is important to develop skills to be able to put meaning to the cues provided and the ability to listen to self. The therapist should try to be aware of the feelings and thoughts going through the patient's mind at the time of consultation.

Responding

Responding is essentially the culmination of listening, attending, and perceiving. Responding means communicating to the patient all that he has said that has been heard. To achieve this, the therapist has to restate the content. The ability to restate the content of the client's message or to paraphrase a client's statement is beginning in the process of learning to listen. Restatement of contents serves three purposes: a) to convey to the patient that you are with him, that you are trying to understand what he is saying, b) to crystallise a patient's comments by repeating what he has said in a more concise manner, and c) to check the interviewer's own perception to make sure he really does understand what the patient is describing.

Reflection of feeling is another skill required for responding. This differs from restatement of content in terms of emphasis. In reflecting on a patient's feeling, the counsellor listens carefully to the patient's statement and responds by paraphrasing the content of the message, but he places the emphasis on the feeling, the patient expressed. By responding to the patient's feelings, the counsellor is telling the patient that he is trying to perceive and understand the patient accurately from the patient's internal frame of reference. The counsellor tries to identify the feeling accurately by listening not only to what the patient says, but also to how the patient says it.

Initiating

Initiating skills refer to those skills the counsellor uses to summarise and clarify the patients' problems and his deficits. With these skills you would be able to elicit more information, solve problems related to diagnosis and management.

Summarising

Summarising enables the counsellor to condense and crystallise the essence of the patient's

statements. The summary of content differs from paraphrasing, in that the summary typically responds to a greater amount of material. A paraphrase normally responds to the client's preceding statement. Ivey (1971) has noted that a summarisation of content is most frequently used in the following situations:
1. When the interviewer wishes to structure the beginning of a session by recalling the high points of previous interview.
2. When the interviewee's presentation of a topic has been either very confusing or just lengthy.
3. When an interviewee has seemingly expressed everything of importance to him on a particular topic.
4. When plans for the next steps to be taken require mutual assessment and agreement on what has been learned so far.
5. When at the end of a session, the interviewer wishes to emphasise what has been learned within it, perhaps in order to give an assignment for the interval until the next session.

The therapist should also try to identify and respond to the overriding feelings of the client, not only the expressed feelings but also the general feeling tone of the phase of the interview being summarised. Summarising a client's feelings forces the counsellor to synthesise the emotional aspects of the client's experience, as such it requires the counsellor to respond in a deep and a perceptive way to the emotional content of the client's experience (Ivey, 1971).

Characteristics of the Counsellor

Counselling is a process of establishing a cooperative relationship and then using it to help the patient. This implies that the counsellor should develop certain characteristics, which can enhance or help to build a cooperative relationship. These characteristics are ability to communicate effectively, develop empathy, respect and positive regard for the patient.

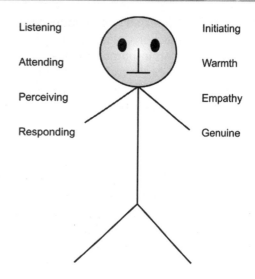

Fig. 19.1: Characteristics of the counsellor

Figure 19.1 illustrates the characteristics and skills of the counsellor.

Communication

Counselling may focus on refining and deepening ordinary communication skills (see Chapter 23). There are difficulties involved in distinguishing counselling skills from general communication and interpersonal skills. Some approaches to counselling particularly person-centred place enormous emphasis on the therapeutic power of certain interpersonal attitudes and skills facilitating the personal growth of the individual. Communication skills used in different professions are different from counselling, as it does not result in enhancement of growth, e.g. a salesman may spend time with customer developing rapport, have empathy with customers concerns, but with an ultimate aim of winning the customer over making a sale than enhancing his autonomy. The counsellor should also develop skills to understand patients communication, which may be disturbed, and manifest not only in terms of spoken or written word but in all interplay of hidden gestures, feelings, bodily reactions, glances, etc. which are constantly going on in human beings. Thereby, an awareness of both verbal and nonverbal factors is essential in order to arrive at a complete understanding of each patient.

Warmth

Warmth is the caring for and accepting of an individual. Warmth is communicated through nonverbal behaviour, such as smile, tone of voice, etc. Warmth does not denote approval or disapproval of the patient, but a caring attitude.

Empathy

Empathy means accurately understanding the individual within that person's frame of reference. This means that you transpose yourself in imagination into your patient's thinking, and feeling, so that you structure the world similar to that of your patient. For example, you have a malnourished child and you are counselling the parents on his food intake, quality, as well as quantity of food that you think that the child should have, may not be feasible for the parents due to poverty, rural set up, etc. If in this case you were able to imagine their context of living, then probably your nature and content of counselling would be entirely different, yet relevant to the patient. This also helps to improve compliance to treatment.

Empathy is feeling with others, not feeling for other. It is communicating an understanding at the deepest level. If we are not able to understand the patient from his internal frame of reference, we will be unable to help that individual.

Respect

Respect is closely related to warmth and caring. Respect can be related to unconditional positive regard, or the patient also has potential, he is worthy of changing himself. Respect should be expressed especially when dealing with elderly patients, women, and colleagues.

Genuineness

Genuineness is the ability to be real and not artificial, to be oneself in a relationship. A major part of genuineness is self-awareness, about yourself and how much help can be provided. It is better to be honest in the relationship with the patient.

Client Expectations

It is important to note whether or not a particular counselling experience will be worthwhile to the client, which will depend on the client's expectations. The counsellor must be aware of her/his expectations and should encourage clients to talk about their expectations. Many clients expect to have something done to/for them as part of the counselling process. Counsellors must communicate to the clients that ultimately it is the client who acts, decides, changes and becomes what he or she should be. In addition, clients often seek counselling in crisis situations, hoping to find remediation. In these situations, counsellors must learn to respond to the immediate needs and working with the client toward some intermediate/ultimate goals through the counselling process.

Influence of counsellors values on the client: Our goals are influenced by our values and which in turn may affect the therapeutic goals.

Therapists should be aware of their values and those of the society (class-caste) and culture in which they live, and must avoid pressing them upon the patient. The values are communicated through direct suggestions, interpretations or building the nature of relationship between the two. The mannerisms of the counsellor indicate the favourable or unfavourable attitude towards patients verbal productions through operant conditioning, e.g. trace of a smile, a pleased look, nod of head, etc. The counsellor must try to be neutral, recognising his morals and values, at the same time express them if he/she feels that the relationship would improve.

Process of Counselling

The goals of counselling can be introduced in the initial session and if acceptable to the client, the counsellor can work toward bringing an end to counselling as soon as clear direction is established. The duration of counselling determines, how long the relationship lasts. This is an important area as it is related to the success of counselling. The processes involved in counselling to bring the minimum change in the person include:

Change of Utilisation

Counselling attempts to bring about the best possible utilisation of what the person already has. We in each case help a person to discover his/her anxieties and conflicts, and gradually move forward. In counselling, the person can be made aware of the directional shifts that are possible for him.

Emphasis on Strength

By and large, our diagnostic thinking rests on the concepts taken from psychopathology. We point out a person's weak spots. Instead, one must place emphasis on 'positive diagnosis'. A person who knows about his/her real strengths and values will be better able to cope with anxieties about certain aspects in life. We can enlist those by asking the patient, through observations from family and friends, etc. This will make the individual aware of assets allowing one to by-pass difficulties.

Counselling Structure

One must try to structure the situation for the client and must take into account his/her expectations and goals, as well as ones own. A counsellor's job is to help the person find out what his/her personality is like, and decide how he can use the assets he has and get rid of obstacles that are blocking his progress. Anything a person wishes to bring up can be considered and analysed.

Necessary Support

Support the patient to look into new possibilities. Support does not mean pep talks, shallow reassurance or encouragement of dependence, but lending one's strength to the patient during which he can be certain about his moves. Once the client has established new direction for himself, one can schedule interview hours a month apart to maintain his/her confidence.

The Closing Phase

Once a clear-direction is established in the client's life, improvement in emotional ties with one's family and a greater willingness to assume responsibility, is an indication of development and time to think about termination, whether it takes two hours or 200, if he succeeds the effort will have been very much worthwhile.

Counselling in Health Care

Counselling is a leading inherent technique in explaining the prevention and management of any illness. Social and psychological factors need to be recognised besides physical problems. Due to increasing health awareness today, educated patients are not satisfied with simple prescription, they wish to discuss about factors that can promote health and prevent further advancement of the disease. One encourages positive behaviours related to change in lifestyle, e.g. eating a balanced diet or exercising regularly. Health education programmes can be given through counselling to provide information related to health, to change attitudes and health

relating behaviours, which are conducive to the same. Counselling is an important adjunct to medical intervention. The role of the counselling in medical settings is twofold.
1. Counselling patients and their relations
2. Work with health professional.

When the individual becomes ill, the concerns, preoccupations and worries have been shown to change dramatically, focussing around the illness and the effect it may have on the daily activities, their work and their family. The most common reaction to an illness is distress and anxiety. Recognising patient's distress is important, as the presence of psychological distress has been found to have a negative effect on recovery from illness. Distress at all stages of illness can be reduced by providing information about the illness and treatment. It is the period of uncertainty, not knowing, which is most difficult to bear. With counselling skills physician can handle the sensitive aspects of the information to be provided, e.g. explanation of treatment of cancer, its side effects and prognosis.

Counselling is increasingly being used to describe a less directive way of helping people especially in dealing with HIV patients. Counselling has been accepted as the control component in the management of AIDS. In developing countries like ours, treatment of AIDS is very expensive; moreover, the prognosis being very poor, prevention is very important. This can be achieved by counselling patients, their relatives, especially the spouses, and high-risk population. The primary prevention of AIDS may involve:
a. Educating people about AIDS
b. Strategies to reduce risk
c. Injecting drug use
d. Promoting safer sex.

The initial sessions one can set goals and gradually provide support directing the individual to recognise and look into his/her behaviour. Counselling process should involve client's expectations, values and motivate patients to aim for improvement in the direction of resolution.

SUMMARY

Counselling is viewed as a relationship, as well as a process. It is designed to help people make choices and resolve problems. It influences change in voluntary behaviour of the client. The purpose is to provide conditions, which facilitate a behaviour change of the clients. As in all relationships, limits are imposed upon clients. Conditions facilitating behaviour change are provided through interviews. Listening is an important component. Counselling is conducted in privacy and discussion is confidential.

Counselling is different from advising, friendship, teaching or psychotherapy. The distinction between these two forms of therapy is not always clear-cut. Instead of viewing them as distinct forms of therapy, these should be viewed on a continuum, with regard to various elements like goals, clients, setting, practitioner and method.

There are five major goals of counselling, namely: facilitating behaviour change, enhancing coping skills, promoting decision making, improving relationships, and facilitating client potential.

The counselling skills include passive listening, accurate understanding, ability to understand the view point of another person, as if from their own perspective, an ability to articulate what one has heard and understood, to summarise the concerns expressed in the conversation and an ability to engage emotionally with others.

Counselling is an important adjunct to medical intervention. The role of the counselling in medical settings is twofold: (i) Counselling patients and their relations, and (ii) work with health professional. Counselling is being used in the prevention of AIDS. The primary prevention of AIDS may involve: (i) educating people about AIDS, (ii) strategies to reduce risk, (iii) injecting drug use and (iv) promoting safer sex.

Behaviour Therapy

All behavioural approaches to therapy have as a common aim the direct modification of observable behaviours, which have been identified as in need of change. These approaches share a common premise, namely, that most behaviour is learned according to basic principles of learning. Behaviour serves as a function in their current context and is maintained by the events, which precede and follow them. These may or may not be the same factors, which gave rise to them in the first place. Behaviour therapy therefore, addresses to those factors that are seen to be maintaining problems rather than those which may have originally caused them to appear. It does not postulate underlying causes, as psychodynamic therapies do, but regards the observed behaviour itself as 'the problem'.

This view of behaviour therapy regards behaviour as functional or goal oriented. The relevant goals are the observable or reportable consequences of the behaviour, which maintain it. Behaviour, which includes thoughts, is therefore, a sample of the difficulties faced by the patient and not merely a symptom of the underlying pathology. These characteristics of behaviour therapy are described as:
  i. Behaviour therapies attempt to modify the problematic behaviours themselves.
  ii. Like the social behaviour theories that guide them, behaviour therapies emphasise the individual's current behaviours rather than the historical origins of his problems.
  iii. Most behaviour therapists assume that deviant behaviour can be understood and changed using the same learning principles that govern normal behaviour.

Though behaviour therapy has been applied since ages for disciplining children's behaviour, rewarding and providing feedback for good academic work, etc. The application of learning principles to the problems occurring within the context of a clinical disorder has been in practice since late fifties in some developed countries. In India, this form of therapy is being practiced since early seventies, and at present this form of therapy is the most popular amongst all psychological therapies.

Foundation of Behaviour Therapy

The historical roots of behaviour therapy are based in the two fundamental learning theories of classical and operant conditioning, (see Chapter 5). The social learning theory of Bandura (1969), which significantly contributed to the recognition of the role of cognitions on overt patterns of behaviour, was followed by the introduction of various therapeutic techniques which affected a change in observable behaviour by focussing on the mental processes or hidden behaviours referred to by Bandura. The role of the mediational processes and the subsequent development of covert treatment strategies are viewed by many practitioners as a complementary extension of traditional behavioural concepts.

In recent years, adopting a behavioural perspective to management of psychiatric problems has grown in popularity. There is the focus on the here-and-now, observable behaviour and the avoidance of dynamic formulations. This form of therapy is objective, structured and can be practiced by nurses, parents, spouse and teachers as cotherapists.

The limitations of the classical and operant models, in terms of their reliance on external, observable phenomena, focussed attention on the role of internal behaviours, thinking, reasoning and imagining, for example, and the way in which such covert processes influence the performance of behaviour. The resultant mediational theories of learning propose that environmental stimuli do not in themselves initiate overt behavioural responses; rather, the nature of the response is additionally influenced by cognitive or information processing elements.

An important feature of Bandura's social learning theory is the suggestion that learning can take place indirectly and not just through direct experience, as proposed by earlier theorists (Bandura, 1969). Indirect or vicarious learning can occur through the observations and experiences of others. The mimicry ability of children is well known and often a cause of adult embarrassment and amusement. Young girls learn how to apply make-up by observing and then imitating their mother, boys through the same process, can replicate their father's shaving ritual. Moreover, as every parent knows, children do not just learn crude approximations, or the mere mechanics of behaviour. Their imitations will include subtle changes in facial expression or body posture; similarly desirable behaviour patterns or maladaptive responses can also be acquired. A child who observes his mother's anxiety response to certain situations is likely to demonstrate equivalent behaviour when faced with analogous situations. Vicarious learning, however, involves more than simply watching. Bandura describes four cognitive processes, while acknowledging that there may be others, which mediate between the external event and the behavioural response, namely, attention, retention, reproduction and motivation. The child for example, must be able to focus his attention on his father's behaviour; he must then retain what he sees, so that he can reproduce the action. Finally, but just as importantly, the child must be motivated to perform the behaviour.

The prominence given by Bandura to the internal or hidden processes generated prolific developments in clinical techniques explicitly directed at these covert behaviours. Mahoney (1974), for example, examined the relationship between perception and behaviour. He suggested that the interpretation of an event might not represent the reality of the situation. A train passenger who thinks an alteration in engine vibration means that the train is about to crash has not authentically interpreted what is happening. The concomitant effective and physiological responses are a consequence of his unrealistic perception of events. A few years later, Meichenbaum (1977) demonstrated how psychotic patients could learn to control disruptive cognitions. Advances in the therapeutic manipulation of these mental processes not only enhanced contemporary knowledge of human behaviour, but also expanded the clinician's skills repertoire. The contemporary practice of behaviour therapy recognises the contribution to individual problems of living of distorted or unhelpful cognitive functioning. Cognitive treatment approaches are increasingly combined with the more traditional behavioural methods of intervention to help people improve their quality of life.

Characteristics of Behaviour Therapy

Genuineness, warmth, empathy and the therapeutic relationship that are important for the counsellors, (see Chapter 19) are also important to behaviour therapists and full recognition is given to their significance as determinant variables of treatment efficacy. The therapeutic approach is based on a model, which views human behaviour largely as a function of the individual's interaction with his environment. Furthermore, it suggests that maladaptive behaviours, are primarily acquired through the process of learning, in the same way as adaptive behaviours are learned. It is the behaviour itself, which is the focus of attention rather than any underlying psychopathology, with the emphasis on the here and now of the problem, which detracts from the individual's quality of life. The characteristics of behaviour therapy can be summarised as follows:

1. Behaviour therapy is an empirical, scientific, client-centred approach to an individual's problems.
2. There is a rigorous systematic assessment process, which precisely defines in operational terms the patient's problem and identifies environmental factors, which influence the problem behaviour.
3. Explicit treatment goals are agreed upon and defined prior to treatment intervention. The degree to which these targets are met allows for accuracy in progress evaluation and treatment outcome.
4. The treatment techniques of behaviour therapy are effective because they are derived from clinical and experimental research. Behaviouralists place great emphasis on scientific validation of their practices and on the individual appropriateness of the treatment methods selected.
5. During the assessment periods, observations are made of the problems behaviour, which provide baseline measurements. These measurements are repeated at regular intervals during the treatment phase and again on completion of the intervention programme. This progress is rigorously monitored from start to end. They are indicators for continuance or modification of the treatment package.
6. The collaborative nature of this style of therapy and the active participation of the patient is strongly emphasised from the very beginning.
7. Change, to have any real value to the individual, must be socially significant. Therapy cannot be said to be therapeutically effective if, on a practical everyday level, the patient experiences no real improvement in his quality of life.
8. It is a fairly common practice of behavioural interventions, to involve the use of cotherapists who will assist in the delivery of the treatment programme. Cotherapists may be parents, nursing staff, spouses, friends or colleagues, who with the agreement of the client, make a structured contribution to the resolution of the problem.

Process of Behaviour Therapy

Behaviour therapy aims to facilitating behaviour change, to achieve this aim the first step is to identify the specific nature of his problem, to identify possible factors that precipitate and maintain the problem behaviour, to assess the baseline functioning of the patient, degree of distress caused by the problem, patients motivation to change his maladaptive behaviour and readiness of key family member to' act as a cotherapist. Behavioural assessment is summarised in the Table 20.1.

Table 20.1: Behavioural assessment

1. Defines problem	Functional analysis
2. Helps	Selection of treatment, e.g. relaxation therapy exposure
3. Assesses	Change in behaviour through self report
	Parent's observation
	Cognitive functioning
	Psychosocial factors
	Baseline and ongoing assessment, e.g. frequency, intensity of panic attacks

Observations made in clinical settings by trained observers can provide useful behaviour data. The programme includes evaluating the behaviour of chronic patients and monitoring the activities of staff members working with them.

In other situations, where observation in the natural setting is not possible, the clinician may construct an artificial observational situation that can provide information about the individual's response to a particular situation. For example, an individual who has a phobia for snakes might be placed in a situation where snake-like objects and pictures are presented.

An often-used procedure that enables the clinician to observe the patient's behaviour directly is role playing. The patient is instructed to play a part, for example, someone asking for his rights. Role-playing in a situation like this not only can provide assessment information for the clinical assessment but also can serve as a vehicle for new learning for the patient.

A type of self-observation which serves as a therapeutic strategy as well as an assessment procedure is self-monitoring. With this technique, patients are asked to observe and record their own problem behaviour. In case of child patient, parents can record the particular behaviour. For example, they might be asked to record the number of times during the week patient had severe anxiety attack.

Treatment Methods in Behavioural Therapy

To modify or change maladaptive behaviours, various treatment methods are used. Some methods help to decrease the maladaptive behaviour, e.g. anxiety, while others tend to increase adaptive behaviours, e.g. assertiveness, some methods build new adaptive responses, e.g. shaping language in mentally subnormal children, others eliminate maladaptive responses, e.g. temper tantrums. Some of the commonly used treatment methods are discussed in this section.

Relaxation Training

Relaxation training is the most effective method of controlling anxiety. Though there are some different methods used in relaxation training like yoga, meditation, autogenic training, but Jacobson's progressive muscle relaxation procedure is used more commonly. The muscle relaxation training involves progressively tensing and then relaxing major muscle groups in the body. This procedure requires about 20 minutes to practice. Initial few sessions are given under the therapist's instructions, later the patient learns on his own and practices at home. At times, audiocassettes are provided to the patient for home practice. The patient continues practicing the relaxation procedure until he or she can relax all the muscles in the body through the recall of the relaxed state. The goal then is to teach the patient to discriminate between tension and the relaxed stage. Relaxation exercises are commonly done in the supine state without pillow. It can also be done while sitting on the chair.

The variations to this form of relaxation are 'savasana' (yoga), brief relaxation, and cue relaxation. Cue relaxation is also used as an adjunct to the standard procedure; it involves imagination of a neutral scene, or listening to some soft musical tune that is relaxing for a particular patient, after the patient has finished relaxation exercises. Later this cue acts as a conditioned response to decrease anxiety.

Biofeedback Training

Biofeedback training typical involves providing information about physiological functions that are normally not in the patient's awareness. The physiological functions used in biofeedback are: GSR, EMG, respiratory, and temperature. A specified target response, such as cervical muscle tension is electronically monitored and information about changes in the functioning of the targeted response is relayed to the patient via various feedback devices, such as a meter reading or an auditory signal or visual signal in form of light. The goal is to use the feedback to teach the patient to relax.

Hypnosis

Hypnosis is also used to decrease anxiety. The actual hypnotic procedure typically varies, depending on therapist or patient, but the goals are generally similar. Goals can include altering the patient's negative perception of the problem, e.g. pain, shifting it to a neutral or a positive one, enhancing positive self-statements, and improving health-related attitudes. Hypnosis is also used in patients with somotoform disorders.

Exposure

Exposure is the main technique used for treatment of phobias. The patient is exposed to anxiety provoking stimuli to decrease his anxiety. It is also used in conditions where anxiety is related to specific situations e.g. anxiety on seeing patients of leprosy. In theory, phobias can be overcome by facing the things that are feared. The therapist should explain the model, using the patient's individual symptoms to illustrate how vicious circles maintain symptoms. For example, an agoraphobic patient described having felt hot and fainted in a bus one day (a physiological symptom), and then taking an alternative mode of transport, walking or hiring taxi to go to work the next day for fear of going on the bus again (an avoidance reaction that maintains the anxiety). Gradually she began to dread journeys (anticipatory anxiety, another reaction), and persuaded her husband or friends to take her to work (behaviour of others maintained her avoidance). With explanation of what has happened, it becomes clear that if the avoidance is reversed, gradually, in manageable steps, then the fear will subside. The patient should be encouraged to think actively about what to do.

The self-help rationale of treatment is that the vicious circle cannot be broken without the active participation of the patient. The therapist should explain that treatment involves learning how to work on the problem effectively and independently. Treatment sessions should therefore, be backed up by regular homework, and improvement will be the result of a collaborative effort. It is necessary to keep a record of practice, and to use this both to monitor progress, and to identify stumbling blocks. The function of practice is the same as when learning a physical skill.

Graded exposure: In practice, it is not always easy to stick precisely to the guidelines for exposure described above, and treatment demands much creativity from both patient and therapist. Various other procedures can be combined with exposure, such as relaxation exercises, distraction, role playing, rehearsal, and modelling.

Devising practice tasks: It is frequently difficult to draw up a graduated list of tasks. A number of useful strategies are available when this happens. If the phobia is circumscribed, as in animal phobias or fears of specific illness, any means of communication can be used as a basis for practice. The patient may thus be able to extend the range of tasks by reading, writing, or talking about the phobic object; by watching relevant television programmes or films, or by listening to radio programmes, and so on.

The greater the variety of available practice tasks the better, even though practice is hard work, and may be boring. Greater variety increases motivation, confidence, and the probability that improvement in one aspect of the phobia will generalise to other aspects (e.g. from waiting in the queue at the bus stand, to waiting in the hospital for the physician, and waiting for someone who is late returning home). Strategies can also be used to break tasks down into smaller steps when the next item on the hierarchy is too difficult. Encouraging patients to search for opportunities to approach instead of avoid, helps them to overcome disruptive types of avoidance. These include feeling reluctant to do something, postponing activities, not thinking about the phobia, and giving excuses or rationalisations.

Real life exposure: A major goal of treatment is to give patients the confidence to face the things they have been avoiding. This is why strong emphasis is placed on homework, and on the realistic setting of practice. Nevertheless, it can be useful to accompany a patient during exposure to begin with. This may reduce anxiety and/or make it easier to move faster up the hierarchy. It may also be a way of demonstrating particular skills, for instance in managing anxiety or social interactions.

Imaginal exposure: In some cases, for example thunder phobia or fear of travelling in trains, it is not easy to arrange real-life exposure, and imaginal exposure has to be used instead. Imaginal exposure should be graduated in the same way as real-life exposure, and the two should be combined whenever possible. So the travelling phobic may have to prepare for a journey in imagination, but will also benefit from reading or talking about train journey, from visits to railway station, and, of course, from regular travel by train. The patient starts by imagining the item vividly enough to induce anxiety, and goes on thinking about it in as much detail as possible until anxiety subsides. Items should be repeated until they provoke little anxiety, before moving on to the next item on the list. There is much variation in the ability to use imagery, so some patients may need a little prompting before they can get a clear image, and others need the therapist to describe the scene to them. For this reason, much of the exposure takes place during part of the treatment, and if the patient notes down the imaginal scenes used, and is shown how to keep a record of anxiety and how it changes during imaginal exposure, it should be possible to continue the exercise at home for half an hour each day.

Audio exposure: It is also used in the treatment of obsessive compulsive disorders, with these patients audio exposure has been found to be successful. In audio exposure the patient is required to write a script about the worst scenario that he fears. Each scenario is like a story and runs for 1-2 minutes. Several such scenarios are written. Then the patient is asked to record the script on an audiotape in his own voice. The patient is required to listen to this tape over and over again, several times in a day till his anxiety related to a particular obsession is reduced. The patient is instructed to listen to the tape as long as it triggers off anxiety. This tape should be listened in the place where he is less likely to be distracted. This is further helped by listening to the tape using a headphone. An inpatient setting, is not likely to be more beneficial than encouraging a self-controlled reduction of rituals (Skeketee et al, 1993).

Procedure

Exposure can be applied in many ways. As treatment has to be adapted to the patient's needs, phobics are frequently treated individually, and about an hour per session is used to review progress, practice of exposure, and planning of tasks to be completed outside the session.

Home-based treatment, in which the partner or a relative of the patient is also taught about treatment and cooperates with the therapist to encourage, motivate, and advise the patient, has been found to be particularly successful with agoraphobics (Mathew et al, 1981). It is also extremely economical of therapist's time, good and lasting results having been obtained during research trials in five brief sessions. Generally, in order to be effective, exposure should provoke anxiety. These techniques do not undermine exposure by removing anxiety completely, but facilitate it by developing skills for controlling symptoms.

Operant Conditioning

Operant conditioning procedure is based on Skinner's principles (see Chapter 5). The basic notion in operant conditioning is that behaviour is determined, in part, by its consequences. If a behavioural response of crying with abdominal pain in a child is followed by parental attention, not going to school or getting demands fulfilled, then it tends to be strenghtened and occur more frequently under the same environmental circumstances, as shown in Figure 20.1. On the other hand, if the response is followed by an aversive stimulus (punishment) or by no stimulus at all (extinction), it tends to be weakened and occurs less frequently under the same environmental circumstances. This kind of conditioning occurs continuously in daily life, because most behaviour operates on the environment; that is, has consequences in it. Behaviour is continually altered and shaped as a result.

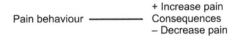

Fig. 20.1: Operant conditioning model

The procedural steps in operant conditioning are given in detail in management of mentally subnormal children, in the later part of this chapter.

Token Economy is for management of psychotic patients in the ward. The systematic applications of this method were first demonstrated by Ayllon and Azrin. This method is based on the principles of operant conditioning, the only difference being in the delivery of rewards. In token economy as the name suggests tokens are given as a consequence of positive response, these tokens are later exchanged for the rewards. This method has also been applied to train mentally retarded adults.

Social Skills Training

Deficits in social skills are frequently seen in psychiatric patients. The indications of social skills training are for those patients who have never learned appropriate social behaviour (ASB) like a severe adolescent stutterer, patient with impulse control disorder. The other type of patients in whom social skills training is indicated, where appropriate social behaviour is not available due to disuse, like chronic schizophrenia. Patients with faulty cognitive evaluative appraisal and high level of anxiety are known to have interpersonal and interactional problems. Thus these individuals also benefit from social skills therapy.

This method places an emphasis on performance not on causation of the problem. Hence, the technique of social skills training consists of, training in assertiveness, personal effectiveness, behavioural rehearsal and structured learning therapy. Modelling, reinforcement prompts, homework assignments feedbacks, instructions and role-play are used to build or enhance socially appropriate behaviours.

This method holds a great promise for a wide range of psychiatric disorders in adults and children both. A very shy adolescent girl having social phobias, or a withdrawn schizophrenic, or a drug addict requiring rehabilitation are some examples for its applications.

Aversion Therapy

Aversion therapy is used to control inappropriate behaviours, such as addictions, and sexual attractions to inappropriate stimuli. A small battery operated apparatus is used to give electrical aversion. In some cases chemical aversion is also used, e.g. antabuse for alcoholics. This technique has also been used by Despande and Mehta (1990) for controlling tricotillomania.

Contingency Contracting

The contingency contracting is based on the operant conditioning principles. In this method a contract is made between the client (as this is applicable for modification of all types of maladaptive behaviour) and the therapist, that on the achievement of the target behaviour, client receives a reward and on failing to achieve the target, he does not receive a reward and like negative marking, he loses one reward from the earlier gained reward. The client maintains a contigency chart to monitor his progress. This method is very effective for self-management programmes, like cessation of smoking, controlling aggressiveness, enuresis, habit disorders, etc.

Applications of Behavioural Therapy

Behaviour therapy has very wide applications to clinical problems; these have been applied not only to the psychiatric problems but also to other fields of medicine. Its application in medicine are dealt in Chapter 22. In psychiatric disorders, this form of therapy is the first choice of treatment for phobias and mental subnormality. It is being used as an independent mode of treatment of anxiety disorders, obsessive compulsive disorders, sexual disorders and addictions. At present, social skills training is given as an adjunct treatment to schizophrenics.

Behaviour therapy has been very effective in the treatment of child psychiatric disorders. In Indian setting, these techniques have been applied for the management of behavioural problems in normal children and in mentally handicapped, habit disorders, enuresis and encopresis, specific learning disability, somatoform disorders, attention deficit hyperactivity disorders, abdominal pain, headache, and infantile autism.

Behavioural Training for Mentally Subnormal Children

The effectiveness of behaviour modification in training in mentally handicapped is now a long established fact. (Matson and Andrasik, 1983, Mehta et al, 1990). A wide range of behaviours, reflecting the diversity of age groups, levels of retardation and treatment settings, have been modified using behavioural techniques. Mostly attention has been devoted to training self-care skills, language, and social behaviour. Problem behaviours of all kinds have been found to respond readily to behavioural intervention.

Usually parents are involved in the management because of advantages such as the proximity and availability of the parents, the greater feasibility of their being able to conduct the training in the home and for an adequately long period of time, and most of all their potential as powerful sources of reinforcement. In addition, behaviour modification techniques are relatively simple and can be readily acquired by almost anyone. The added benefits are also of easier generalisation and persistence of learned behaviour.

In India, numerous programmes have been explored and developed. One of the models (Mehta et al, 1990) is represented in Figure 20.2.

This model of behaviour training can be used by all those concerned with the mentally handicapped persons. The training programme involves parents as cotherapist. The training is imparted in various steps listed in the Figure 20.2.

Assessments of parents: It is important to carefully assess parents before involving them in a training programme. This is not to say that a complete personality profile is what is required but attitudes, traits or behaviour patterns likely to facilitate training should be explored. The most

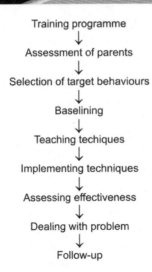

Fig. 20.2: Treatment plan for mentally retarded children

important of these are perception of the problem and motivation to train the child. Assessment of the parent's daily routine and the home situation needs to be made. Many parents would like to spend time training their children but in fact have built up a routine, which does not allow for this. It would be pointless in such a case, to push parents straight into a training programme unless some changes in routine are first established.

The measurement of such, parameters as perception of the problem and the motivation to deal with it is both difficult and time consuming. Moreover, measurement devices to suit the varied situations likely to be encountered do not exist and would need to be prepared. Despite this, it is pointless to proceed with training unless there is some previous knowledge of its likely benefit with a particular set of parents. It may prove helpful to assess parental attitude toward the problem by preparing a brief questionnaire for this purpose. Motivation may be rated by two or more persons, independently while talking to the parents. A trial task may be carried out as a demonstration. A monitoring task in which each parent in turn monitors target behaviour, or a neutral behaviour can be set up and the extent and quality of compliance be used as a rough indicator of the parent's future compliance in training tasks. A similar task can be set up for the parents to carry out at home.

Behavioural Training

Selection of target behaviours and reinforcers: This stage is best dealt within individual sessions with the parents. It is recommended that more than one target behaviour be selected so as to allow the parents to be trained in varied techniques and be equipped to deal with a variety of target behaviours.

Obtaining baseline information: Importance must be given to the necessity of baselining and monitoring target behaviour. Baselining for different kinds of behaviours must be demonstrated using charts. The parent must try a baselining task in the clinic to ensure that the procedure has been adequately learned. The process of baselining and monitoring is important for assessing the effectiveness of the training.

The target behaviours to be worked with must be recorded for a period of three days to one week depending, of course, on the apparent frequency of the behaviour.

Teaching behavioural techniques: The various techniques used in the training are based on operant conditioning. To build new behaviours contigency management, task analysis, prompting, fading and shaping are used. To decrease or eliminate undesirable behaviours, time out from reinforcement and overcorrection methods are used. In task analysis, target behaviour is broken in small steps, which are easy to learn for the retarded child. Prompting is used to guide and help the child to learn and as the learning progresses, the prompts are gradually faded. Shaping is gradual forming of behaviour through establishing various chains of tasks. The common example for this is teaching dressing to a retarded child. Each part of dressing, wearing undergarments, shirt, pants, socks, shoes and combing of hair can be developed step by step and then chaining the entire process. Time out simply means depriving child from the reward. The most effective time out from reinforcement is inattention froth parents. Overcorrection is used with children who have lesser degree of retardation. The child is forced to do corrections of his undesirable behaviours, like messing or throwing things and the child is also forced to correct others things in the environment. For severely retarded children for maladaptive behaviour at times restraint is also used.

Practical demonstrations of the use of various techniques appears more effective than lectures or discussions as a training medium, particularly when training aids such as films, slides, posters, etc. are used.

Implementing the techniques: Training tasks must be allotted to the parents so as to give them the opportunity to implement the techniques learned.

Assessing the effectiveness of training: Both the progress made by the parents, and that made by the child must be assessed. Since a positive change in the child's target behaviour is the strongest indicator of progress made by the parents, this must be assessed carefully by scrutinising, monitoring records and by observation and ratings made separately by trainers.

Dealing with problems encountered: Group sessions may be scheduled for handling the difficulties with training encountered by the parents and to allow trainers to monitor the progress made by parents and children. Such group meetings must allow discussion, catharsis and sharing of experiences.

Home visits: Whenever possible home visits by trainers should be made to ensure that parental training is effective and is being generalised.

Duration of training: The duration of the training programme and the number of session will depend on the availability of personnel, the convenience of the parents and the numerous other considerations, and hence will have to be tailored to suit each situation.

Follow-up: Ideally, follow up immediately after the training should be intensive and frequent, phasing out gradually. Ensuring follow up when parents often come from distant places has always posed a problem, which will often be the case since help services are usually concentrated in the larger cities. At times postal contact may have to be resorted to for the lack of an alternative.

Limitations of behavioural techniques: Though behavioural therapy may seem very simple and straight forward process but in practice one comes across problems like getting cooperation from the patient or his family members. Many of our patients do not understand the value of home assignment, or regular practice, or keeping appointments. Majority of the patients get more satisfaction by taking medicine, as they do not wish to put in any efforts. They want therapist to do magic to make them symptom-free.

As behaviour therapy has various applications and it holds promise in successful treatment of many disorders, we need to develop methods to enhance generalisation of the learned behaviour, as once the schizophrenic patient has learned to socially interact with other patients in the ward, after going home he should also be able to interact with his family members.

There are not many trained personnel to take the tremendous load of patients requiring behaviour therapy. Development of different training programmes, for professionals like psychologist, psychiatrist, nurses, parents and teachers is required. The training modules should be made according to the need, intensity of involvement, and duration of the training.

Documentation of improvement requires maintaining records, which is not very easy with all classes of patients, especially the illiterate. There are certain behaviours, which are easy to record, some are not feasible as in case of child patient, and behaviour occurring at school cannot be measured. In such cases the patient, his family and the therapist should try to find an alternative solution of recording.

SUMMARY

Behaviour therapy regards behaviour as functional or goal orientated. Most behaviour is learned according to basic principles of learning and behaviours serve a function in their current context and are maintained by the events, which precede and follow them. Behaviour therapy therefore, addresses to those factors that are seen to be maintaining problems.

The historical roots of behaviour therapy are based in the two fundamental learning theories of classical and operant conditioning. Later it has also adopted techniques from the social learning theory of Bandura.

In recent years, adopting a behavioural perspective to management of psychiatric problems has grown in popularity. Behaviour therapy is an empirical, scientific, and a rigorous systematic assessment process which precisely defines in operational terms the patient's problem and identifies environmental factors which influence the problem behaviour.

Explicit treatment goals are agreed upon and defined during the assessment periods, where observations are made of the problem behaviour, which provide baseline measurements. The collaborative nature of this style of therapy and the active participation of the patient is strongly emphasised. Cotherapists may be parents, nursing staff, spouses, friends or colleagues, who with the agreement of the patient, make a structured contribution to the resolution of the problem.

Behaviour therapy aims to facilitate behaviour change, to achieve this aim the first step is to identify the specific nature of the problem, to identify possible factors that precipitate and maintain the problem behaviour, to assess the baseline functioning of the patient, the degree of distress caused by the problem, patients motivation to change his maladaptive behaviour and readiness of key family member to act as a cotherapist. Observations may be made by trained clinicians or individuals may be asked to maintain a type of self-observation. To modify or change maladaptive behaviours, various treatment methods are used. Some of the commonly used methods are relaxation training, biofeedback, hypnosis, exposure, operant conditioning, social skills training and aversion therapy.

Behaviour therapy has been very effective in the treatment of a wide variety of psychiatric disorders. Various studies have reported its efficacy in the treatment of phobias, anxiety disorders, obsessive compulsive disorders, sexual disorders and addictions. Social skills training are given as an adjunct treatment to schizophrenics. In severe problems, behaviour therapy is also used as an adjunct to pharmacotherapy. This form of treatment has been especially effective in the management of child psychiatric disorders. It has been used in the management of behavioural problems in normal children, the mentally handicapped, in habit disorders, enuresis, encopresis, specific learning disablity, somatoform disorders, attention deficit hyperactivity disorders, abdominal pain, headache and infantile autism. Behavioural methods are used extensively in the management of mentally subnormal children.

Cognitive Behaviour Therapy

Cognitive therapy is a system of psychotherapy, which has been derived from cognitive psychology, information processing theory and social psychology. A set of therapeutic principles and techniques, are based primarily on empirical investigations.

Cognitive therapy implies that psychological disturbances frequently stem from specific, habitual errors in thinking. For example, a depressed patient may have self-defeating assumptions, he may incorrectly interpret his life situation, have high expectation from himself, which are difficult to achieve hence, and he may blame himself for not doing and may jump to inaccurate conclusions. He may also fail to use effective strategies to solve his problems related to external world.

Cognitive behavioural therapy is a recent development toward the integration of cognitive and behavioural approaches to therapy. The new perspective, which has been emerging, combines the behavioural emphasis on experimentation with the cognitive emphasis on the client's unique and influential interpretation of the world. Cognitive behaviour therapy fills a gap between purely behavioural therapy, and the dynamic psychotherapies.

Theoretical Basis of Cognitive Therapy

Cognitive behavioural therapy has its origins in two models.

i. Developed by Ellis based on rational emotive behaviour therapy (REBT)
ii. Developed by Beck's cognitive model.

Rational Emotive Behaviour Therapy: In REBT, Ellis has developed a model of therapy based upon the idea of using reason in the pursuit of short-term and longer-term hedonism. In his view people have a strong innate (biological) tendency to think irrationally, which is supported (reinforced), especially in childhood development, by the irrational ideas of parents and society. Ellis has proposed that human thinking and emotions are not two different processes, but for all practical purposes, they overlap. Ellis has identified several irrational (dysfunctional) beliefs. These include demandingness where the person mistakes preferences or choices for demands or commands. Such beliefs inevitably include reference to words like must, should, and ought. Ellis has also referred to this belief in terms of perfectionism or intolerance (Ellis, 1973). Although he has identified as many as 11 or 12 irrational beliefs, in his view every disturbed feeling is closely linked to one or other of the following irrational, or self-defeating, beliefs (iBs):

1. I must do well and must win approval for everything I do; otherwise I am a useless person.
2. You must act kindly, considerately and justly towards me or else you are a louse.

3. The conditions under which I live must remain good and easy, so that I get practically everything I want without too much effort or discomfort, or else the world turns damnable, and life hardly seems worth living (Ellis, 1977).

These three core beliefs are examples of what Ellis has called 'musturbation'. In Ellis's view, there is no escape from individual responsibility. This approach aims to minimise the person's self-defeating outlook, and to attain a more realistic, tolerant philosophy of life. His therapeutic tactics emphasise disarming the patient on a conceptual level, often using punchy, direct language.

Beck's Cognitive Model

The conceptual model upon which Beck's cognitive therapy is based represents a synthesis of five distinct theoretical elements, each of which has been used to explain the genesis and maintenance of specific problems of behaviour. Four functions within the individual (cognition, behaviour, mood and biology/biochemistry) interact with each other; all four interact with the person's environment. Such reciprocal interactions can lead, from the perspective of this model, to the genesis of problems such as anxiety and depression.

This model acknowledges the role of predisposing and precipitating factors. Hereditary characteristics are accepted as potential predisposing factors, as are physical illness, which might generate neurochemical abnormalities. From a developmental perspective, inadequate exposure to experiences essential for the formation of adequate coping mechanisms would constitute a learning deficit, which might predispose the person to psychological problems in later life. Equally, the acquisition of rigid, dysfunctional belief systems, such as values and assumptions, would represent further predispositions toward psychological problems in later life.

The cognitive triad or three specific thinking patterns are common in emotional disorders. These involved a negative view of self, a negative interpretation of life experiences (the world); and a tendency to take a negative view of future events. In the depressed patients, these thinking patterns appear to revolve around ideas of loss and deprivation. They perceive themselves as deficient in important qualities, unworthy or generally inadequate. Such dysfunctional thoughts intertwine with a range of fairly discrete thinking errors, which involve faulty information processing. Among the errors identified are: dichotomous reasoning (black-and-white thinking): 'If I do not succeed at everything I do, then I am a total failure', arbitrary inference (jumping to conclusions); 'we had a fight, this means he does not love me any more'; selective attention (discounting the positive); 'but I always do that anyway, that is not important'; magnification /minimisation (catastrophising); 'this is awful and there is nothing I can do about it'; personalisation; 'why does this always happen to me?'

The term schema designates relatively stable cognitive patterns. These form the basis of the person's interpretation or organisation of experience. Schemata represent the person's interpretation or organisation of experience, and the person's beliefs about himself. They are commonly construed as unspoken premises, rather than conscious thoughts. Burns (1980) has classified seven discrete 'silent assumptions' expressed in terms of needs. The need for: approval, love, achievement, perfectionism, entitlement, omnipotence, and autonomy.

Cognitive Approaches

Two broad categories of cognitive approaches can be distinguished: covert conditioning therapies and cognitive learning therapies.

Covert Conditioning Therapies: As the name implies, the covert conditioning therapies attempt to apply a conditioning model to private events. Thoughts, mental images, and memories are viewed as covert behaviours, which conform to the same laws of learning that, were developed through observation of overt behaviours. Thus, thoughts are considered to be stimuli, responses, or consequences, and principles such as reinforcement, punishment, and extinction are said to affect their frequency and intensity.

A good example of a covert conditioning therapy is Cautela's technique of covert reinforcement. In this procedure, the client is instructed to imagine performing some difficult task (e.g. refraining from drinking alcohol) and then to reinforce himself by imagining some pleasant activity (e.g. watching a cricket match) A long involved task may be broken down into a series of discrete steps, each of which is covertly reinforced. A number of other covert conditioning techniques are available, including exposure and thought stopping. By now most of the principles of learning, which have been applied to overt behaviours, have been incorporated into some covert technique.

Cognitive Learning Therapies

The second class of cognitive approaches is those, which have been labelled "the cognitive learning therapies". They are a much more heterogeneous set of strategies, sharing a few assumptions but differing widely in their derivation and procedure. Though a precise model unifying these approaches has yet to be developed, one or more of the principles appear to be fundamental to most of them.
1. That human beings respond not to environments *per se* but to their cognitive representations of those environments.
2. That thinking, emotion and behaviour are all causally interrelated.
3. That human learning involves the active acquisition of complex rules and skills (deep structural changes) rather than the passive conditioning of simple habits or responses (surface structural manifestations).
4. That the task of the clinician is to teach skills and offer experiences which replace maladaptive cognitive representations with more adaptive cognitive systems.

Process of Cognitive Behavioural Therapy

The process of cognitive therapy involves five main goals. The person learns to:
1. Identify, evaluate and examine his thoughts in relation to specific life events.
2. Judge the validity of such thoughts using objective evidence as a guide.
3. Identify the silent assumptions (unspoken schemata), which underpin his negative thoughts.
4. Practice a range of behavioural and cognitive strategies, which can be applied *in vivo* when confronted by new or unexpected stresses.
5. Develop alternative, more adaptive, thoughts about himself, the world and the future, as well as less dysfunctional schemata.

Cognitive Behavioural Assessment: Assessment in cognitive behaviour therapy is used to devise an initial formulation and treatment plan. The formulation is tested out in subsequent homework and treatment sessions, and modified if necessary. Cognitive behavioural approach is largely self-help, and that the therapist aims to help the patient develop skills to overcome not only the current problems, but also any similar ones in the future.

A cognitive-behavioural assessment also has a general educational role and focusses the patient on internal and external variables, which may not have been seen as relevant to the problem. The patient is asked about situations, physiological states, cognitions, interpersonal factors, as well as overt behaviour, and about how each of these groups of variables relates to the problem.

The assessment interview has an important role in beginning the process of therapy. Patients frequently present with an undifferentiated array of difficulties. As the therapist helps to clarify and differentiate between problems, so the difficulties are frequently reduced to manageable proportions, and the patient begins to believe that change is possible. For example, a patient who presents with a series of problems including mood disturbance, self-dislike, hopelessness, feels relieved to learn that these are all common symptoms of one problem (i.e. depression), for which there are well-established treatment approaches.

The assessment emphasises the possibility of change, by helping the patient to think of what may be achieved, rather than dwelling continually on problems. It also sets reasonable limits on what might be achieved through treatment; for example, it is unreasonable for an agoraphobic patient to aim never to experience unpleasant emotions, but it should be possible to undertake a train journey in comfort. The assessment also allows the patient to see that variations in the intensity of distress are predictable in terms of internal and external events, and are not just arbitrarily imposed by fate. It is implicit that if the variations are predictable, they may also be controllable. The therapist should offer non-judgemental sympathy and concern about the patient's problems and distress; this may provide enormous relief, especially if the patient has felt embarrassed, guilty, or hopeless, as is often the case.

Finally, an important function of the assessment is to establish whether there is anything, which needs dealing with as an emergency. For example, if the patient is depressed, suicidal intent must be assessed; if someone is complaining of difficulties in managing children, the possibility of physical abuse must be explored.

In summary, the main goal of the cognitive-behavioural assessment is to agree a formulation and treatment plan with the patient. In addition, it allows the therapist to educate the patient about the treatment approach, and to begin the process of change. It also allows emergency factors to be assessed (Table 21.1).

Table 21.1: Methods of assessment

- Behavioural interview
- Self-monitoring
- Self-report (questionnaires, global rating scales)
- Information from other family members.
- Interviews and monitoring by key others (parents, spouse)
- Direct observation of behaviour in clinical settings
  - role-play
  - behavioural tests
- Behavioural by-products
- Physiological measures.

Behavioural Analysis

To discover how the problem is currently maintained, in what way it is interfering with the patient's life, and whether the problem is serving any useful purpose for the patient. There are two commonly used approaches, first is the method, which is also used in Behavioural Therapy and discussed, in the previous chapter. In this method each problem can be analysed in terms of consequences. Each of these factors may increase or decrease the probability that the behaviour will occur.

Second approach though similar but more straightforward way of carrying out a behavioural analysis is to describe the contexts in which the problems arise, to look at the factors which modulate the intensity of the problems, and to assess the consequences, including avoidance, of them.

Detailed description of problem: As a first step, it is useful to ask the patient for a detailed description of a recent example of the problem. This gives more specific information than is obtained from a general description and provides clues about maintaining factors.

Context and modulating variables: A detailed assessment of contextual triggers is required because treatment plans often include manipulation of the contexts in which problems occur. In addition, treatment frequently involves variations in the modulating variables associated with particular cues. The range of possible triggers is almost infinite: for example, an obsessional patient may constantly ritualise at home but never at work, an agoraphobic patient may be anxiety-free if in a town where she is unknown, a compulsive gambler may only gamble when angry.

The patient may not be aware of the contexts in which the problem occurs, nor of the modulating variables. It is generally necessary for further information to be collected, either through self-monitoring or a behavioural test. These contexts and modulating variables could be situational, behavioural, cognitive, affective, interpersonal or physiological. Similarly, the same variables could be responsible for maintaining a particular behaviour.

People differ in their methods of coping with problems and distress, and in the extent to which they rely on themselves rather than on other people. This ranges from the individual's familiarity with specific strategies, like relaxing the shoulders when tense, through to more general assets, like being able to communicate distress to others.

A description should be obtained of previous history, particularly of similar episodes. The patient's response to previous treatment is particularly important. This is partly because it may predict current response to treatment, and, in the case of poor outcome, might give information about pitfalls to avoid. Patients are unlikely to engage in treatment, if the approach the therapist offers is not congruent with their beliefs about the nature of the problem.

Most cognitive-behavioural treatment demand a high level of commitment on the patient's part, and many treatments fail because the patient does not apply the agreed procedures. It would be useful to identify those people who are most likely to fulfill their side of the treatment bargain. It is helpful to discuss with the patient some of the components, which make up a desire for change, correct any misconceptions, and together make an informed decision about whether it would be worthwhile continuing with treatment.

The assignment of homework and its completion is necessary component of cognitive behaviour therapy. Hence, patient's attitude towards homework should be elicited and problems should be discussed related to incompletion of homework.

Self-monitoring

These techniques involve monitoring or recording of certain behaviour. Monitoring one's behaviour in this way also has a direct effect on the behaviour itself. For example, individuals who record negative behaviours, such as overeating, usually reduce the amount of their food intake over the period of self-observation. Thus, the assessment technique of self-monitoring has become a major strategy in the treatment of problem behaviour.

Techniques used in Cognitive Behavioural Therapies

There are some specific therapeutic techniques used in cognitive behaviour therapy.

Thought Stopping

To deal with intrusive thoughts, which are persistent patterns of negative thinking and disrupt the fulfillment of everyday living can be overcome by the procedure known as thought stopping. Thought stopping eliminates perseverative thinking which characteristically is unrealistic, unproductive, anxiety provoking or otherwise disruptive. At times this procedure has been used to control negative ruminative thoughts or auditory hallucinations. The procedure involves the patient to relax and think about the negative thought. As soon as the negative thought is produced the patient signals the therapist by raising his forefinger. The therapist shouts STOP. This interrupts the thinking process after few sessions the patient is asked to repeat this exercise on his own. Sometimes, the family members also can take the role of the therapist when the trials are to be practiced at home. Initially, the patient may say STOP loudly on his own or he can use audio tape recorder. The patient is instructed to gradually change from verbal STOP to subvocal and then to imagery of STOP.

Self-statements

Self-statements are thought which a patient has about specific events and their meaning for the person concerned. The manipulation of negative statements is used to enhance confidence, assertiveness and self-esteem in the patients. This is the simple and effective method, it involves following stages.
1. The person is helped to recognise the occurrence of such thoughts through use of self-monitoring.
2. The person is helped to generate challenges to the negative thoughts, as well as production of alternative self-statements.
3. The person is helped to assess his reaction to be manipulation of self-statements, in terms of his eventual behaviour and concomitant emotions. This approach has been used most successfully in depression, anger management, and impulse control in children.

Problem Solving

The focus upon the importance of cognition in understanding, mediating and resolving interpersonal and interpersonal problems. Problem-solving abilities are directly related to adjustment in children, adolescents and adults. People who do not have such skills have problems like depression, anxiety, substance abuse, and marital discord. Problem-solving approach has five stages.
1. Recognition and understanding the nature of interpersonal problems.
2. Identifying the realistic targets and specific goals. This involves problem definition and formulation.
3. Generation of a range of possible solutions.
4. Arriving at a decision making out of the list of possible solutions.
5. Implementation and evaluation of the selection solution.

Problem-solving approach has been found effective in management of number of psychiatric problems both in children and adults. This approach has a preventive value as once learned this strategy can be applied to the future problems also.

Distraction

A variety of distraction techniques can be used as immediate symptom management strategies. Early in therapy, training in distraction can be a very useful way of combating patients' beliefs that they have no control over their anxiety. Later in therapy, distraction can be a useful symptom-management technique in situations where it is not possible to challenge automatic thoughts, for example, while talking to someone. In this situation, the distraction exercise would involve becoming outwardly directed, perhaps moving closer to the person so that they feel the patient's field of view, and concentrating on the conversation itself rather than on thoughts concerned with evaluation of his or her own performance. Distraction can also be used to provide a potent demonstration of the cognitive model of anxiety.

Activity Schedules

In an activity schedule patients record their hour-by-hour activities, rating them (on 0-100 scales) for salient features such as anxiety, fatigue, pleasure, and mastery. Activity schedules intense time pressure, they can be used to plan activities in such a way that they are likely to be able to engage in one task at a time (trying to do brief breaks between tasks).

Time pressure and other anxious concerns can lead some patients to stop engaging in leisure and social activates which they previously enjoyed. Often these activities contributed to their sense of worth and perceived control over their environment. Therefore, dropping activities often increases anxiety and perceived vulnerability. Once this problem is identified, the therapist and patient can use an activity schedule to reintroduce pleasurable activities. Inspection of activity schedules can also help to identify periods of anxious rumination, problems with perfectionism (suggested by highly polarised mastery and pleasure rating—everything is either rated 10 or 0), and anxiety triggers.

Verbal Challenging of Automatic thoughts, Beliefs and Assumptions: In Beck's model of depression, dysfunctional beliefs is cardinal feature of depression.

Challenging irrational or dysfunctional beliefs is important to bring change in the patient's cognition. Hence in cognitive behavioural therapy the patient is helped to identify, challenge and subsequently classify specific forms of thinking errors, in the form of specific self-statement. A series of questions are used to help patients to evaluate negative automatic thoughts and to substitute more realistic thoughts. Within sessions, patients and therapist work collaboratively to identify rational responses to automatic thoughts. Between sessions patients attempt to put into practice the questioning skills they have learned in the sessions by recording and challenging automatic thoughts as they arise. One particularly convenient way of doing this is to use the daily record of dysfunctional thoughts.

Behavioural Experiments: In addition to discussing evidence for and against patients' negative thoughts, therapists should also attempt to devise behavioural assignments, which help patients to check out the validity of their negative thoughts. These assignments can be one of the most effective ways of changing beliefs.

Learning New Behaviours and Skills: For some patients, part of the reason why they find social situations difficult is that they either lack, or have difficulty using social and conversational skills. When this is the case, brief training in appropriate social skills can be helpful. Once a problematic situation has been isolated, role-plays and discussion of what the patient actually did in the situation are used to identify inappropriate behaviours. Once these behaviours have been identified, alternatives are suggested, modelled by the therapist and then practiced by the patient, initially in the safety of a role-play in the therapy session and later in real-life situations.

Role-playing

Role playing and rehearsal are more often used in the treatment of social phobias than of other Phobias, and a role-play may itself be a type of exposure. For example, a patient who finds it difficult to say no, or to be assertive, can practice being assertive during a role-play with the therapist. This has many advantages. It may reveal a lack of skill or knowledge, such as difficulty in moderating responses, or being unable to be assertive without being aggressive. The role-play can then be repeated in various ways, until the patient discovers how he or she wishes to change. Role-plays are particularly useful in preparation for events such as interviews. Video (or audio) recordings, if available, allow patients to make the most of this type of practice. Watching the video provides accurate feedback as well as new information: for instance that they may feel much worse than they look.

Rehearsal

This is a way of preparing for exposure, many phobics find that their minds go blank when they are faced with phobic objects or situations, or when feeling panicky. Techniques for managing the symptoms of intense anxiety, especially panic attacks, should therefore be rehearsed. When this 'blankness' occurs in social situations it creates awkwardness, which rapidly increases anxiety. It is less likely to happen if appropriate strategies are rehearsed, and appropriate material prepared, such as lists of questions to ask, or topics to talk about. Social skills can be separately rehearsed and may improve with practice. Rehearsing difficult events, such as speaking in public, making a request, or introducing someone, both increases confidence and reduces anticipatory anxiety. Lastly, detailed rehearsal helps to reveal 'blocks' that might prevent exposure.

Modelling

This is a less direct technique, in which the therapist demonstrates how to approach the phobic object, for example a snake or the edge of a high building, while being observed by the patient. Modelling is most effective when the model exhibits, and overcomes, anxiety, and it is suggested that observation of such a 'coping model' facilitates the patient's own coping skills. These might be poor either because patients do not know what to do, or because they are unable to think what to do at the time.

Clinical Applications

Cognitive approaches to treatment probably came to the attention of most clinicians in the management of depressive disorders. However, cognitive behaviour therapy has much wider applications, many of which relate to conditions, which often cannot be treated easily, and effectively in other ways. These conditions include anxiety and obsessional disorders, eating disorders, certain somatic problems, aspects of the disabilities of patients with chronic mental illness, as well as sexual and marital problems.

Treatment of depression, anxiety and stress management are dealt in some detail, in this section.

Treatment of Depression: The main treatment strategies used in the treatment of depression are given in Table 21.2. Depressed patients lack in activity, have no interest and do not derive pleasure from their activities. There are a number of reasons that can explain the low rates of positive reinforcement and/or high rates of punishment experienced by depressed patient: (1) the limited availability of immediate environment; (2) the lack of skill that prevents the individual from obtaining available positive reinforcing and/or coping effectively with aversive events; and (3) a diminishment of the potency of positively reinforcing events and/or a heightening of the negative impact of punishing events. Thus, the first step in the treatment is aimed towards increasing activity, and increasing sense of mastery. These aims are achieved using the first two strategies given in the table, cognitive and behavioural strategies.

Table 21.2: Strategies for treatment of depression

1.	Cognitive strategies	Distraction techniques
		Counting thoughts
2.	Behavioural strategies	Monitoring activities, pleasure and mastery
		Scheduling activities
		Graded task assignment
3.	Cognitive-behavioural strategies	Identifying negative automatic thoughts
		Questioning negative automatic thoughts
		Behavioural experiments
4.	Preventive strategies	Identifying assumptions
		Challenging assumptions
		Use of set-backs
		Preparing for the future

The patient may also be urged to identify, and question negative automatic thoughts. Patient may also try to elicit automatic thoughts by imagining in detail the distressing situations that trigger the emotional response and then role-playing them with the therapist, for instance, if they are interpersonal. Testing automatic thought by operationally defining a negative construct, reattributing it, and generating alternatives is the next stage of therapy. The therapist and patient define, in operational terms, what the patient means by a particular word or expression (e.g. failure). Once the patient and therapist agree upon the criterion for "failure", they examine past evidence to assess whether the label "failure", is indeed a valid one. The goal of this procedure is to teach the patient to recognise the arbitrary nature of his self-appraisal and to make the patient more aware of more common-sense definition of these negative terms.

Another technique used in the therapy is that of reattribution, whereby patient and therapist may review the situations in which patient and therapist may review the situations in which patients unrealistically blame themselves for unpleasant events and explore other factors that may explain what happened other than, or in addition, the patients behaviour. Finally, a problem-solving approach may be adopted, whereby the patient and therapist work to generate solutions to the problems that had not been considered previously.

The therapist also attempts to identify, with the patient's help, underlying assumptions responsible for automatic thoughts. Underlying assumptions may be viewed as the rules or the "rights", and "wrongs" of the patient in judging himself or herself and other people. One of the major goals of therapy is to identify and challenge these rules, which are typically couched in absolute terms are unrealistic, or are used inappropriately excessively. One strategy, for example, used in testing the validity of maladaptive assumptions may be for the therapist and patients to generate lists of the advantages and disadvantages of changing an assumption and then discuss and weigh these lists, the patient is also assigned homework to facilitate the transfer of learning of new skills from therapy sessions to the home environment.

Verbal challenging of automatic thoughts is followed by behavioural experiments through which new ideas are put to test. The practice of preventive strategies can reduce the risk of relapse.

Treatment of Anxiety

Cognitive behaviour therapy aims to reduce anxiety by teaching patients how to identify, evaluate, control and modify their negative danger-related thoughts and associated behaviours. A variety of cognitive and behaviour techniques are used to achieve this aim.

Identifying negative thoughts: Some patients find it easy to identify their negative thoughts at the start of therapy. However, others require some training before they can confidently identify their key anxiety-related thoughts. Shifts in mood during a session can be particularly useful sources of automatic thoughts.

Finding alternatives: The Cognitive techniques for identifying and then examining the thoughts associated with anxiety can be used to control symptoms, for example of panic, as well as to challenge thoughts about the phobia. They are particularly useful for dealing with worries about future events or anticipatory anxiety, during which patients often underestimate their capacity for coping, and over-estimate the likelihood or disaster.

Discussing a recent emotional experience: Patients are asked to recall a recent event or situation which was associated with anxiety and for which they have a fairly clear memory. The event is described in some detail and the therapist elicits the thoughts associated with the onset and maintenance of the emotional reaction.

Distraction: Paying attention to symptoms of anxiety perpetuates the vicious circle, and makes the symptoms worse. Distraction can reverse this process. This is a useful short-term strategy, but can be unhelpful in the long-term if used as a way of avoiding symptoms, or of disengaging from exposure. There are many distraction techniques, most of which involve focussing on external factors, and many patients like to devise their own.

Role-play or use of imagery: When simple direct questioning fails to elicit automatic thoughts, it can be useful to ask patients to relive the recent emotional events by either replaying it in great detail using imagery or, if it is an interpersonal interaction, by role-play.

Determining meaning of an event: Sometimes, skillful attempts to elicit automatic thoughts are unsuccessful. The therapist should then attempt to discern, through questioning, the specific meaning of the event for the patient.

Modifying negative thoughts: A wide range of procedures are used to help patients evaluate, control, and modify their negative thoughts and associated behaviours. When choosing specific procedures to use with a particular patient, the therapist is largely guided by the assessment interview and, in particular, by the hypotheses which he or she developed about the main cognitive and behaviour processes maintaining the patient's anxiety state.

As an adjunct to these cognitive strategies, relaxation exercises are also used with some anxious patients.

Management of Stress/Pain: Cognitive-behavioural approaches have been utilised in the form of stress/pain inoculation training (Meichenbaum and Turk, 1976), to help patients manage their pain experience. Typically, a patient would initially be given information to enhance his or her understanding of the pain and the stressors that accompany it. The patient would then be trained in a variety of coping strategies (e.g. relaxation, distraction, imagery techniques) and finally would be asked to rehearse these strategies while conceptualising the pain and stress at each phase of the total pain experience. Based on such a hypothesis, illness behaviour accordingly is seen to develop as a result of: (1) vicarious learning through models, particularly in childhood; (2) direct social reinforcement of illness behaviour by family, friends, and physicians; and (3) avoidance learning (secondary to a social skill deficit or social anxiety).

Cognitive strategies for pain management are used for all types of pain, but these have been reported to be especially very effective in management of chronic pain, cancer pain, and psychogenic pain.

SUMMARY

Cognitive therapies are an offshoot of cognitive, and social learning theories. They imply that psychological disturbances stem from specific, habitual errors in thinking. These theories have originated from two models, Ellis' Rational emotive therapy and Beck's cognitive model. Both the models have identified irrational beliefs, which are linked to depression or any maladaptive behaviour. Beck has proposed a cognitive triad, which involves a negative view of self, others, and of future events. This model is commonly referred to, in the treatment of depression.

There are two broad approaches used in cognitive therapy: Covert conditioning therapies and Cognitive learning therapies. There are various specific techniques used in cognitive behavioural therapies, such as thought stopping, problem solving, distraction, identifying negative assumptions, automatic thoughts and their modification, role playing, rehearsal, modelling, etc.

Though cognitive behavioural therapy has wide applications, it has been specially claimed to be very effective in the treatment of mild depressive disorders, management of anxiety, pain and stress. This form of therapy is also being used in medical disorders, which are discussed in the next chapter.

Behaviour Medicine

Behavioural medicine is the interdisciplinary field concerned with the development and integration of the behavioural and biomedical science, knowledge and techniques relevant to health and illness. The application of this knowledge and these techniques are used in prevention, diagnosis, treatment and rehabilitation.

As an interdisciplinary approach this science draws the knowledge and skills from a variety of research and clinical practitioner who bring to the analysis and treatment of health-related behaviour their own perspective and expertise and collaborate with one another. It includes disciplines such as medicine, sociology, psychology, epidemiology, nutrition, biochemistry, and many other related fields.

Behavioural medicine emphasises the role of psychological factors in the occurrence, maintenance and prevention of physical illness. It extends our conception of disease beyond the traditional medical preoccupation with physical breakdown of organs and organ systems. To put it simply, it seeks to understand the relationship of behaviour and biology and effectively promotes individual's health. In contrast to psychosomatic medicine, which is influenced by psychodynamic theory and biological psychiatry and emphasises the aetiology and pathogenesis of disease; behavioural medicine is influenced by conditioning and learning theories, and emphasises the treatment and prevention of disease.

Examination of Biopsychosocial Contexts of Problems

Behavioural medicine examines the broad biopsychosocial context of the following problem areas.

Aetiology

How do critical life events, characteristic behaviour and personality organisation predispose an individual to physical illness, e.g. a person with anxious personality are more prone to hypertension.

Host Resistance

How are the effects of stress mitigated by resistance resources like coping style, social support and certain personality traits. Persons with good coping skills can manage stressful situations without many negative effects on their health.

Disease Mechanism

How is human physiology altered by stressors, particularly those arising from maladaptive behaviour? For instance what effects are produced in immune gastrointestinal and cardiovascular system due to stress?

Patient-Decision Making

What are the processes involved in the choices individuals make with respect to matters such as hasardous lifestyles, excessive smoking and consumption of alcohol, seeking of health-care and adherence to preventive regimens.

Compliance

Which factors like biomedical, behavioural, self-regulative, cultural, social and interpersonal (physician-patient relationship) determine compliance with medical advice?

Intervention

How effective are psychological measures like health education and behaviour modification in altering unhealthy lifestyles and in the direct reduction of illness and illness behaviour at individual and community levels.

Techniques used in Behavioural Medicine

Behavioural medicine is not restricted to a set of techniques or particular principles to change behaviour. A wide variety of procedures are employed like contingency management operant conditioning, desensitisation, conditioning and cognitive-behavioural approaches. Details of these techniques you have already read in the previous Chapters (20 and 21). The common goal of all these techniques is to alter bad living habits, distressed psychological state and aberrant physiological processes in order to have a beneficial impact on are individual's physical condition.

As you read earlier that before focussing on the treatment programme, one needs to do a detailed assessment. It is important to take information from various sources into account. The medical problems along with the complications they present need to be understood. The effects and side effects of the medications should also be understood. Assessment of the disability status can provide a feedback about motive behind patient's illness, (also refer to chapter on Illness Behaviour).

In behavioural medicine, some of the common methods used to modify behaviour are described here.

Self-monitoring

This is an effective treatment strategy and it involves systematic observation of behaviour. The patient is given instructions to maintain comprehensive daily record of fluctuation of symptoms. This helps the patient to sharpen self-observational skills and become more aware of the symptoms. Self-monitoring helps the patient to receive immediate feedback regarding factors that contribute to an increase and/or decrease of symptoms. It can also help the patient to develop internal performance standards that guide behavioural change.

Stimulus Control

In this, the patient learns to identify the cues in the environment that foster adaptive or maladaptive behaviour and then alter the environment and behavioural routines. The attempt is to modify behavioural routines and eliminate emotional cues that maintain behavioural problems. This method is especially useful in treatment of obesity, addictive behaviours and insomnia. Many obese individuals admit that they eat more while watching TV, so by changing behavioural routine of watching TV, like doing some simple activity simultaneously can break the habit of eating with watching of TV.

Self-control of Internal States: Both relaxation training and biofeedback procedures are used to achieve self-control of internal states, like anxiety. Relaxation exercises are known as behavioural aspirin. These are used as basic step in almost all problems related to behavioral medicine. Details of Jacobson's Progressive Muscular Relaxation and biofeedback have been given in the previous chapter.

The behavioural scientists may also use cognitive restructuring, behavioural counselling, contingency management, stress management and systematic desensitisation to bring about the desired changes.

Applications of Behavioural Medicine

Behavioural medicine techniques have been applied to such diverse topics as alcohol and tobacco use, exercise, AIDS, diabetes, hypertension, stress and immunisation. It can also be applied to diverse health problems like cancer, heart disease, infections and pain. Some of the important applications of behavioural medicine are in the management of headache, chronic pain, psychophysiological disorders, insomnia, and gastrointestinal disorders.

Headache

Headaches represent one of the two types: muscle-contraction headaches and migraine headaches. The former are thought to be due to increased levels of tension and latter due to changes in cerebral blood flow.

Relaxation training and biofeedback techniques are commonly used for the treatment of headaches. EMG biofeedback is generally used for muscle-contraction headaches and is typically conducted by attaching electrodes to the forehead muscles.

In case of migraine headaches, thermal biofeedback training is used more commonly. The procedure involves attaching a sensor to the finger. The sensor measures the blood flow to the periphery.

Cognitive behavioural therapy has also shown some promise in the treatment of headaches. Psychosocial factors, stressful life events and daily hassles play an important role in the causation of headache. In children headache is related at times to negative family environment.

Chronic Pain

Chronic pain is generally described as pain that persists for more than 6 months and has little likelihood of remission. Thus it is important that patients learn to manage pain and pain-related impairment effectively. Before starting the treatment regimen it is necessary that thorough assessment be done. It is essential to obtain a description of pain and its onset, evaluation of pain-related impairment, emotional distress and marital and vocational factors. The assessment is aimed to identify specific activity goals and appropriateness of the patient for rehabilitation. Most benefit is obtained from rehabilitation programme if the patient has pain-related impairment, some emotional distress and a significant other willing to attend treatment sessions. The answer to the question 'why is impairment essential?' is that the aim of the treatment is to get the patient to engage in activities in spite of pain. Treatment of chronic pain involves reconditioning through physical therapy, exercises, cognitive restructuring, reprogramming the patients' environment and addressing vocational issues. The aim of cognitive restructuring is to help the patient and significant others set reasonable goals and limits. The environmental reprogramming involves including the significant others. The significant others are involved so that they do not undermine the treatment by prohibiting patients from engaging in health promoting behaviours or pushing them beyond reasonable limits.

Psychophysiological Disorders: According to ICD-10 psychophysiological disorders are physical problems that have a known or suspected pathophysiological mechanism and may be influenced by psychological factors.
1. *Asthma*—is a complex disorder of bronchial tubes, caused by hyperreactivity to various stimuli like exercises, cold air, respiratory infections. It leads to difficulty in breathing. Behavioural scientists have found that emotions and certain situations trigger asthma attack in some individuals. It also appears that asthma attacks are conditionable, i.e. having an asthma attack may predispose an

individual to have another attack when exposed again to that particular situation.

Behavioural treatment of asthma includes EMG Biofeedback and relaxation training to help patients overcome fear and panic. Deconditioning of stimuli thought to produce asthma attack, has also been attempted. Asthmatics are taught about self management which includes gathering information about the attack, what prompts their occurrence, and management skills. Management skills emphasise that the patient should avoid triggering stimuli adheres to medication regimen, and use positive coping strategies. Mehta and Chawla (1984) reported effectiveness of systematic desensitisation in the management of frequent asthma attacks.

2. *Insomnia*—is a subjective feeling of not having obtained enough sleep along with objective verification of sleeping difficulties and/or daytime fatigue. Insomniacs may complain of difficulty falling asleep, frequent awakenings during night, awakening much earlier in the morning and inability to sleep again.

Behavioural medicine specialists emphasise on sleep hygiene behaviour. It includes avoidance of caffeine, alcohol before sleep, avoidance of daytime napping and maintenance of regular sleep schedule. Patients are instructed to use the bed for sleeping only. Relaxation and biofeedback have also been used as treatment procedures.

3. *Raynaud's disease*—This disease is characterised by episodic attacks of vasospasm in finger and/or toes. Due to lack of blood flowing to the periphery, the tips become cold. Relaxation therapy and thermal biofeedback are carried out in an effort to increase flow of blood to the periphery.

4. *Gastrointestinal disorders*—These include problems associated with stomach and intestines. Peptic ulcers, irritable bowel syndrome, ulcerative colitis and Crohn's disease are the most common type of gastrointestinal disorder, which are affected by emotional state of the individual. The intervention includes stress management, anxiety management, assertiveness training, relaxation and biofeedback. The effectiveness of this treatment in case of Crohn's disease is inconclusive. Bowel movement biofeedback is found to be successful in management of Crohn's disease.

Health Promotion

Health promotion activities aim at reducing the risk of developing disease. It includes exercise adherence, smoking cessation, weight management, stress management, medication adherence and AIDS prevention.

Exercise Adherence

Physical activity is recognised as an accepted form of treatment for a variety of disorders like— diabetes, obesity, hypertension, coronary heart disease, depression and chronic pain conditions. Individuals may begin an exercise programme but some find it difficult to adhere to it for long duration. Behavioural medicine specialists use the following intervention techniques for exercise adherence:

i. have the patient monitor the amount of physical exercise performed and establish some kind of reward system for completion of a prescribed amount of exercise.
ii. use feedback and social support from family members, friends and treatment staff.
iii. focus on identification of primary impediments to maintenance of exercise and develop ways to cope with such impediments.

Smoking Cessation

Addiction of smoking can be maintained by physiological, social and behavioural conditioning factors. Behavioural strategies for smoking cessation include use of self-monitoring and administration of rewards. Patients set a criterion number of cigarettes to smoke and a reward for meeting that criterion. Patients generally reduce the number of cigarettes until total abstinence is achieved. Use of social support increases the likelihood of change and maintenance of cessation. Relaxation training is incorporated to combat the physiological arousal that may result from craving. Efforts are also made to eliminate the settings associated with smoking.

Management of Stress

Stress results in illness through two mechanisms: (a) directly by the effect of stress on immune system and other physiological function and (b) indirectly by reducing the likelihood of engaging in healthy behaviours such as relaxation, reading, and increasing the likelihood of engaging in unhealthy behaviour, such as drinking alcohol, smoking. The aim of stress-management programmes is to teach the individuals to cope with daily demands in an effective manner. To help cope with physiological effects of stress, individuals are taught some method of physical relaxation-like progressive muscle relaxation, yoga, meditation, or biofeedback assisted relaxation. To reduce the relative importance attributed to potentially negative situations, cognitive therapies are used. It may also involve training in social skills or problem-solving (refer to Chapter 10).

Medication Adherence

Behavioural medicine specialist help in improving a patient's nonadherence to prescribed medication. Factors that contribute to non-adherence are lack of understanding about medication, need for medication, potential side effects and benefits of adhering to treatment regimen (also see Chapter 17). The behavioural medicine specialist focusses on: (1) enhancing patient's understanding about the need for and benefit of medication (2) teaches the physicians the strategies that will increase patient adherence. He also helps him to develop effective communication patterns. This involves: (a) Explaining to the patient, the physical and or psychological problems that they have, (b) to help the patient accept that they have a problem that needs treatment. No acceptance may be due to fear or denial or other factors, (c) explaining the specific treatment strategies, including the side effects, intended effects, benefits of adhering and possible complications of nonadhering, and (d) lastly the patient needs to adhere to the treatment, and he may be provided with reinforcement for complying.

AIDS Prevention

As AIDS is becoming one of the major concerns for health workers, and prevention of AIDS is on the top priority, behavioural medicine can contribute significantly in the achievement of this task. In this context behavioural medicine specialists serves as a primary health care professional. HIV is transmitted via certain life-style behaviours, especially involvement in unsafe sexual practices and use of infected needles for intravenous drug use.

AIDS prevention efforts include use of educational programmes emphasising the importance of abstinence from high-risk behaviour. Stimulus control procedures are used which focus on identification of situations that serve as cues to engage in high-risk behaviour and making attempts to avoid these situations. Modelling may also be used, since having a model that is perceived to be similar to oneself may increase the likelihood of engaging in similar behaviours.

Type A Behaviour and Hostility Reduction: Type A behaviour has been described as consisting of competitiveness, achievement orientation, impatience, hostility, interpersonal dominance and control. Research has shown that type A behaviour pattern places an individual at risk for coronary heart disease. Behaviour treatment involves some kind of character procedure to combat the physiological effects of cardiac hyper-reactivity. It may also include marital therapy, time management, stress management techniques or individual therapy aimed at reducing negative attributions.

Diabetes

Behavioural medicine research emphasises on weight reduction, diet restriction and exercise to aid in diabetic control. The role of stress and efficacy of stress management techniques in controlling blood glucose is also being examined. It is hypothesised that stress increases the amount of glucose in the blood. Biofeedback and relaxation strategies have been used successfully for the treatment of diabetes. In a diabetic clinic (AIIMS) yoga has been introduced as an adjunct to medical treatment.

SUMMARY

Behavioural medicine is the diverse field concerned with the development and integration of the behavioural and biomedical techniques relevant to health and illness. This knowledge and these techniques have been applied in prevention, diagnosis, treatment and rehabilitation. Behavioural medicine uses a wide variety of behavioural techniques based on conditioning both classical and operant, and cognitive behavioural therapies. These include relaxation procedures, continency management desensitisation techniques, stimulus control, self-monitoring. Assessment is concerned with redefinition of symptoms in observable and measurable terms and how the symptoms are experienced and function in the life of the individual. Behavioural medicine has made significant advances in treatment of psychophysiological disorders (asthma, chronic and acute pain, headache, diabetes, hypertension), behavioural and habit disorders (smoking, overweight, addictive behaviours). It has contributed to preventive medicine through identification and counteraction of health risk factors involved in smoking, stress, Type A behaviour pattern. Behavioural medicine identifies factors that contribute to health or risk of illness and develop intervention to alter' lifestyle in direction of health. Development of health promotion strategies especially in AIDS prevention, adherence to medication and exercise regimen are also part of behavioural medicine. As life-threatening diseases are becoming curable, rehabilitation of patients with such problems can be planned on these behavioural principles.

PART 6: Applications of Behavioural Sciences to Health

23. Communication Skills

When a patient seeks medical help, the clinician's first task is to ensure that he behaves in such a manner that the patient is able to trust him and disclose why he has presented, otherwise the clinician may not determine the true nature and extent of the patient's current difficulties. Once the diagnosis is made, the clinician has to discuss that with the patient and explain any action he plans to take. Unless he does this adequately, the patient will probably feel dissatisfied and fail to comply with advice or treatment.

The patient may be extremely worried about the possible diagnosis, investigations and treatment. His fears can be allayed only if the clinician is able to clarify exactly what they are and reassure him. The history, physical examination and investigations may reveal a potentially life-threatening or fatal illness. The clinician has then to decide whether, when and how to break the news to the patient and close relatives. Failure of the clinician to correctly identify what they wish to know about the disease and prognosis may hinder their attempts to cope and lead to serious psychological problems. Doctors can discharge these important tasks effectively only if they possess the relevant skills. Unfortunately, many do not appear to acquire them during their professional training.

Communication skills (Hess 1969; Ivey 1983) are those skills by which—
- The clinician-patient relationship is created and maintained.
- Verbal information relevant to the clarification and solution of the patient's problem is gathered.
- The solution to the problem is negotiated.

The quality of the clinician-patient relationship is positively related to the communication skills using which the clinicians keep patients informed about the how and why of their actions. It is necessary to establish an effective working relationship. Communication skills are one of the most important skills that a clinician must have. It is not enough to have the scientific knowledge alone, but also the skill to bring that knowledge to bear in the diagnosis and treatment of illness. Clinicians must be able to communicate not only with the patients, but also with colleagues, nursing staff and administrators. Difficulties in clinician-patient communication are often reported as a major barrier to an effective patient care. It has been found (Evans et al, 1991), that after taking part in a communication skills course, medical students were more efficient at detecting the patient's verbal and nonverbal cues. They could elicit more relevant information from the patients.

A fundamental requirement for effective communication is an understanding of the patient as an individual. Since most of the medical students are educationally and socially different from their patients, they have difficulty in understanding their patient's problems. In a survey conducted at AIIMS by D' Monte and Pande (1990), students had expressed the need for training in communication skills especially for management of outpatients. The patients expect the clinicians to listen to their complaints, to encourage them to ask about their illness and advise about their prognosis and subsequent preventive measures.

Fletchner (1973) emphasised that for optimal benefit, effective communication must depend on clinician's understanding of the patient, as an individual who has an illness, rather than as a disease process alone. Clinicians should communicate in such a manner that it matches the patient's knowledge, social background, interests and needs.

It has also been shown that better informed patients cope better with their disease, are more compliant to treatment, less anxious and generally more functional. On the basis of the available evidence, open communication appears to be of great benefit, giving the patient an avenue for information and support.

Components of Communication Skills

A good communication in medical practice comprises of certain skills. A basic level of competence and consideration for the patient in the following areas can enhance effectiveness of clinician patient communication.

Appropriate Physical Environment: An appropriate physical environment should be established to enhance privacy, comfort and attentiveness. Even in the crowded room, a suitable environment can be created by arrangement of seating, or having a curtain. A sense of privacy tends to improve the outcome of the interview.

Greeting Patients

Greeting patients in a manner acceptable within the cultural norms relating to age, sex, etc. will help maintain their dignity and encourage their participation.

Listening

This involves using both verbal and nonverbal communication techniques. The clinician should clearly indicate that he is attentive to the patient, by looking at the patient, by offering acceptance and nods. A willingness to listen actively is best indicated by asking open-ended questions.

Empathy, and Warmth

The clinician should also learn to show empathy, warmth, respect, interest, and support. This will also involve being nonjudgemental in attitude. Development of these skills is dependent upon the attitude. Clinicians should clearly signal their interest in how the patient's problem is perceived by them, how it affects their life, what their hopes and expectations are.

Language

While communicating with the patients, clinicians should be careful in selecting words and the use of a particular language. If the patient is illiterate, use of english language and technical words should be avoided. Similarly, for educated patients, if very simple language is used, then they feel offended. Most clinicians find difficulty in explaining diagnosis and the reasoning behind it and suggestions for management.

Nonverbal communication: Skills in non-verbal communication like eye contact, physical proximity, and facial expression need to be monitored with feedback to the students, to help them improve their interactions. This should convey to the patient that the clinician is attentive and interested.

Closing the Interview

In addition to the skills of setting up, beginning and continuing an interview, the way of closing the interview is also important. The clinician should close the interview by summarising what has been said and what has been negotiated.

Communication Skills in Specific Situations

Core communication skills can be taught as a way to improve clinician-patient communication in medical interviews. Communications skills are required to express oneself, and to be able to understand what patient is communicating. Often patients may not be able to communicate clearly, which creates problems in history taking. To be able to cope with such difficult situations, the clinician may require higher levels of competence in core communication skills, for which additional training may be required.

Information Gathering

A critical part of all clinician-patient interaction involves eliciting information from the patient. The core skills, which are needed to facilitate the process of information gathering, are skills, which help to facilitate the patient's involvement in the medical interview in a way that enables the clinician to arrive at an accurate diagnosis of a patient's problem or symptoms.

Deficiencies in History-taking Skills: Studies of medical students have found that they experience considerable difficulty when obtaining a patients' history, presenting either physical or psychiatric problem. They generally assumed that the problem was more likely to be organic than psychological, despite the psychiatric setting in which they were conducting their interviews. Very few students followed a predictable sequence of questions, apart from those directed at a review of the major physical systems of the body, there was not any consistency in the way they began, conducted or terminated their interviews.

There was often little connection between consecutive topics and it seemed more often matter of chance which areas they covered. Only rarely did they try to establish how any problems had affected the lives of their patients and their families.

Similar deficiencies were found by Heifer (1970), when he used stimulated parents of sick children to assess the interviewing skills of senior medical students. He noted that they used techniques, which hindered the collection of relevant information, relied on leading questions, used unfamiliar medical jargon, cut off patients' communications and neglected to pursue important psychological and social aspects.

Over half the clinicians used complicated medical words, which the mother did not understand. They wasted much unnecessary time through needless repetition or getting into unhelpful battles with the mother. Many even failed to introduce themselves before they asked questions and substantial proportion were perceived by the mothers as cold and uncaring.

This failure of clinicians to respond to cues given by patients or relatives about their main concerns was also found in a study of communications between surgeons and women attending a breast clinic. Although most (95%) of those who had rated themselves as very distressed on a self-rating scale just before the consultation gave clear verbal or nonverbal clues that they were upset, these were heeded and clarified in only 5 per cent. In 20 per cent of cases, the surgeons appeared to have realised that the woman was worried, but dealt with it by bland general statements such as 'Don't worry, there is nothing to be bothered about' or 'we will sort it all out for you'. In the remaining 70 percent, there was no evidence that they had picked up the cues. Only rarely did any of the surgeons inquire directly about how the women had reacted emotionally to the discovery of breast disease and possible cancer. Consequently, many of these who had been distressed before the clinic were just as distressed afterwards (Maguire, 1980).

The failure of clinicians to enquire systematically how patients and relatives are adapting psychologically and socially to serious physical disease may partly explain why so much of the associated psychiatric morbidity, remains hidden. In a recent study of patients who underwent mastectomy for cancer of the breast, the surgeons detected only a fifth of those who had developed psychiatric problems. They also commonly failed to realise the extent to which women were suffering pain, swelling and disability in the arm affected by surgery or adverse physical toxicity when treated with cytotoxic drugs (Maguire, 1980).

There has been much less study of the ways in which clinicians give patients information and advice about their disease and treatment. Even so, there is considerable indirect evidence that many clinicians are equally deficient in these skills.

Survey of patients in hospital and the community reveal that many feel dissatisfied with the amount of information they are given about their condition and treatment. They commonly complain that they did not understand what their clinician said to them and had insufficient opportunity to ask questions and discuss any worries. In hospital studies, the proportion expressing dissatisfaction with the information given has ranged from 5 to 65 per cent (Ley, 1977). For example, even insulin, which could be life-saving for diabetics, was found to have been taken in the wrong dose by half of them. Moreover, 34 per cent had no knowledge of how to test their urine and so had no proper basis on which to estimate the insulin dose.

Inadequate Preparation for Major Investigative and Surgical Procedures: These deficiencies in the explanations given to patients have been especially apparent in patients undergoing major investigations or surgery. They have complained that they were not given enough information beforehand, and that this made them much more fearful than they would otherwise have been. It has caused some patients to claim that they would not have agreed to surgery, had they fully realised what it entailed. Inadequate preparation has been commonly given as an explanation by patients, who fail to adapt psychologically to major surgery such as mastectomy or colostomy.

In patients who are diagnosed as having cancer, there is commonly a serious mismatch between the patient's wish for information and the clinician's willingness to provide it. Still, many clinicians debate whether to share or not to share the diagnosis with the patient, it often depends on their judgement of the patient's capacity to cope rather than on the patient's own wishes, even when these are openly expressed. Doctors may also go against the patient's wish to know by agreeing with the relatives' request that they should not be told.

Motivating Patients for Compliance: Information giving skills described earlier, will contribute to patient compliance to treatment plans by making sure that the patient has understood the relevant information about the diagnosis and proposed treatment. Poor compliance with advice and treatment has been linked to perception of the clinician as business like rather than warm and friendly, neglect of psychological and social aspects of illness, lack of feedback from the clinician, poor explanation of diagnosis and failure to meet patients' expectations. It represents a major problem in medical practice, since it renders much of the offered treatment and advice ineffective. Some of the strategies to enhance patient compliance are skills for the promotion of behaviour change, since realistic compliance with treatment plans may require patients to make significant changes to their diet, lifestyle or daily routine on a short-term or long-term basis (also see Chapter 17). Table 23.1 lists strategies for promoting compliance.

Table 23.1: Strategies for promoting compliance

- Provide a rationale for behaviour change
- Tailor the treatment to suit the patient's lifestyle
- Counter barriers to change
- Provide examples of role models
- Allow opportunities for verbal rehearsal of the treatment
- Feedback (positive reinforcement of constructive behaviour changes)
- Understanding how the patient explains the illness

Preparation for Major Investigation and Surgery: The systematic provision of information and support to patients, who are to undergo surgery or special investigations appears to have beneficial effects (Ley, 1977). Egbert et al (1964) compared a control group, who received only the care routinely given with patients, who were also told what pain to expect, given instruction about postoperative exercises and visited more regularly by the anaesthetist. The experimental group recovered sooner, required fewer analgesics and was discharged earlier. In another study, Schmitt and Wooldridge (1978) compared the effects of routine preparative care with those of giving information, advice and clarifying any worries or misconceptions. The experimental group was much less anxious, discharged sooner and showed less physiological disturbance than control subjects.

These and other similar studies, which have found a positive link between preoperative preparation and outcome of surgery, have used several approaches at once. It is therefore still not clear, what contributions of the ability to provide needed information and support and to clarify and correct misconceptions before surgery make to this improved outcome. Moreover, the beneficial effects have so far been shown only in relation to less serious surgery. Indeed, in a recent study of the effects of providing advice and information before mastectomy it was found that while the women welcomed this help, it did not prevent the later development of psychological and social problems (Maguire et al, 1980c).

Other work has suggested that whatever approaches are used, they should be tailored to the individual needs of the patient. Patients who were experiencing low levels of anxiety were actually harmed by the presentation of a leaflet, which told them about the surgical procedures which were shortly to be performed. Patients who had high levels of anxiety benefitted from the leaflet. Patients, who cope by not facing the outcome of their disease and its implications, may fare less well, if forced to accept information. Those who cope best by knowing about what is happening to them may not improve faster if information is withheld. Skills in assessment are clearly required, if clinicians are to determine how patients best cope. Communication skills should be applied in routine practice to improve preparation of patients before surgery.

Communicating with the Dying and Bereaved: Studies of patients dying in hospitals or at home have found that many of their problems continue unabated because they are not recognised by their clinicians or disclosed by the patients. Even problems like nausea, breathlessness, pain, anxiety, depression and mental confusion, which cause much distress to patients and relatives, are often unknown to the clinicians (Cartwright, et al, 1973). There has been little systematic study of how clinicians relate to the recently bereaved. However, it seems likely that they often feel inadequate when called upon to do so, especially when faced with strong feelings of sadness or hostility and when they feel upset by the death.

There is no doubt that many clinicians feel especially inadequate when confronted with communication with seriously ill patients, especially those suffering from cancer, the dying and bereaved. They have usually emphasised the use of listening skills, clarification of the patient's feelings, needs and wishes, and the importance of being alert to verbal and nonverbal cues. Thus, training in this area is very important for all clinicians.

Recent work by Hinton (1979) suggests that willingness to communicate more frankly with patients who are dying leads to a reduction in their anxiety, depression and irritability. Moreover, he found that patients prefer this openness and appeared less troubled by thoughts of dying and more prepared to discuss it than patients who had been spoken to less honestly. Attempts to counsel those bereaved people who are at high risk of developing psychosomatic or psychiatric illness have also had encouraging results (Parkes, 1980). They appear to reduce the risk of a poor outcome to that of low-risk groups. Therefore, it would seem worthwhile to give clinicians and medical students more training in the relevant skills (also see Chapter 14).

Breaking Bad News

Few responsibilities demand more of the clinician than that of breaking bad news to patients. It calls for sensitivity, gentleness, honesty and willingness to be available and to be vulnerable, done in the right way, it can facilitate the patient's adjustment to his/her situation by relief of uncertainty, in itself therapeutic, and by clarification of what must be faced.

There is also evidence that although clinicians may think that they have broken the news, the message may not have been received or at least, retained by the patient. The truth may be marked by language, may be too technical for the patient to understand. Again, a single communication may be insufficient for a listener distracted by pain or anxiety to take in. A recent study of a group of dying patients who were aware of their condition revealed that only 13 per cent had received the news from their clinician. Anxiety and fear generated in patients when they were given insufficient information, and makes a plea for better clinician-patient communication. Thus, there is reason to believe that clinicians may not be communicating as much to patients as the literature suggests or as they imagine themselves to be.

Given that the communication of bad news is an integral part of medical practice, how does the student or practicing physician acquire the requisite knowledge to manage these situations? A search of the literature in the area is discouraging; little seems to be known about the actual process of giving bad news. There is, however, much more information concerning the needs and wants of patients and the effect that receiving bad news has on them.

There are at least three distinct positions on what information to convey to patients who have a serious illness. The first position is that patients should always be given full information regardless of their individual perceptions or needs. Second view states exactly the opposite; that under no circumstances should patients be informed that they have acquired a fatal disease, and that falsehood and deception should be used if necessary, on the basis that the patient needs protection from the terrible reality of terminal illness. A third view suggests a more flexible approach, with a variety of psychological and sociological factors to be taken into consideration, but without guidelines as to how this might be done.

In difficult situations like informing about the fatal diagnosis, the clinicians often have doubts regarding the manner, extent, place, and time, when the clinician should communicate with the patients. Here are some guidelines for communication in such situations.

What to tell? The truth if at all possible. Establish the diagnosis by histology (e.g. malignant disease) or radiological or biochemical evidence. Try to use clear nontechnical language. Tell the truth calmly while sitting at the same levels as the person to whom you are speaking. Also discuss treatment options.

When to tell? When all relevant results are available, a full diagnosis with implications of treatment and prognosis can be given. It may be easier to give the diagnosis in stages; a clinical impression in the first stage, the results of relevant investigations or histology later when you have the reports, and the operative findings once the patient has recovered sufficiently to understand. Try to tell the patient and relatives as soon as possible.

Whom to tell? Tell the patient but use discretion when the prognosis is very poor. Permit the patient to ask questions, related to his illness, treatment, and stay in the hospital if required. He has a right to know what is happening to him. Discuss the clinical implications of the diagnosis with the closest relatives. Reassure them that a truthful approach will permit maximum cooperation from the patient and also justify future admissions, treatments, or continued follow-up at hospital, etc.

Where to tell? Speak to the patient or his relatives in privacy not in the corridor. If in the open ward, draw the screens and ask the nurse allocated to the patient's care to accompany you.

Who tells? Junior resident, senior resident, consultants, or staff nurses. Every consultant has his own policy of communicating to the patient, so it is advisable to follow his policy. Nurses are often asked about the diagnosis or result of an operation during the delivery of care, so they should be involved. After telling the patient, be prepared to talk to him again. When the initial shock has passed there may be many questions. Others may be relieved to have a diagnosis for their troublesome symptoms. Some may accept the situation without further discussion.

Communication skills to break bad news: In the absence of formal training, it is likely that whatever communication skills physicians have acquired by the time they enter practice have either been self-taught or patterned on those of their clinical teachers. Opportunities to observe instructors communicating bad news are rare. Furthermore, it is likely that these teachers learned their skills in the same way one generation earlier. Considering the issues in this perspective, it may not seem quite so unreasonable that patients do not see their physicians as possessing adequate communication skills.

Without formal training or an awareness of the scientific information that exists in the area, there is little else left to do than improvise and develop strategies based on personal social experiences acquired before becoming a professional. Physicians approach communication with patients in different manner from their approach to clinical problems-solving, the latter is much more likely to be managed through the use of rational strategies that depend on the conscious mobilisation of scientific knowledge than the former. Professional communications are often managed in the same way as social communications that were developed prior to professional training and without reference to scientific information.

Strategies to communicate bad news
1. *Have a plan in mind before starting*—The communication of bad news is a difficult activity and cannot be properly executed by relying on the rules of communication utilised in social encounters. Patients will almost

certainly be handicapped to some degree during the encounter because of fear, and the introduction of uncertainty into their lives. The patient will likely look to the physician to provide support and guidance to a greater degree than usual. Indeed, a few patients may require very directive advice until they regain their equilibrium. Emotions are contagious, and intense emotions interfere with clear thinking. In the face of a very upset patient, the physician who has not thought through his management plan before introducing the bad news begins to feel the pressure of having to solve problems as well as attend to a distressed patient. Having a set of general rules about how to manage communication of bad news and having tentative management plan for the specific problem before beginning the process, leaves the physician free to deal with what happens in the here and now, rather than having to think about routine matters. It is however, probably very important to provide the patient with a management plan of some kind during an encounter in which bad news is broken. Recent evidence suggests that health-related problems favour emotion-focussed coping, and that situations assessed as unalterable—or where no action can be taken—also favour this kind of response.

2. *Give the patient control over the quantity and timing of the information he receives*—Even the patient who wants to know everything usually does not want to hear it all at once. A strategy commonly used by experienced physicians is to start the communication with very vague terms and become more specific as the patient asks for more information. It is also important to tailor information to each patient's concerns, knowledge and experience, because this reduces the risk of causing unnecessary worry or discomfort. A patient who is told he has a carcinoma of the transverse colon, may have more concerns about having a colostomy than having cancer *per se*. It is only by asking the patient about his specific concerns that this can be determined.

3. *Allow the patient time to integrate information*—Even in situation where non-fatal illness is being discussed, there is a limit to the amount of information that patients can incorporate at any given time. As the seriousness of the illness becomes greater, so does the potential impact on the patient, which in turn will diminish the individual's ability to hear and incorporate new information.

4. *Soften the bad news with good news by providing some hope*—Patients want and are appreciative of any information that provides hope. Certainly, the more advanced the disease the poorer the prognosis, but no one can be sure which patient will do well in spite of the severity of the disease. For each individual, the distance between being and not being on this earth in infinite. Making the journey from immortality to mortality is painful and takes time. One of the commonly used mechanisms to better this process is denial, which is an essential and normal adaptive mechanism under certain circumstances. It can buy time and comfort for the patient while he completes his underlying grief work and is thereby better able to confront the realities of the situation. Supporting a patient's denial while he is incorporating bad news may be not only humanitarian, but also constructive.

5. *Never tell the patient a falsehood*—Patients need information to make intelligent decisions about their own treatment, but they do not need to know all the details about the course, the prognosis of their disease to do so. Patients also need more general information about their illness and how it

might affect them, so that they can plan for the future.

Every patient physician and situation is different. The flexible use of any strategy will be the only appropriate basis on which to approach the problem. The communication of bad news will never be pleasant, but it can be rewarding for the physician who knows that his planning, and his communication skills have made the situation a little less unpleasant for the patient.

Communication in Other Important Situations

In a document prepared by WHO, there is a list of special situations where communication skills play a very important role. These are:
1. Special groups of population: with language and cultural differences, with families or couples.
2. Special groups of disorders: disabled (blind, deaf, paraplegic, etc.), mentally retarded, chronically ill, terminally ill, depressive and/or suicidal patients, AIDS, STDs, chronic pain, speech impediments, problems of addiction, somatoform disorders, neurotic disorders.
3. Special personality problems: noncooperative patients, hostile patients, overdependent patients, inhibited patients, overdefensive patients.
4. Special clinical situations: giving bad news, dealing with sensitive issues (sexual, etc.), telephone contact, preparation for threatening diagnostic, treatment procedures, vaginal examination, surgery, etc. when speaking to others (e.g. relatives) about a patient.

Assessment of Communication Skills

Assessment of communication skills comprises an evaluation of the student's:
1. ability to understand his patient;
2. ability to communicate his view point to the patient and his family members;
3. ability to explore and answer patient's questions keeping in mind the patient's frame of reference which includes the psychological connotations of patient's complaints, his wishes, expectations and fears, i.e. everything that patient has thought and felt about his problem.
4. ability to propose solution to the problems and to motivate patients for compliance with treatment.

Assessment of communication skills has the dual function of educational feedback for the student and evaluation of his skills or performance. Ideally, the assessment should be linked with the teaching of communication skills. The context in which communication is to take place, should be kept into consideration during the assessment.

The commonly used strategies to assess communication skills are as follows:
1. Observation in routine setting, e.g. during clinical rounds.
2. Observation in a structured situation: 10-15 minutes interview session on a preselected topic; a checklist can be prepared to assess the various components of communication used/unused by the candidate.
3. Listening triad: A role-play exercise in which 3 students take the role of clinician, patient and an 'observer'. The observer records the ensuing interviews, which form the substance for discussion and feedback.
4. In many Western Universities, closed circuit TV monitors are used to assess the manner in which a student interviews the patient. In our set up, use of this method would require few years to become feasible.
5. Communication skills have also been assessed through OSCE (Objective structured clinical examination) stations. OSCE may be used to gather specific information from the patient, or telling mother the advantages of breastfeeding to her newborn child. Simulated or real patients may be used in

the OSCE stations. The assessment can be objectivised using a rating scale or a checklist.

6. Students may be asked to maintain a 'log book', recording write-up of the various exercises and activates related to communication. This is constantly supervised by the teaching staff.
7. The students may view the videotape of an interview situation and point out or answer to the specific questions, such as nonverbal behaviour of the patient.

SUMMARY

Communication is an act of imparting knowledge or exchanging thoughts, feelings or ideas by speech, writing or gestures. Communication in medical practice means interaction between two people—the clinician and the patient. It is recognised that in some hospitals the amount of time a patient clinician have in contact with each other is extremely limited. Constraints may also include lack of space and lack of privacy, with number of patients crowding a room or crowding around the clinician's table. Doctor-patient communication skills can help a clinician be more efficient and effective particularly when such constraints exist. Using communication skills and being innovative can enhance the outcome of the consultation, e.g. using a curtain/screen, or a specific chair to single out the patient currently being seen, focussing full attention on that patient, using appropriate nonverbal communication, and clarifying comments. One may have to priorities patients for additional interviewing and call them back at a more convenient time. More effective use of paraprofessional staff may promote better communication.

Components of communication skills include: appropriate physical environment, greeting patients, listening, empathy and warmth, respect and interest, language, nonverbal communication and closing of the interview. Communication is used for gathering information, but the studies have shown lots of deficiencies in history taking due to lack of communication skills.

There are specific situations in which communication skill are necessary, some of these situations are: motivating patients for treatment compliance, talking to seriously ill, dying patients and bereaved, preparing patients for major investigations, patients with specific disorders like suicidal, depressed, breaking bad news to the family. Special training and use of strategies can be helpful in developing these skills.

Assessment of communication skills can be helpful to students in providing feedback to improve upon these skills.

24
Illness Behaviour

A 50-years male patient is admitted with GI bleeding. On detailed examination, it is observed that this patient has multiple painful disorders like arthritis, diabetes, chronic renal failure, yet this patient is very calm and does not complain of distress or pain. You find him cooperative and his compliance to treatment is good.

A forty-five-year-old male has a minor injury on left leg, he is screaming with pain. He is preoccupied with his injury, and demands full attention from his wife and children. He does not even look after his personal care and is also fed by his wife.

These two cases illustrate the extreme types of behavioural response to illness often encountered in clinical practice. There would be many patients responding in between these two extremes of behaviours. Responses to symptoms and illness can vary considerably in individuals. Illness behaviour is the manner in which persons monitor their bodies, give meaning to their symptoms, and their perceptions of the illness. This has implication on utilisation of various sources of help and health care system. When response to illness is disproportionate to the extent of symptoms or illness, a maladaptive behaviour is presumed. This chapter will help you to understand variations in illness behaviour, how an individual develops an abnormal illness behaviour, its modification and prevention strategies.

Illness Behaviour

The concept of illness behaviour, according to Mechanic (1978), refers to the ways in which an individual perceives, evaluates and reacts to their symptoms. Pilowsky (1977) has defined illness behaviour as 'the way in which individual's react to aspects of their own functioning, which they evaluate in terms of illness and health'. Illness behaviour also refers to any behaviours that involves help seeking and contact with health care provider. As the help seeking behaviour is different amongst patients and can influence the treatment, so it is important to understand the variety of responses to illness—both normal and abnormal. Understanding the nature of human behaviour in health and disease has greater utility in clinical practice as no two patients respond to their illness in the same manner. By understanding the patients' interpretation of illness, his fears and anxieties associated with his interpretation of the illness can be reduced. There are several determinants of help seeking behaviours. These are related to perception of the symptoms, individual needs, available alternate interpretations of the symptoms, treatment availability and cost. Mechanic has described two different levels at which the determinants can operate—'other-defined 'and 'self-defined'. Other-defined refers primarily to situations in which other people evaluate the person's illness behaviour. Like how family members and close associates evaluate abdominal pain in a six years old child. Usually, others defined is applied to children and people with major psychiatric problem. Self-defined refers to situations in which the individual perceives and evaluates his or her own symptoms. When self-defined and other-defined levels differ significantly, then the concerned individual may be forced into treatment. The expression of illness behaviour is both influenced by cultural patterns or norms and social learning at home.

Sick Role

The sick role, a related term was formulated by Parsons (1964). This involves an exemption from normal duties and obligations, provided that the sick person is neither responsible for his disability nor able to terminate it by an act of will. Pilowsky (1978) has defined illness as a 'state of the organism which fulfils the requirements of an appropriate reference group for admission to the sick role'. An appropriate reference group means that group, which is most able or willing to meet the social cost of the illness. Disease on the other hand, is the constellation of objective data, which doctors believe, ought to qualify as an illness. Illness is characteristic of an individual with distinct social significance.

Whenever a person cannot fulfil social roles adequately, he can adopt a sick role, e.g. when a person is not able to work, by adopting sick role he gets an excuse from the society for not working. There are four basic components to the sick roles:

1. *Absence of responsibility*—The patient's inability to perform social roles is not considered to be under that person's volitional control, he needs some treatment or curative process before he can engage in expected social roles.
2. *Exemption from performing social roles*— The type of exemption depends on the severity and nature of the illness. The person suffering from cancer has different exemption of social roles, as compared to person having diabetes.
3. *Being sick is undesirable*—So, the person is obligated to seek help and cooperate with others to recover. He has a responsibility of getting well as soon as possible.
4. *Seeking adequate help*—The person adopting the sick role must seek out and comply with the prescribed treatment.

The sick role gives the possible benefit of exemption from role obligations but in return, the person is expected to recover by seeking help and complying with treatment. At the onset of illness, the individual may adopt the sick role by resting and not performing his social roles. But if the illness is prolonged, it gradually affects other family members, children, friends and work associates. These other people also play a very important role in granting the sick role. Illness behaviour also includes the ways in which individuals react to aspects of their own functioning, which they evaluate in terms of health and illness. In our Indian context, these factors play a very important role, as family members tend to overprotect and encourage sick role.

Abnormal Illness Behaviour

Abnormal illness behaviour is diagnosed when individual illness behaviour does not follow the socially accepted sick role process. These are generally psychiatric illness where no apparent organic cause is present or in cases in which the sick role is no longer adaptive. These disorders are generally labelled as somatoform disorders, conversion reaction or hypochondriasis. Pilowsky had classified abnormal illness behaviour (AIB) as "illness affirming" and "illness-denying syndromes". Both of these categories are important as in illness affirming, the patient becomes convinced of the disease underlying the disorder, e.g. for persistent cough patient assumes that he has tuberculosis or cancer. In contrast, patients with 'illness denying' type, minimise or negate the existence of a significant illness. A patient with heart attack presumes that the chest pain was due to gastric upset. The other factors important in classification are motivation for AIB, which could be conscious or unconscious in both the illness affirming and illness-denying categorists.

Causes of Maladaptive Illness Behaviour

Why some individuals react to illness in an adaptive manner whereas others react in a maladaptive manner depends on various factors. These factors generally originate from interaction between personal and environmental factors. Some of the important causes of maladaptive behaviour are disposition, sociocultural, psychodynamic and social learning (Fig. 24.1).

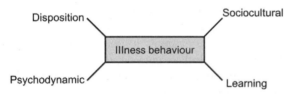

Fig. 24.1: Factors influencing illness behaviour

Disposition

Some patients seek care readily for even minor symptoms; others are reluctant to seek care for even life-threatening illnesses. There can also be considerable variability in an individual's responses from one situation to another and over time.

Illness behaviour is related to patient's appraisals of their symptoms, the assumptions they make about causes, and responses to medical advice are conditioned by patients understanding of their bodily responses. Studies consistently demonstrate major inconsistencies between physicians' expectations and assumptions and patients' responses, resulting in poor communication and difficulties in treatment. Leventhal and his colleague (1985) found, for example, that while physicians assume that patients with hypertension cannot make judgements of their blood pressure, many patients feel confident in their abilities to assess when their blood pressure is high or low, and they adjust their treatment regimens accordingly. Knowing the physicians view, they withhold communicating their assumption or information about modifications or regimen. Understanding illness by patient's perspective offers potential for improved communication and more appropriate therapeutic instruction.

The variability in patient behaviour in a given subculture despite similarity of symptoms also reflects major differences in psychological orientations and predispositions.

At a simple level, people vary in their tolerance for discomfort, the knowledge, information and understanding they have about the illness progress, and the specific ways bodily indications affect needs and ongoing social roles. People seem to vary great deal in their subjective response to pain and discomfort, although there appears to be much less difference in physical thresholds.

Sociocultural Influences

The extraordinary differences among cultures and characterisations, illness conceptions of causation, and modes of treatment are substantially documented in the anthropological literature. Even in modern populations, one finds a blend of sophisticated scientific ideas and folk wisdom. Such cultural content affects the recognition and conceptualisation of symptoms, the vocabularies for communication, modes and content of expression, and the range of remedial efforts attempted.

Sociocultural influences on illness behaviour are transmitted through families. The expression of illness through psychological and social vocabularies is a relatively modern phenomenon coexistent with growth of personal self-awareness and broad self-expression.

Psychodynamic

According to psychodynamic view, conceptualisation of illness behaviour relates to an unconscious gratification and measuring for bodily symptoms and physical suffering. The symptoms and suffering can represent (1) an alternative channel to deflect sexual, aggressive, or oral drives or (2) an ego defense against guilt or low self-esteem (Nemiah, 1980). Physical suffering can serve as a defense against guilt, providing well-deserved punishment for past wrongdoing. Support for these mechanisms is searched for in the early developmental stages of life, and such factors as parental care during illness or identification with a chronically disabled sibling or parent are important candidates for research.

Social Learning

Illness behaviour represents a complex set of behaviours that evolve and are maintained through learning processes like modelling and reinforcement. The social learning model generally conceptualises chronic illness as a function of two major factors: the consequences of illness behaviour and the premorbid state of the individual. In terms of the consequences of behaviour, the concept of reinforcement or secondary gain is crucial. The patient, who adopts or develops the illness behaviour pattern, may receive environmental support for this continuing disability or sick role. Another major hypothesis that the social learning model proposes is that abnormalities in the individuals before the report of the symptoms or disorder may play a role in maintaining the illness behaviour. That is, the premorbid state of the individual or his or her behavioural style may affect the types of illness behaviour the individual subsequently engages in. A common clinical observation with patients experiencing chronic disability uncorrelated with organic disease is that these patients very often lack the social skills that would assist in facilitating recovery.

Cognitive perceptual abnormalities have also been suggested as the cause of abnormal illness behaviour. These possible mechanism are indicated by: (1) patients amplify and augment normal bodily sensations; (2) patients misinterpret bodily symptoms of emotional arousal and normal bodily function; and (3) a constitutional predisposition to think and perceive in physical and concrete terms in contrast to emotional terms, setting the stage for symptom preoccupation. According to Barsky and Klerman, these mechanisms suggest that perceptual defect is the primary underlying disorder, not the illness behaviour itself.

Psychosocial Adaptation to Illness

Physical illness is perceived as a stress and individuals differ in their ability to cope up with stress. Physical illness is considered as a major life crisis that causes physical and psychological disorganisation. A crisis should be resolved in short life span, as any illness makes the individual sensitive he loses key life roles and undergoes changes in appearance and bodily functioning. He may feel helpless and develops unpleasant feelings as anger, guilt and at times, depression.

Adaptation to illness depends on background, personal characteristics, factors related to illness, and physical and social environment. The patient and his family face special problems related to illness like dealing with pain, then they have to adjust to hospital environment and have to develop relationship with the doctors and nurses. The patient has to cope with aversive treatment like frequent pricks, waiting for and undergoing investigations, etc. Many patients do not express their feelings of sadness, anger and hopelessness; they keep these feelings to themselves but it is manifested in their behaviour.

Family members also do not know how to help the patient to overcome these feelings. The patient needs to achieve a reasonable emotional balance, perception of an adequate self-image and feeling of competency. During serious illness, social support to the patient and the family is important. It helps the patient to recover faster with less medication.

During illness, various individuals use different types of coping strategies, these may be adaptive or nonadaptive. Moos and Tsu (1977) have described several types of coping skills. These are: (1) denying or minimising the illness, e.g. heart attack is taken as gastric problem by the patient, (2) seeking relevant information, e.g. learning about the seizures/cause and course of a renal failure, can help the patient feel more in control and know better what to expect, (3) seeking reassurance and emotional support from family, friends and health care professionals. Some patients join special group, national group for haemophiliacs, cancer, alcoholic anonymous, (4) learning specific illness relevant procedures, setting concrete goals, rehearsing alternative outcomes and finding a general purpose or pattern of meaning are also skills that can help patients to cope with their illness.

The journey to recovery is influenced by many factors like age, intelligence, beliefs, past coping experience, and personal characteristics of the individual patient. Religious beliefs are very crucial in Indian culture as a source of coping. Developmental factors should be considered in case of child patients.

Besides providing the medical/surgical illness, it is critical to evaluate the biopsychosocial environment of the patients, an individual assessment to understand the particular patient, is mandatory to develop a good doctor-patient relationship understanding and application of these factors help in speedy recovery and can prevent many consumer protection problems for the physician.

Management of Abnormal Illness Behaviour

Abnormal illness can be modified by psychological techniques. The use of cognitive therapies in the modification of illness behaviour is based on the rationale that faulty or irrational patterns of thinking modulate maladaptive emotions and behaviours. Wooley, Blackwell, and Winget (1978) reported a treatment programme that focussed on enhancing the patient's ability to take independent action in coping with his or her illness. Wooley et al (1979) targeted specific goals to alter a patient's illness behaviour. These goals included (1) having the patient assume responsibility for his or her care, (2) decreasing the care-taking response by others, especially physicians and family members, (3) altering the social contingencies that supported illness behaviour, (4) decreasing the frequency of complains throughout hospitalisation and increasing achievement orientation, and finally, (5) collecting one-year follow-up data on the generalisation of success from target to nontarget behaviours. The treatment programme emphasised the elimination of social reinforcement for illness behaviour (through group therapy) by teaching the patient techniques directed at reducing physical symptoms (e.g. relaxation, distraction, biofeedback, and self-control programmes), initiating therapy directed at helping family members reconstruct the learning process that led to the development of illness behaviour in the patient, and establishing contingencies to support the patient's emerging sense of autonomy and independence. Anxiety and depression is often seen as a manifestation of illness behaviour, and chronically ill patients may show many of the features of a major depressive episode.

Rational emotive behaviour therapy is aimed at helping the patient identify irrational thoughts or beliefs that have self-defeating or self-destructive consequences and testing or challenging these beliefs in therapy sessions and in actual extra therapeutic situations (Ellis, 1977). This heightened perceptual sensitivity to bodily sensations, and their subsequent misinterpretation by the patient, may lead the patient to believe that he or she is the victim of some disease process (e.g. stomach cancer). Such a conviction may often precede the development of illness behaviour. Rational emotive behaviour therapy, therefore, would focus on the therapist first eliciting the precipitating external stimulus events, then determining the specific thought patterns (and underlying beliefs) that constitute the internal response to these events that generate negative emotions (e.g. anxiety, depression), and finally helping the patient modify these beliefs and thought patterns.

Lewinsohn et al (1982) have provided guidelines for implementing a treatment programme that attempts to assist the patient in (1) decreasing the frequency and the subjective aversiveness of unpleasant events in his or her life and (2) increasing the frequency of pleasant events in his or her life. The five steps suggested in accomplishing this goal include (a) daily monitoring of unpleasant and pleasant events, (b) relaxation training, (c) managing aversive events, (d) time management, and (e) increasing pleasant activities. The treatment programme is presented to the patient as problem solving, task oriented, and education. Compliance with the programme is facilitated through the use of contingency contracts, and an effort is made throughout treatment to keep the intermediate goal meaningful and specific for the therapist and the patient. The final stage of the treatment programme involves the therapist and patient planning tactics that would help the patient resist the pressure of the old environment and facilitate the practice of new skills. In order to gradually fade out therapist support and to assist the patient in an easier transition to the home environment, sessions toward the end of the treatment programme are spread out over several weeks. This latter approach is a common procedure in clinical behaviour therapy.

The patient is faced with the task of adapting to the numerous changes in his or her social and physical functioning. Moos and Tsu (1977) have delineated a model of coping with chronic illness, in which psychosocial intervention may be beneficial. These psychosocial interventions may be targeted at helping the patient both with illness related and general adaptive tasks. Often in the context of medical settings, psychosocial teams are consulted (consultation-liaison teams) to facilitate the patient's coping within this framework. Such an approach is believed to serve as a preventive measure for further medical complications, as well as the occurrence of illness behaviour.

At times, some additional procedures may also be used in the management of maladaptive illness behaviour. These techniques are primarily related to decrease anxiety or stress and to enhance social and interpersonal skills. The family should be included in the management programme because many maladaptive illness behaviours are reinforced and maintained by the family members.

Clinical Applications

The different perceptions, evaluations and responses to illness have, at times, dramatic impact on the extent to which symptoms interfere with usual life routines, chronicity, attainment of appropriate care and cooperation of the patient in treatment. Variables affecting illness behaviour usually come into play well before any medical scrutiny and treatment (Mechanic, 1978a).

An illness behaviour model permits the compatible integration of current social and behavioural science concepts regarding individuals as social organisms. It also allows for the future incorporation of new information of the interaction between biological state, psychological processes and social functioning. As these aspects of illness behaviour are considered an equally important dimension, with none having a prior superiority in understanding the nature of human behaviour in health and disease. An illness behaviour model may have greater utility for present and future interdisciplinary research, education and clinical practice than that which exists at present.

Illness behaviour is a dynamic process in which the sick person defines problems, struggles with them, and attempts to achieve a comfortable accommodation. Such processes of adaptation are partly learned and partly shaped by the social situation and influences in the immediate environment. The health professional thus can help to guide the process by suggesting constructive alternatives for the patient and by avoiding the reinforcement of distorted meanings and maladptive responses.

SUMMARY

Illness behaviour is a dynamic process in which the sick person defines problems, struggles with them, and attempts to achieve a comfortable accommodation. Illness behaviour involves the manner in which persons monitor their bodies, define and interpret their symptoms, take remedial action and utilise various sources of help. Whenever a person cannot fulfil social roles adequately, he can adopt a sick role, e.g. when a person is not able to work, by adopting sick role he gets an excuse from the society for not working. The basic components to the sick role are: (1) absence of responsibility, (2) exemption from performing social roles, (3) being sick is undesirable, and (4) seeking adequate help.

Abnormal illness behaviour is diagnosed when individual illness behaviour does not follow the socially accepted sick role process. Illness experience is shaped by disposition of the patient, sociocultural and social-psychological factors irrespective of their genetic, physiological and other biological bases. Psychodynamic and social learning also influences illness behaviour.

Cultural definitions, social development and personal needs shape the experience of illness and meanings attributed to physical factors that serve as its basis. While magnitude, severity, persistence and character of symptoms all effect and establish limits for personal and social definitions, there is great variability in what is perceived, how it is defined, the interventions that are considered and used, requests for support and special consideration and illness outcomes.

Physical illness is perceived as a stress and individuals differ in their ability to cope up with stress. Physical illness is considered as a major life crisis that causes physical and psychological disorganisation. A crisis should be resolved in short life span as any illness makes the individual sensitive, he loses key life roles and undergoes changes in appearance and bodily functioning. He may feel helpless and develop unpleasant feelings as anger, guilt and at times depression.

Abnormal illness can be modified by psychological techniques. The use of cognitive therapies in the modification of illness behaviour is based on the rationale that faulty or irrational patterns of thinking modulate maladaptive emotions and behaviours.

The different perceptions, evaluations and responses to illness have, at times, dramatic impact on the extent to which symptoms interfere with usual life routines, chronicity, attainment of appropriate care and cooperation of the patient in treatment.

Psychology of Pain

Try the following experiment in your class. Ask 10 students to prick their left index finger with a fine needle. Observe each student's facial expression and rate intensity of pain experienced by all the five. Some students would prick without feeling much pain, whereas some might scream and may not even prick the finger. After the prick, again observe the different behaviours of these students. Some may report pain long after the prick, others may keep looking and pressing the finger, yet others may not even bother about the prick. These differences in pain can be understood by learning psychology of pain.

Pain varies greatly in terms of duration, severity, quality, and the degree to which it interferes with adaptive functioning. There are several patterns of pain: pain may be acute, chronic-periodic, recurrent, chronic intractable-benign, or chronic-progressive (Turk, Meichenbaum and Genest, 1983). This differentiation is important because the pattern of pain may provide helpful information in formulating hypotheses regarding mechanisms involved in the development, exacerbation, and maintenance of the pain problem, and the pain pattern also relates to intervention planning.

Not all individuals suffering with chronic or recurrent pain find it impossible to cope with persistent pain. Many individuals are able to accept and cope with such disorders as arthritis, migraine, and back pain without abuse of medication, invalidism, and overuse of the health care system. Others however, develop a complex cluster of symptoms independent of the type of pathophysiology. These individuals display a constellation of problems, including personal and social difficulties as well as patterns of health care use that are quite consistent across pathologies. This cluster of problems has been called the chronic pain syndrome.

The recognition of the important role that psychological and social factors play in the maintenance of chronic pain complaints, has led to the systematic investigation of the utility of psychosocial parameters as predictors of treatment response in a wide variety of chronic pain conditions, and with different pain treatments.

It is commonly observed that chronic pain patients vary widely in their level of psychological and behavioural dysfunction. All too often, chronic pain becomes associated with psychological distress, especially depression (Romano and Turner, 1985); martial difficulties (Maruta et al, 1981; Ahern et al, 1985), vocational dysfunction, decreased ability to perform normal activities. Yet some chronic pain patients do continue to work, have minimal disruption of normal activities, and are not clinically depressed.

Now there is evidence that how a patient appraises and copes with his pain problem has a major impact on his psychological distress and physical disability. If causal relations between certain now pain-coping strategies and physical and psychosocial adjustment can be identified, then treatment programme can work with patients to increase the use of adaptive strategies and decrease the use of maladaptive coping efforts.

Gate Control Theory

Pain signals can be altered by a variety of psychological processes as they are transmitted within the nervous system. Pain is more than a simple transmission of sensory signals from a pain source ascending the spinal cord to the brain. Rather, it is the net result of a series of complex interactions of neurophysiological and neurochemical processes permitting such psychological processes as motivation, emotion, and cognition to modulate the pain experience. Melzack and Wall (1965) proposed a model that helps to explain the role of such psychological factors in CNS modulation of pain. The gate control theory of pain has had a profound influence on the conceptualisation and treatment of pain over the past two decades. It has been particularly important in stimulating interest in empirical research on psychological processes in pain and the use of psychological techniques in pain management. It has emphasised the need for the use of an integrative psychobiological approach to theory and practice in the area of pain and pain control.

Physiological and Psychosocial Models of Pain

Scientists have proposed various models to understand pain perception and tolerance. Initial attempts to understand pain were mainly from a physiological perspective. Later models have included the psychological or experiential aspects in modelling the human experience of pain.

The specificity model, or stimulus response model, was one of the original theories proposed. This model claimed that when peripheral sensory receptors are stimulated as a result of injury to the body, nerve impulses travel through the spinal cord to the brain. The intensity of pain is assumed to be a direct reflection of the activation of 'pain receptors'. Various treatment techniques that followed this model were effective for acute type pains, but not chronic pains.

The learning theory of pain distinguishes between the initial psychological reaction to a painful stimulus and the resultant behaviours. Respondent pain behaviours are actions that result from the actual nociception. Operant pain behaviours are actions that develop when the pain experience is linked to forms of reinforcement such as receiving pain medication, or attention, or being allowed to avoid unpleasant situation. The reinforcements encourage the pain behaviour to linger on and become separated from the original painful stimulus. If respondent pain behaviours last long enough, learning will occur and behaviours will then be controlled by the operant pain behaviours. In chronic pain, both respondent and operant pain behaviours may exist. Certainly, learning theory can contribute much to our understanding of cross-sectional (birth cohort) differences in response to stressors, including pain.

It is the psychological aspects of pain that adds complexity to understanding pain mechanisms and is an area of current debate. Pain may begin with the noxious stimulus that can lead to tissue damage, but it does not stop there. There also is cognitive appraisal of the stimulus as well as evaluation of the context in which the stimulus occurs. Finally, there is the affective dimension of pain.

Recently one pain model proposed that the affective dimension of pain is composed of two stages. The first of these stages is related to the immediate unpleasantness of the pain. The second is dependent upon subsequent ramifications of experiencing pain that are strongly influenced by subject variables.

According to Loeser (1982), the phenomenon of human pain can be divided into four categories: nociception, pain, suffering and pain behaviour. Nociception is the detection of tissue damage by transducers in the skin and deeper structures. Pain is the perception and interpretation of the nociceptive input by the highest parts of the brain. Suffering is the negative response to pain or to other emotion-laden events such as fear, anxiety, isolation, or depression. Pain behaviour is what a person says or does or does not do or say, which leads the observer to infer that the patient is suffering from pain.

The literature that addresses the psychological aspect of pain primarily examines people who experience chronic pain, as opposed to acute pain. Regardless of the classification, pain that persists can inhibit the person's functional capacities, emotional state, psychological condition, and socioeconomic status. The longer a person experiences chronic pain, the more the pain is likely to affect the psychological and social factors. Psychological conditions that are often found in people with chronic pain include depression anxiety, adjustment disorder, dysthymia, and personality disorder. For people with chronic pain of an organic nature, it is estimated that 20 to 40 per cent have major depression and 40 per cent have dysthymic disorder. Furthermore, the cause-effect relationship between pain and depression may go in either direction. Being depressed may lead to higher levels of pain, and high levels of pain may cause a person to become depressed.

People who have an internal Locus of Control (LOC) believe that they can affect their experiences/outcomes by their own behaviour. Studies have shown that chronic pain patients, who have external LOC as perception of pain, are more depressed than are those people with internal LOC (Skevington, 1983). In addition, locus of control in patients with chronic pain is significantly correlated with the use of pain coping strategies and psychological distress. People with more external or chance LOC are more likely to have increased pain and functional impairment because of ineffective use of coping strategies and avoidance of activity. Being sensitive to individual differences in personality factors may be beneficial in both the assessment and treatment of pain.

How pain perception affects the person's functional abilities. Research on people with spinal cord injuries has shown that the amount of distress associated with pain, is correlated to the extent to which the pain interferes with expected functional activities. Comparing paraplegic patients and quadriplegic patients with similar levels of chronic pain, paraplegics perceived the pain as more unpleasant or disturbing than did quadriplegic. This may reflect the greater potential for self-care in relation to functional activities among paraplegic. In another study of the effect of pain associated with menstruation, it was found that pain-related emotional distress was positively correlated with the perceived inference with functional activities.

Another factor that has been found to affect a person's pain experience is social support. Overall, the presence of social support is viewed as beneficial for recovery, rehabilitation, and adjustment to chronic disease. Research on the influence of social support on pain behaviour has demonstrated interesting results. The number of people available for support was not a significant factor, but the level of satisfaction with the support did influence pain behaviour of chronic pain patients. People who reported high levels of satisfaction with their support, demonstrated higher level of pain behaviour. The social support for these patients worked as a reinforcement to continue pain behaviours.

Psychological models of pain are not adequate to explain why pain experience varies from one individual to another. Locus of control, interference with functional activities, and social support are examples of psychological and social factors that influence the affective dimension of pain and pain behaviours. These examples are certainly not the limit of psychosocial factors influencing pain-related suffering and behaviour. Other examples include cognitive models, expectancies, socioeconomic status, cultural background, gender, religious beliefs, and social roles. Any of these may be influenced by chronological age in the later years of life. Furthermore, both actual and perceived social support are likely to be factors mediating chronic pain-related suffering resulting from degenerative processes in the elderly. This is likely as true in the long-term care setting as in the community dwelling.

Despite the great advances in our understanding on mechanisms of pain, there is still no single model or schema which completely describes the nature of the human pain experience.

Coping with Chronic Pain

Research has shown that people appraise pain in diverse ways and develop a variety of cognitive and behavioural strategies to help them cope with pain. Pain-coping strategies that are adopted and used over prolonged time periods, may significantly affect physical and psychological functioning. Behaviour therapists have developed treatment programmes designed to decrease maladaptive and increase adaptive pain-coping strategies. Such programmes have been developed from theoretical and common sense perspectives on what is maladaptive and what is adaptive, with little empirical testing of these ideas.

The Lazarus and Folkman (1984) model of stress, appraisal and coping provides a focus for clinicians and researchers in the identification of important variables to assess in studying adjustment in chronic pain problems.

Turner et al (1987) conducted analyses to learn more about how patients' beliefs about their pain related to the strategies they used for coping with pain. Patients, who believed they must accept their pain and that pain did not require them to hold back from what they would like to do, were more likely to use problem-focussed coping. These beliefs may be associated with low frustration, which may in turn allow far more objective and problem rather than emotion-focussed coping. Accepting one's pain was also associated with less seeking of social support, and it may be that acceptance of the pain leads to less frustration and distress and thus less need for information or support. Patients were also more likely to seek social support if they had not experienced previous episodes of pain. This points out the importance of viewing coping with a stressor as a process, with different coping strategies used at different phases. Seeking social support may be most useful in the early stages of coping with a pain problem, when uncertainty and anxiety are likely to be highest. Finally, Turner et al (1987) found that patients, who believed their pain would be resolved in four years, used significantly less avoidance. This is consistent with previous research indicating avoidance is expected when one perceives few alternatives for resolution.

Methods to Assess Pain Profile

Recent advances on the pain have led to greater appreciation of the multidimensional nature of pain. The critical role of motivational, affective and environmental factors in determining the behaviour of many chronic pain patients is being recognised. Learning and cognitive factors play an important role in changing human behaviour in response to environmental situation. Some models have been suggested that nociceptive input from tissue or the nervous system is not the sole determinants of individual pain behaviour. Motivational, affective, and environmental events should also be considered to be relevant factors in all chronic pain patients; particularly those in whom operant and psychological mechanisms are predominant.

Assessment methods are similar for both acute and chronic pain. Sometimes a distinction between pain as a state and pain as a trait is made. A state is a situation—specific condition of pain like postoperative pain. On the other hand, a trait is a relatively enduring tendency to feel or behave in a certain way of most of the times and across all circumstances. An example of this is chronic low back pain. As the patient endures pain for years, this pain affects his behaviour and activities.

To understand the complex nature of pain and successful remediation, good assessment is a prerequisite. One needs to quantify pain and also requires assessing illness behaviour, which may be normal or abnormal. It is important to assess the disability, suffering, behavioural and psychological factors involved in persistent, pain, in order to provide an appropriate intervention for altering pain behaviour.

Patients with chronic pain problems require comprehensive and time consuming assessment. What a patient with pain thinks or feels or behaves, might not be well-communicated to the doctor. Assessment of pain profile might serve the following functions:
1. To provide baseline material against which the progress and treatment can be compared.
2. To provide the therapist, with a detailed information about the nature of patient's medical condition, previous treatments, patient's perceptions of their pain, expectations about treatment, and patient's resources for handling pain.
3. To assist in the establishment of appropriate and objective treatment goals.
4. To examine the important role of significant factors in the maintenance of maladaptive behaviours and as resources in the changed process.

There are various methods to assess pain, depending upon the aim of the assessment, a combination of methods can be used, e.g. to assess the severity of pain one needs a method which can quantify the pain, on the other hand to understand the pain behaviour, psychological tests are used. List of all the methods used in the assessment of pain are given in Table 25.1.

Table 25.1: Methods of pain assessment

History of pain	Psychological evaluation
Quantification of pain	Life stress
Self-report	Psychological dysfunction
Questionnaire	Depression, somatisation
Behaviour analysis	Family

History of Pain

History of pain should include onset and course of pain, subjective feeling of distress and disability, finding of physical investigations, previous treatments, drug and alcohol use as well as abuse; perception of pain by family members, their expectations and history of pain in other family members; presence of psychiatric problem should be asked. Assessment of patient's adjustment at home and at work can provide clues regarding psychological implications for the individual.

Quantification of Pain

The aim of quantification of pain is to assess objectively severity intensity and duration of pain periods. Quantifiable scales are also used to evaluate the efficacy of different therapeutic treatments. Quantitative pain scales are broadly grouped as self-report on single dimension scales, which usually measures the intensity of pain. These include category rating scales, both verbal and facial scales, numerical scales and visual analog scales. The second group of scales intend to measure multidimensions of pain including the experience of pain. McGill Pain Questionnaire is the example of this group of scales.

Self-report: Patient's subjective report of intensity, frequency and duration of pain is elicited. This is the most commonly used method in clinical practice, but it has its limitations because of memory lapses on the part of the patient to report correctly.

Verbal descriptor scales: Verbal descriptors have been used for simple reporting of subjective pain. Melzack and Torgetson (1971) introduced the following scale for pain intensity: *Instructions*: Choose the word below; which best describes how your pain feels at this time.

Mild Discomforting Distressing Horrible Excruciating. Category judgement is not limited to words only; facial expressions of pain of varying intensity are placed on eight-point scale for assessment (Frank et al, 1982). The major advantage of such scales is that categories can be formed in native languages and is easy to use in clinical setting. The disadvantage of this scaling form is to remember or have a written form for the words and limited number of response categories. It also lacks statistical manipulations of categories.

Numeric rating scale: The simplest and most frequently used approach to assessing subjective pain is a numerical rating scale. Patients are asked to rate their pain on a scale from 0 to 10 or 100, on which 0 represents no pain and 100 indicates the worst pain. This approach is very commonly used in clinical practice by all of us. It is easily understood by a majority of our patients. By this approach, only intensity of pain is measured. An example of this approach is as follows:

Instructions: Choose a number from 0 to 10, which indicates how strong your pain is right now.

Visual analog scale: The visual analog scale (VAS) is considered to be one of the best methods available for the estimation of pain. It provides a continuous scale for magnitude estimation and consists of a straight line, the ends of which are defined as the extreme limits of pain. Having the patient mark the line to indicate pain intensity, and then measure the mark on either a 1-10 or 1-100 scale does scoring. An example of visual analog scale is: *Instructions*: Mark on the line below how strong is your pain right now. No pain the worst pain.

Pain maps: Measures of pain location can be made using pain maps (Keele, 1948), which are a simplified human outline. The patient is asked to shade those body areas in which pain is experienced. Pain maps have been reported (Mooney et al, 1976) to help identify those patients who complain of anatomically implausible pain and those who may exaggerate pain. As pain maps only help in locating the pain, additional scales to measure intensity of pain should be used.

It is important that the patients should clearly understand the two end points and they are free to indicate a response at any point in the scale. High correlation has been reported for VAS and numerical/verbal scales and is considered valid and sensitive. However, it has been reported that the completion of the scale is difficult for some patients. The other disadvantages are that measurement is too subjective, not suited for statistical procedures—unidimensional in nature, yields estimates of pain intensity only.

The primary limitations of the above-mentioned, unidimensional subjective scaling of pain resides in the strong risk of subjective bias and inability to assess the complex nature of the experience of pain. These simple scales can fail to yield reliable and valid measurement if care is not taken to ensure accurate reporting. In spite of these limitations, pain intensity measurements are the most commonly used tools as they are simple, inexpensive, easily understood and with culture fairness.

Questionnaires

As an alternative to single or unidimensional scales, multidimensional scales have been developed. The most widely used scale of this category is McGill Pain Questionnaire.

McGill pain questionnaire (MPQ): This questionnaire scales pain in three dimensions: sensory, affective, and evaluative (Melzack, 1975). The test consists of 20 sets of words that describe pain. The first 10 sets represent sensory qualities, the next 5 are affective, only one set numbered 16 is evaluative, and the last 4 sets are miscellaneous words. Patients have to select the sets that are relevant to their pain and circle the words that best describe it within each selected set. Each set has 2 to 6 words in varying intensity. One can score each dimension and a total score can also be obtained. It requires 5 to 15 minutes to complete the questionnaire.

At times Dartmouth Pain Questionnaire (Corson and Schneider, 1984) is used as an adjunct to McGill Pain Questionnaire. The advantage of using Dartmouth Pain Questionnaire is to get additional information on the quality of pain and on positive functioning or assets of the patient, instead of only deficits in functioning. MPQ though statistically is a sound tool, yet in our culture many patients cannot understand the vocabulary. As a clinical tool, MPQ helps in understanding the quality of pain, both in sensory dimension and in its impact on the affect (mood) of the patient.

Brief pain inventory (BPI): The Brief Pain Inventory has been reported as a quick, multidimensional, valid scale for measuring pain in cancer and arthritis patients (Daul et al, 1983, Cleeland, 1985). It measures analgesic medication, relief in pain, qualitative descriptions of pain and beliefs about the cause of pain, and areas of interference with quality of life. It also measures location of pain and intensity of pain on scales from 0 to 10.

West Haven-Yale multidimensional pain inventory (WHYMPI): This inventory is much briefer than McGill Pain Questionnaire (Kerns et al, 1985). It has 52 items divided in three parts:

i. Five general dimensions of the experience of pain, suffering, interference with normal family and work functioning and social support.
ii. Patient's perceptions of the response of others to displays of pain and suffering.
iii. Frequency of engagement in common daily activities. This scale has a much broader approach in assessment than the other scales. It is also linked to cognitive-behavioural theory and assesses on dimensions beyond subjective distress.

Pain perception profile (Tursky et al, 1982): It measures sensation threshold, uses magnitude—estimation procedures to judge induced pain, measures pain on intensity, reaction and sensation dimensions using psychophysical scaling of verban pain descriptions, and the three dimensions of psychophysically scaled verbal descriptors in a diary format for repeated assessment over time. This method is shorter and simpler than MPQ and more valid than VAS. For research purposes this method requires more validation work.

Memorial pain assessment card (MPAC): The MPAC scales pain, pain relief, and mood on visual analog scales and adds a set of adjectives reflecting pain intensity. Advantages of this method are that it is easily administered, takes no time and correlates highly with other scales.

Behavioural Analysis

In behavioural analysis, also known as Behavioural Assessment, pain is viewed as a set of behaviours. Pain states are characterised by certain consistent patterns, e.g. sighing, guarding, movements. Pain behaviour is operationally defined and measures are employed to assess pain by objectively recording the frequency, occurrence and setting of their pain-related behaviours. Behavioural methods for assessing pain generally include observational procedures in which independent raters record patient's physical behaviours by tallying over time and score in terms of frequency. Observations also include activities, which evoke pain.

Self-monitoring of pain related the patients themselves could do behaviours. Semi-illiterate patients in our setting can be trained to record intensity, frequency and duration of pain. In our psychosocial milieu, significant family members should also be involved in maintaining records of pain. The following information should be elicited during behavioural analysis: changes in patient's activities because of pain, changes in significant persons (spouse/parent/children) activities because of pain, patient's behaviour when in pain, family members responses to pain behaviours and well (no pain) behaviours, factors that increase or decrease pain, impact of pain on patient's personal, vocational, family, social and leisure-time activities.

Pain diary is useful in maintaining records of pain. A pain diary should include pain-relevant activity broken down into small blocks of time, such as hourly segments. Activities are categorised as walking, sitting, resting. Pain can be rated on 0 to 10 scale. It is also useful to record medication taken. An example of pain diary is as follows:

Activity, Pain Assessment Record Form

Date   Activities   Pain Level
Time   Sitting Walking Resting Thoughts Medication 1-10

The use of pain diary with pain patients offers several advantages:
i. It is not subject to distortion, as it is filled out at the time of pain.
ii. It provides information on patterns of normal activity related to pain.
iii. It is expensive.
iv. It provides information about patient's behaviour at home and at work.
v. It provides feedback to the patient at home as to which activities increase or decrease pain.
vi. It is possible to correlate behavioural patterns with severity of pain.

If systematic records are maintained, behavioural assessment can provide important information on various dimensions. One can also get information regarding reinforcing factors for pain behaviours.

Psychological Evaluation

To understand any persistent pain problem, for a number of reasons, comprehensive psychological evaluation is required. A pain problem originally can be caused by certain processes (e.g. trauma), but can persist for entirely different reasons (Fordyce, 1983). With continuation of pain for a longer period, the chances of psychological and behavioural processes increase, as pain and disability have profound effects on mood, vocational and interpersonal relationship. The aim of a psychological evaluation is to determine specific psychological factors causing pain and suffering. Psychosocial factors elicited can be correlated to the patient's problem and can also be useful in the selection of particular therapeutic approaches for a given patient.

Psychological evaluations of chronic pain patients are indicated in the following situations:
a. Medical evaluation fails to reveal a physical cause of the pain.
b. Physical findings are insufficient to explain the degree of pain behaviour.
c. Physical findings are only speculative or inferred.

A psychologic evaluation can be useful in all those cases in which the pain interferes significantly with the patient's ability to engage in normal activities or has disturbed interpersonal relationships, shows sign of psychological distress like depression, or secondary gains out of illness rederived.

Life Stress

Current stressors in the patient's life can contribute to psychophysiologic dysfunction, such as increased levels of muscle tension, illness behaviour and disability. Patient might use maladaptive coping strategies such as use of medication or alcohol. Pain, inability to engage in normal social, recreational, vocational, household activities and worry about the prognosis or cause of the pain often acts as a source of major stress. These stresses affect the patient's emotional functioning and interpersonal relationships.

Basic research is being directed to study the underlying psychophysiological processes, adaptational and coping mechanisms thought to mediate stress responses. Often, an association between pain and life stresses is seen in our clinical experience, although patients can initially deny or minimise the contributions of stress to their pain problems. The interview with the other significant family members frequently reveals information about stresses affecting the patient. It is difficult to identify stress factors in an initial interview and many patients might not have experienced major stress in the recent past. Interview during subsequent visits should be directed to elicit stress in the patient's work, marriage, children and other areas of his functioning. Treatment can be directed on the effects of stress on pain, suffering and family functioning.

Psychological Dysfunction: The emotional impact of chronic pain, disability, or progressive diseases can result in changes in psychologic functioning. Identification of psychologic dysfunction is often missed out in a large number of patients suffering from pain. This is probably due to a host of factors such as lack of clinician's knowledge concerning psychological disorders and lack of time spent with patients in discussing psychosocial issues. On the other hand, patients may deny or minimise psychological symptoms. The common psychologic dysfunctions are depression, anxiety and somatisation disorders. Another important concept that has recently emerged in relation to psychologic dysfunction is abnormal illness behaviour.

Depression: It is one of the commonest problems seen in pain patients. Therefore, this should be routinely assessed as part of the psychological evaluation. Assessment of depression should not be limited to asking about depressed mood. One should enquire about symptoms such as persistent irritability, fatigue, insomnia, lack of interest in day-to-day activities, and inability to participate in entertainment and leisure time activities. At times depressive symptoms can occur as a side effect of medication. Identification of depression can be done on the basis of clinical interview and brief rating scales such as Beck Depression Rating Scale and Zung Depression Scale. Depression can be easily treated by medication or cognitive therapy.

Anxiety: It is often associated with acute pain. If the patient has not been communicated by the treating doctor about the cause, pathology, treatment and prognosis, he fails to make an accurate appraisal of his condition. This often gives rise to anxiety. Some patients are anxious by temperament and acute pain symptoms are perceived as a threat to personal integration.

Somatisation disorders: The unconsciously motivated forms of abnormal illness behaviours are often manifested as somatisation disorders. These differ from hypochondriasis, as the patient denies preoccupations or fears about illnesses, but rather complains of pain and the consequences of the symptom. Often, patient enjoys secondary gains from pain, as he gets a sick role. Somatisation disorders can be assessed through clinical interview and on MMPI. These disorders are best managed by behaviour therapy.

Illness behaviour: This refers to the ways in which individuals think, feel and act in relation to their health status. Illness behaviour constitutes patient's total experiences in relation to pain, which are shaped by biological, psychological, and sociocultural influences. Illness behaviour can manifest as abnormal psychopathological state, in some patients. Abnormal illness behaviour (AIB) is defined as the persistence of an inappropriate or maladaptive more of perceiving, evaluating and acting in relation to one's own state of health (Pilowsky, 1978).

Assessment if illness behaviour is not required for acute pain problems. Illness behaviour is determined by psychological and behavioural factors operating upon the patient and his environment.

Family

In India, because of our strong bonds, family plays an important role in maintaining, reinforcing illness behaviour and also in providing a social support system necessary for treatment and rehabilitation of pain patients. To assess the probability of social reinforcement of pain behaviours it is important to ask from family members how they respond to the patient's pain. If family members are frequently responding to pain behaviours and providing 'sick role' to the patient, then these problems should be addressed in treatment. Research findings have indicated the role of family as a model for tolerating pain (Mehta and Dutta, 1993). The meaning of pain behaviours should be understood within the context of family and culture. Expectations of family regarding prognosis should also be elicited. In situations where patient activity is discouraged by family members, or excessive fear and anxiety are experienced by the spouse or other significant family member then counselling to family members should be given.

The psychologic evaluation of chronic pain problems is highly complex task involving a broad range of clinical questions and issues. Psychologic and behavioural factors involved in persistent pain disability and suffering, with a view to prescription of appropriate interventions for altering these patterns are needed. The outcome of this evaluation is a synthesis of the information gathered resulting in a list of problems reflecting contribution of specific psychologic and behavioural processes to the maintenance of suffering and pain behaviours.

Psychological Approaches to Pain Control

Pain is a prevalent and costly health problem. When pain persists beyond the "natural" course of an illness, extends beyond the typical time required for an injury to heal, or is associated with a progressive illness such as arthritis, the pain is designated chronic. Such costs are related to hospitalisation, outpatient treatment, medication, health care, surgery, loss of work productivity, and loss of income, disability payments and litigation settlements. The social impact of pain is also considerable.

An increasingly greater number of psychological treatments are available for the management of chronic pain. Different psychological treatment approaches are based on different theories and attempt to intervene according to those aspects emphasised by the theory. Interventions can be grouped in one of the four major areas: focus on pain behaviour, modulation of the pain experience, modulation of mood, and cognitive-behavioural functioning.

Operant Therapy

Operant therapy attempts to intervene at the level of pain behaviour and applies learning principles to the treatment of chronic pain.

Fordyce (1976) pioneered the operant treatment approach to chronic pain. The focus of this approach is on changing overt pain behaviours rather than on the patient's subjective experience of pain. Pain behaviours include avoidance of physical activity, medication use, verbal pain complaints, grimacing, and groaning. Thus, behaviours that can be observed and measured are the targets of intervention.

Pain behaviours are not assumed to solely reflect underlying pathophysiology, but rather are subject to influence of a variety of factors, including systematic environmental consequences of the patient's actions.

The goal of this form of treatment is to reduce pain behaviours, while simultaneously increasing well behaviours. Contingencies of pain behaviour are modified. Behaviours incompatible with pain behaviour, such as increased physical exercise, time spent on hobbies, and work are reinforced, and the patient's well behaviours are praised and attended to. In approaching chronic pain patients with this operant treatment procedure, it is recognised that the patient is experiencing subjective distress, but it is explained to the patient that this focus on the pain (defined by each individual's pain behaviour observed and reported) will be reduced if physical and social activities are increased, despite the presence of pain. The use of selective reinforcement for non-pain behaviour and extinction of pain behaviour by staff, in the case of inpatients, of family, in the case of inpatient and outpatient cases, is a major component of this approach.

The operant approach is also helpful for the management of medication abuse whereby a patient is taking narcotic analgesics contingent upon exacerbations of pain. The approach assumes that such a contingent relationship (increased pain-increased medication) reinforces pain and pain behaviour because of the positive consequence of the medication (pain relief or expected pain relief). The patient is, therefore, given medication at fixed intervals (e.g. every four hours), regardless of pain level.

Biofeedback Training

Biofeedback training typically involves providing information about physiological functions that are normally not in the patient's awareness. A specified target response, such as cervical muscle tension, is electronically monitored and information about changes in the functioning of the targeted response is relayed to the patient via various feedback devices (see Chapter 20). The goal is to use the feedback to teach the patient to pain problem.

Relaxation Training

Another treatment that attempts to modulate the pain experience is relaxation training (see Chapter 20). The goal is to teach the patient to discriminate between tension and thoughts that cause muscular skeletal pain or contribute to pain associated with some other type of health problem when tense. The relaxation approach has been used with a variety of chronic pain problems.

Hypnosis

Hypnosis is also used to modulate the pain experience. The actual hypnotic procedure typically varies, depending on therapist or patient, but the goals are generally similar. Goals can include altering the patient's negative perception of the pain, shifting it to a neutral or a positive one, enhancing positive self-statements, improving health-related attitudes, and instilling feelings of deep relaxation potentially incompatible with certain pain behaviours.

Cognitive-Behavioural Approach: Pain Inoculation

A cognitive-behavioural approach conceptualises chronic pain problems in terms of coping skill deficits in either the cognitive or behavioural domains. The goal is to help the patient develop more adaptive cognitive and behavioural responses to the physical problem. When discussing the cognitive approach, the patient is taught to identify negative, habitual thoughts related to pain; recognise the connection between thoughts and consequent feelings and pain; substitute more adaptive thoughts; and use coping strategies (such as relaxation, distraction, imagery), to reduce suffering. Often in conjunction with these cognitive strategies, the patient is introduced to operant conditioning principles, and a programme is established to reinforce nonpain-related behaviour, such as medication use. These methods have been reported to be very effective in all types of pain, all ages and in all cultures (Mehta, 1993).

Pain in Elderly

The beliefs and attitudes of the elderly pain patient have an important effect in shaping relationships with physicians. The patient's beliefs about his pain and its causes, perceptions of his physicians' beliefs, and his general attitudes towards health professionals, all directly affect the relationships and their outcomes. This is clearly reciprocal process: The physicians' beliefs, perceptions, and attitudes are equally important in determining the quality of the relationships and their outcomes. A commonly encountered popular belief is the linkage between aging, illness and impairment.

There is considerable variance in the beliefs of both elderly pain patients and their physicians. When there is a discrepancy in beliefs between the elderly patient and his physician, it influences the effectiveness of the patient-physician relationship. There is a substantial research literature in support of positive outcomes related to agreement between patient and physician about the importance of various aspects of an illness and its treatment. For chronic pain, views about appropriateness of certain kinds of treatments are often closely associated with beliefs about the origins of the pain. The redeeming effects of such patient-physician agreement have been found to include positive health outcomes. Greater conformity to prescribed treatment regimens and greater patient satisfaction.

Pottes and Silverman (1990) demonstrated the potency of physician beliefs and their effects on some areas of patient outcome. The patients of physicians, who viewed psychological concerns as important, were found to be less depressed and anxious than were patients of physicians who attached less importance to these factors. Similarly, patients of physicians who viewed a broad range of treatment components as important were found to have experienced less sleep disturbance and less general disability.

Many elderly pain sufferers have negative and even contemptuous views of the health care system. These views can represent substantial barriers to treatment if not addressed by the health professional. In a study of reasons for refusal of hospitalisation among elderly patients, negative perceptions of the health care system were the primary reason given by the refusers (Barry, Crescenzi, Radovsky, Kern, and Steel, 1988). These negative perceptions included previous negative experiences, fear of hospitals, and a mistrust of the medical system.

SUMMARY

There are individual differences in coping with persistent pain. Many individuals are able to accept and cope with such disorders as arthritis, migraine, and back pain without much of medication. Others however, develop a complex cluster of symptoms independent of the type of pathophysiology. These individuals display personal and social difficulties as well as patterns of health care use that are quite consistent across pathologies. This cluster of problems has been called the chronic pain syndrome.

Melzack and Wall (1965) proposed a model that helps to explain the role of such psychological factors in CNS modulation of pain. It has emphasised the need for the use of an integrative psychobiological approach to theory and practice in the area of pain and pain control.

Analysis of patient's appraisals and coping strategies is useful in understanding functional disability and distress in chronic pain patients. Attempts have been made to measure appraisals and coping strategies for chronic pain. Studies have consistently yielded certain important findings. First, passive coping strategies, catastrophising, and little perceived control over pain are associated with greater pain, depression and functional disability.

Psychological models of pain are not adequate to explain why pain experience varies from one individual to another. Locus of control, interference with functional activities, and social support are examples of psychological and social factors that influence the affective dimension of pain and pain behaviours.

Patients with chronic pain problems require comprehensive and time consuming assessment. To understand the complex nature of pain and successful remediation, good assessment is a prerequisite. One needs to quantify pain, assess illness behaviour, the disability, suffering, behavioural and psychological factors involved in persistent pain, in order to provide an appropriate intervention for altering pain behaviour.

Behavioural treatment for pain is related to decreases in patient catastrophising and increases in perceived control over pain, and these changes are associated with decreases in pain rating and disability. Finally, there is evidence that attention-diversion techniques, which are taught in many pain programmes, may not be useful for chronic pain. These findings suggest that the effectiveness of pain management programmes may be increased by interventions targeted at patient's sense of control over pain. This may be more important than training in specific coping strategies.

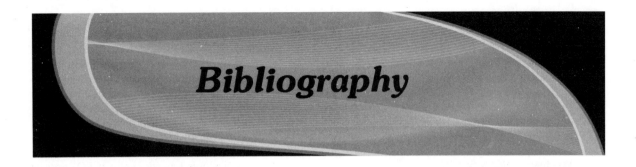

Bibliography

1. Ackerman NW. Treating the Troubled Family. New York: Basic Books 1966a.
2. Agras WS, Kazdin AE, William GT. Behavior Therapy: Toward and Applied Clinical Science (Ed) W.H. Freeman & Co. San Francisco 1979.
3. Ahern DK, Adams AE, Follick MJ. Emotional and marital disturbance in spouses of chronic low-back pain patients. Clin. J. Pain, 1985;1:69-74.
4. Allen KE, Harris FR. Elimination of a Child's Excessive Scratching by Training the Mother in Reinforcement Procedures. Behaviour Research and Therapy, 1966;4:79-84.
5. Allport GW. Pattern and Growth in Personality. London: Holt, Rinehart and Winston 1961.
6. Aman U, Khan MD. Clinical Disorders of Memory. New York: Plenum Medical Book Company 1986.
7. American Psychiatric Association. Diagnostic and Statistical Manual of Mental Disorders (Third Edition Revised). Washington, DC: American Psychiatric Association 1987.
8. Anastasi A. Psychological Testing. New York: Macmillan Publishing Company 1988.
9. Anderson and Anderson. An Introduction to Projective Techniques. New York: Prentice-Hall, Inc. 1951.
10. Anthony J, Marsella Velma A, Kameoka. Ethnocultural Issues in the Assessment of Psychopathology in Measuring Mental Illness. In S. Weltzer, Psychometric Assessment for Clinicians (Eds). Washington, DC 2005.
11. Apley J. The Child with Abdominal Pains. Oxford: Blackwell Scientific Publications 1975.
12. Atkinson JW, Birch DC. An introduction to motivation (2nd ed.). New York: D. Van Nostrand 1978.
13. Atkinson RC, Shiffrin RM. Human memory: A proposed system and its control processes. In K.W. Spence & J.T. Spence (Eds.), The psychology of learning and motivation (Vol.2). New York: Academic Press 1968.
14. Ausubel DP, Novak JS, Hanesian H. Educational Psychology: A Cognitive View (2nd Edition).New York: Holt, Rinehart, and Winston 1978.
15. Ausubel DP, Novak JS, Hanesian H. Educational Psychology: A Cognitive View. New York: Holt Rinehart Winston 1990.
16. Baile WF, Engel BT. A behavioural strategy for promoting treatment compliance following myocardial infarction. Psychosomatic Medicine, 1978;40(5):413-9.
17. Bandura A, Walters RH. Social learning and personality development. New York: Holt, Rinehart and Winston 1963.
18. Bandura A. A social learning interpretation of psychological dysfunction. In P. London & D. Rosenhan (Eds), Foundations of abnormal psychology. New York: Holt, Rinehart and Winston 1968.
19. Bandura A. Aggression: A social learning analysis. EngleWood Cliffs, N.J: Prentice-Hall 1973.
20. Bandura A. Principles of Behaviour Modification. New York: Holt, Rinehart and Winston 1969.
21. Bandura A. Social learning theory. Englewood Cliffs, NJ: Prentice-Hall 1977.
22. Baron RA. The reduction of human aggression: A field study of the influence of incompatible reactions. Journal of Applied Social Psychology, 1973;6:260-74.
23. Barrett J, Rose R. Mental Disorders in the Community. Progress and Challenge. New York: Guilford Press 1986.

24. Bateson G. Mind and Nature: A Necessary Unity. New York: Dutton 1980.
25. Beck A, Ward H, Mendelson M, et al. An inventory for measuring depression. Arch Gen Psychiatry 1961;4:561-71.
26. Beck A, Weissman A, Lester D, et al. Measurement of Pessimism: The Beck Hopelessness Scale. J Consult Clin Psychol 1974;42:861-65.
27. Beck AT, Ward CH, Mendelson M, et al. An inventory for measuring depression. Arch Gen Psychiatry 1961;4:561-71.
28. Beck AT. Cognitive Therapy and the Emotional Disorders. New York: International Universities Press 1976.
29. Beck AT. The development of depression: a cognitive model. In R.J. Friedman & M.M. Katz, The Psychology of Depression: Contemporary Theory and Research. New York: Wiley 1974.
30. Becker MH, Haefiner DP, Kasl SV, Kirscht JP, Maiman LA, Rosenstock IM. Selected psychosocial models and correlates of individual health-related behaviours. Medical Care, 1977;15 (Suppl.5) 27-46.
31. Bellak L. Psychological aspects of normal aging. In: Bellak L, Tosko BD (Eds). Geriatric Psychiatry. New York: Grune and Stratton 1976.
32. Benton A, Hamsher K, Varney N, et al. Contributions to Neuropsychological Assessment. New York: Oxford University Press 1983.
33. Berkowitz L, LePage A. Weapons as aggression eliciting stimuli. Journal of Personality and Social Psychology 1967;7:202-07.
34. Bigga JB. Learning strategies, student motivation patterns and subjectively perceived success. In JR Kirby (Eds). Cognitive Strategies and Educational Performance. Orlando: Academic Press 1984.
35. Billings AG, Moos RH. The role of coping responses and social resources in attenuating the stress of life events. Journal of Behavioural Medicine, 1981;4:139-57.
36. Blumer D, Hilbronn M. Chronic pain as a variant of depressive disease: The pain-prone disorder. The Journal of Nervous and Mental Disease, 1982;170(7):381-406.
37. Bonivs JI. Importance of the problem. In JJ Bonica, V Ventafridda (Eds). Advances in pain research and therapy (Vol. 2). New York: Raven Press 1979.
38. Bouchard TJ, Lykken DT, McGue M, Segal NL, Tellegen A. Sources of human psychological differences. The Minnesota study of twins reared apart. Science, 1990;250:223-28.
39. Bradley RH, Caldwell BM. Early home environ-ment and changes in mental test performance in children from 6 to 36 months. Developmental Psychology, 1976;12:93-97.
40. Brink TL. Geriatric Psychotherapy. In E Busse, E Pfeiffer (Eds). Behavior and adptation in later life (2nd ed.) Boston: Little, Brown 1977.
41. Broadbent D, Cooper P, Fitzgerald P, et al. The cognitive Failures Questionnaire (CFQ) and its correlates. Br J Clin Psychol 1982;21:1-16.
42. Brown GK, Nicassio PM. Development of a questionnaire for the assessment of active and passive coping strategies in chronic pain patients. Pain, 1987;31:53-64.
43. Bruner JS. Toward a Theory of Instruction. Cambridge, Massachusetts: Harvard University Press 1966.
44. Bush B, Shaw S, Cleary P, et al. Screening for alcohol abuse using the GAGE questionnaire. Am J Med 1987;82:231-35.
45. Butters N, Albert M. Process underlying failures to recall remote events. In LS Cermak (Eds). Human Memory and Ammesia. Hillsdale, NJ: Lawrence Erlbaum Associates 1982.
46. Cannon WB. The The James - large theory of quotions: A critical examination and an aternative theory -American Journal of Psychology, 1927;39:106-24.
47. Caprara GV, Barbaranelli C, Borgoni L, Perugini M. The Big Five Questionnaire –a New Questionnaire for the measurement for the five factor model. Personality and Individual differences 193;15:281-88.
48. Carver CS, Scheier MF. Control theory: A useful conceptual framework for personality-social, clinical, and health psychology. Psychological Bulletin, 1982;92:111-35.
49. Cattell RB. Abilities: Their structure, growth and action. Boston: Houghton Mifflin 1971.
50. Cattell RB. The Handbook for the 16 Personality Factor Questionnaire. Champaign, 1llionois: Institute for Personality and Ability Testing 1986.
51. Cattell RB. The Scientific Analysis of Personality. Penguin, Harmondsworth 1965.
52. Chambers WJ, Puig-Antich J, Hirsch M, et al. The assessment of affective disorders in children and adolescents by semi-structured interview: Test-retest reliability of the Schedule for Affective

Disorders and Schizophrenia for School-age children, present episode version. Arch Gen Psychiatry 1985;42:696-702.
53. Charney E, Bynum R, Eldredge D, et al. How well do patients take oral penicillin? A collaborative study in private practice. Pediatrics 1967;40:188-95.
54. Charney E. Patient-doctor communication: Implications for the clinician. Pediatr. Clin. North Am. 1972;19:263-79.
55. Chesney MA, Eagleston JR, Rosenman RH. The Type A structured interview: A behavioural assessment in the rough. Journal of Behavioural Assessment, 1980;2:255-72.
56. Cinciripini PM, Williamson DA, Epstein LH. Behavioural treatment of migrain headaches. In JM Ferguson, C Barr Taylor (Eds). The Comprehensive Handbook of Behavioural Medicine (Vol. 2). New York: Spectrum Medicial, 1981.
57. Copp LA. The spectrum of suffering. Am. J. Nursing, 1974;74:491-95.
58. Costa PT Jr, McCrac RR. Revised NEO Personality Inventory (NEO-pi-R) and NEO-five factor inventory (NEO-FFI) Professional manual. Odessa; FL; Psychological Assessment Resources 1992.
59. Craig KD. Social modeling influences on pain. In RA Sternbach (Ed). The psychology of pain. New York: Raven Press 1978.
60. D'Monte B, Pande JN. The use of Inquiry-driven strategies for innovations in medical education, AIIMS experience In: Verma K, D'Monte B, Adkoli BV, Nayar U (Eds). Inquiry driven strategies for innovations in medical education in India. AIIMS 1991;49-53.
61. Davidson PD. Issues in patient's compliance. In TI Millon, C Green, R Meagher (Eds). Handbook of Clinical Health Physiology. New York: Plenum Press, 1982.
62. Davis MS. Physiologic, psychosocial, and demographic factors in patient compliance with doctors' order. Medical Care, 1968;6:115-22.
63. De Benedittis G, Lorenzetti A, Fieri A. The role of stressful life events in the onset of chronic primary headache. Pain, 1990;40:65-75.
64. Derogatis L, Lipman R, Covi L. SCL-90: An outpatient psychiatric rating scale: Preliminary report. Psychopharmacol Bull 1973;9:13-27.
65. Derogatis LR. The Symptom Checklist-90 Manual. Towson, MD: Clinical Psychometric Research 1983.
66. Despande SN, Nehta M. Aversion Therapy in the treatment of tricollotomania J of Per and Clinical Studies 1990;6(1):145-47.
67. Dowling J. Autonomic indices and reactive pain reports on the McGill Pain Questionnaire. Pain, 1982;14:387-92.
68. Dunbar J, Stunkard A. Adherence to diet and drug regimen. In R Levy, B Rifkind, B Dennis, N Ernst (Eds). Nutrition, Lipids, and Coronary Heart Disease. New York: Raven Press, in press.
69. Eaton W. The epidemiology of Schizophrenia (Volume 1). G Burrows, T Norman, G Rubinstein (Eds). Epidemiology, Etiology, and Clinical Features. New York, Elsevier 1986.
70. Edelbrock C, Costello AJ, Dulcan MK, et al. Parent- child agreement on child psychiatric symptoms assessed via structured interview. Child Psychol Psychiatry 1986;27:181-90.
71. Edwards PW, Zeichner A, Kuczmierczyk AR, Boczkowski J. Familial pain models: The relationship between family history of pain and current pain experience. Pain, 1985;21:379-84.
72. Egbert LD, et al. Reduction of postoperative pain by encouragement and instruction of patients. J Med 1964;270:825-27.
73. Ellis A. Humanistic Psychotherapy: The Rational-Emotive Approach, Julian Press, New York 1973.
74. Ellis A. Irrational ideas (hand-out), Institute for Rational Living, New York 1977.
75. Ellis A. The basic clinical theory of rational-emotive therapy. In A Ellis, R Grieger (Eds). Handbook of Rational-Emotive Therapy. New York: Springer 1977.
76. Endicott J, Cohen J, Nee J, et al. Hamilton Depression Rating Scale: Regular and change versions of the schedule for affective disorders and schizophrenia. Arch Gen Psychiatry 1981;38:98-103.
77. Endicott J, Spitzer R, Fleiss J, et al. The global assessment scale. Arch Gen Psychiatry 1976;33:766-71.
78. Endicott J, Spitzer RL, Fleiss JL, et al. The Global Assessment Scale: A Procedure for measuring overall severity of psychiatric disturbance. Arch Gen Psychiatry 1976;33:766-11.

79. Endicott J, Spitzer RL. A diagnostic interview: The schedule for Affective Disorders and Schizophrenia. Arch Gen Psychiatry 1978;35: 837-44.
80. Entwistle NJ, Hanley M, Ratcliffe G. Approaches to learning and levels of understanding. Br J Educ Res 1979a;5:99-114.
81. Epstein NB, Bishop DS. Problem-centered systems therapy of the family. In AS Gurman, DP Kniskern (Eds). Handbook of Family Therapy. New York: Basic Books, 1981.
82. Erikson EH. Identity Youth, and Crises. New York: WW Norton 1968.
83. Eron LD. Prescription for reduction of aggression. American Psychologist, 1980;35(3):244-52.
84. Evans BJ, Standley RO, Mestorovic R, Rose L. Effects of communication skills training on students diagnostic efficiency. Med Educ 1991;25:517-26.
85. Eysenck HJ. Trait theories of personality. In AM Colman (Ed) Companion Encyclopedia of Psychology (Vol. 1) London: Routledge 1990.
86. Feuerstein M, Bush C, Corbisiero T. Stress and chronic headache: A psychophysiological analysis of mechanisms. Journal of Psychosomatic Research, 1982;26:167-82.
87. Fleming R, Baum A, Gisriel MM, Gatchel RJ. Mediating influences on social support on stress at Three Mile Island. Journal of Human Stress, 1982;8:14-22.
88. Fletchner CM. Communication in Medicine. London: Nuffieldi Provincial Hospital Trust 1973.
89. Fordyce WE. Behavioural methods for chronic pain and illness. St. Louis: Mosby 1976.
90. Fordyce WE. Learning processes in pain. In: RA Sternbach (Ed). The Psychology of Pain. New York: Raven Press 1978.
91. Freud S. Morning and Melancholia. Standard Edition, Vol. 14. London: Hogarth Press 1917.
92. Freud S. Three Essays on the Theory of Sexuality. Standard Edition, Vol. 7. London: Hogarth Press 1905.
93. Friedman EH. Systems and ceremonies: A family view of rites of passiage. In: EA Carter, M McGoldrick (Eds). The Family Life Cycle. Gardner Press, New York 1980.
94. Friedman M, Rosenman RH. Association of specific overt behaviour pattern with blood and cardiovascular findings. Journal of the American Medical Association, 1959;169:96-106.
95. Gagne RM. Essentials of Learning for Instruction. Hinsdale, Illinois: Dryden Press 1974.
96. Garb IR, Garb JL, Stunkard AJ. Effectiveness of a self-help group in obesity control. Arch. Int. Med. 1974;134:716-20.
97. Gardner H. Multiple intelligence: The Theory in Practice. New York: Basic Books 1993.
98. Gillum RF, Barsky AJ. Diagnosis and management of patient non-compliance. J Am Med Assoc 1974;228:1563-67.
99. Goldberg EL, Comstock GW. Epidemiology of life events: Frequency in general populations. American Journal of Epidemiology, 1980; 111(6):736-52.
100. Goldberg JO, Shaw BF, Segal ZV. Concurrent validity of the Millon Clinical Multiaxial Inventory Depression scales. J Consult Clin Psychol 1987;55:785-87.
101. Goldman SR, Hogaboam TW, Bell LC, Perfetti CA. Short-term retention of discourse during reading. Journal of Educational Psychology 1980;68:680-88.
102. Goleman D. Emotional intelligence. New York: Bantam Books 1995.
103. Gorer G. Death, Grief and Mourning. London: Crescent Press 1965.
104. Guilbert JJ. Educational Handbook for Health Personnel. WHO offset Publications No.35. World Health Organization. Geneva 1992.
105. Guilford JP. The structure of intellect. Psychological Bulletin 1956;53:267.
106. Haggerty RJ, Bloom SW, Mechanic D, Pardes H. Report of the commission's subcommittee on the Behavioural Sciences: In Medical Education in transition, Commission on Medical Education: The Sciences of Medical Practice. The Robert Wood Johnson Foundation 1993;74-78.
107. Haley J. Problem-Solving Therapy. Jossey-Bass, San Francisco 1976.
108. Hamilton M. Development of a rating scale for primary depressive illness. Bri J of Social and Clinic Psychol 1967;6:278-96.
109. Hamilton M. Rating depressive patients. J Clin Psychiatry 1960;41:21-24.
110. Harris, Louis, Associates. Inc. The public and high blood pressure. Unpublished survey conducted for the National Heart and Lung Institute, June 1973.
111. Hathaway SR, McKinley JC. Minnesota Multiphasic Personality Inventory (MMPI).

Minneapolis, University of Minnesota Press 1943.
112. Haynes DL, Sackett RB (Eds). Compliance with therapeutic regimens. Baltimore: Johns Hopkins University Press 1976.
113. Haynes SG, Feinleib M, Kannel WB. The relationship of psychosocial factors to coronary heart disease in the Framingham Study. American Journal of Epidemiology, 1980;lll (I),37-58.
114. Hebb DO. Textbook of Psychology (3rd Ed). Philadelphia: Saunders 1972.
115. Hefler RE. An objective comparison of the paediatric interviewing skills of freshman and senior medical students. Paediatrics, 1970; 45:623-27.
116. Heider F. The Psychology of Interpersonal Relations. New York: Wiley 1958.
117. Heilman KM, Valenstein E. Clinical Neuropsychology (IIIrd Ed) UK Oxford University Press 1993.
118. Helzer JE, Robins LN, McEvoy LT, et al. A comparison of clinical and Diagnostic Interview Schedule diagnoses: Physician reexamination of lay-interviewed cases in the general population. Arch Gen Psychiatry 1985;42:657-66.
119. Helzer JE. The use of a structured interview for routine psychiatric evaluations. J Nerv Ment Dis 1981;169:45-49.
120. Hess JW. A comparison of methods for evaluating medical student skills in relation to patients. J Med Educ, 1969;44:934-8.
121. Hill R. Family under stress. New York: Harper & Row 1949.
122. Hinton JM. The physical and mental distress of the dying. Quarterly Journal of Medicine 1963;32:1.
123. Holm JE, Holroyd KA, Hursey KG, Penzien DB. The role of stress in recurrent tension headache. Headache, 1986;26:160-67.
124. Holmes TH, Masuda M. Life change and illness susceptibility. In BP Dohrenwend (Eds). Stressful life events: Their nature and effects, New York: Wiley 1974.
125. Holmes TH, Rahe RH. The social readjustment rating scale. Journal of Psychosomatic Research, 1967;11:213-18.
126. Horn JL, Wanberg KW, Foster FM. The alcohol Use Inventory. Baltimore, Psych Systems 1983.
127. Hudson L. Contrary Imaginations, Methuen, London 1966.
128. Hughes JR, O'Hara MW, Rehm LP. Measurement of depression in clinical trials: an overview. J Clin Psychiatry 1982;43:85-88.
129. Hulka BS, Cassel JC, Kupper LL, Burdette JA. Communication, compliance, and concordance between physicians and patients with prescribed medications. Am J Public Health 1976;66:847-53.
130. Ilfeld FW Jr. Coping styles of Chicago adults. Description. Journal of Human Stress, 1980;6(2), 2-10.
131. Ivey A. Intentional interviewing and counselling. California: Brooks/Cole Publishing Company 1983.
132. Jackson H, Cooper J, Mellinger WJ, et al. Streptococcal pharyngitis in rural practice: Rational medical management. J Am Med Assoc 1966;197:385-88.
133. James W. What is an emotion? Mind, 1884;9: 188-205.
134. Janis IL, Mann L. Decision making: A psychological analysis of conflict, choice, and commitment, New York: Free Press 1977.
135. Jenkins CD. Recent evidence supporting psychologic and social risk factors for coronary disease. New England Journal of Medicine, 1976;294(18):987-94.
136. Jensen AR. The nature of the black-white difference on various psychometric tests: Spearman's hypothesis. Behavioural and Brain Sciences 1985;8:193-263.
137. Kagan A, Levi L. Adaptation of the psychosocial environment to man's abilities and needs. In: L Levi (Ed). Society, stress and disease. London: Oxford University Press 1971.
138. Keefe FJ, Block AR. Development of an observation method for assessing pain behaviour in chronic low back pain patients. Behaviour Therapy, 1982;13:363-75.
139. Keefe FJ, Caldwell DS, Williams DA, Gill KM, Mitchell D, Robertson C, Martinez S, Nunley J, Beckham JC, Crisson JE, Helms M. Pain coping skills training in the management of osteoarthritic knee pain: a comparative study. Behav Ther, 1990;21:49-62.
140. Khan AU. Clinical Disorders of Memory. New York: Plenum Publishing Corporation 1986.
141. Kohler W. The mentality of apes. New York: Harcourt, Brace & World 1927.

142. Kubler-Ross E. On Death and Dying. New York, MacMilan Publishing Co 1969.
143. Lambert MJ, Hatch DR, Kingston MD, et al. Zung, Beck, and Hamilton rating scales as measures of treatment outcome: A meta- analytic comparison. J Consult Clin Psychol 1986;54:54-59.
144. Lange C. The emotions. Baltimore: Williams & Wilkins. (Ongoing published 1885) 1922.
145. Lazarus RS, Folkman S. Stress, appraisal and coping. New York: Springer-Verlag 1984.
146. Lazarus RS. Patterns of adjustment. New York: McGraw- Hill 1976.
147. Lazarus RS. Positive denial: The case for not facing reality. Psychology Today. 1979;13:44-45.
148. Lazarus RS. Psychological stress and coping in adaptation and illness. International Journal of Psychiatry in Medicine, 1974;5:321-33.
149. Lazarus RS. Psychological stress and the coping process. New York: McGraw-Hill 1966.
150. Lazarus RS. Thoughts on the Relations between emotions and cognition. American Psychologists 1982;37:1019-24.
151. Levy RL. The role of social support in patient compliance: A review. In RB Haynes, ME Mattson, TO Engebretson (Eds). Patient compliance to prescribed antihypertensive medical regimens: A report to the National Heart, Lung, and Blood Institute, Bethesda, MD: National Heart, Lung and Blood Institute 1980.
152. Lewinson PM, Sullivan JM. Distraction and coping with pain. Psychological applications. In AJ Rush (Ed), Short-term psychotherapies for depression. New York: Guilford Press 1984.
153. Lewis CE, Resnik BA, Schmidt G, Wazman D. Activities, events and outcomes in ambulatory patient care. N Engl J Med 1960;280:270-273, 291.
154. Lewis CE, Resnik BA. Nurse and progressive ambulatory patient care. N Engl J Med 1967;277: 1236-41.
155. Ley P. Giving information to patients. In: Eiser JR (Ed). Social Psychology and Behavioural Medicine. London: John Wiley 1983;339-74.
156. Lindemann E. The symptomatology and management of acute grief. American Journal of Psychiatry 1944;101:141.
157. Linton SJ, Melin L. Applied relaxation in the management of chronic pain. Behavioural Psychotherapy, 1983;11:337-50.
158. Luria AR. The frontal lobes and the regulation of behaviour. In KH Pibram, AR Luria (Eds). Psychophysiology of the Frontal Lobes. New York: Academic Press 1973.
159. Maguire GP, Rutter DR. History-taking for medical students: Deficiencies in performance. The Lancet 1976;556-58.
160. Mahoney M. Cognition and Behaviour Modification. Ballinger, Cambridge MA 1974.
161. Malik SL, Manchanda SK, Deepak KK, Sunderam KR. The attitudes of medical students to the objective structured practical examination. Med Educ. 1988;22:40-6.
162. Mannuzza S, Fyer AJ, Jlein DF, et al. Schedule for Affective Disorders and Schizophrenia-Lifetime Version modified for the study of anxiety disorders (SADS-LA): Rationale and conceptual development. J. Psychiatr Res 1986;20:317-25.
163. Marcotte DB, Held JP. A conceptual model for attitude assessment in all areas of medical education. J. Med. Educ. 1978;53:310-4.
164. Marlatt GA. The Drinking Profile: A questionnaire for the behavioural assessment of alcoholism. In EJ Mash, LG Terdal. Behaviour Therapy Assessment. New York: Springer 1976.
165. Marlon F. Describing conceptions of the world about us, Research Report from the Institute of Education, University of Gothenburg 1978.
166. Marlon FS. On qualitative differences in learning oulcome and process. Br J Educ Psychol, 1976b;46:4-11.
167. Marsella AJ, Sartorius N, Jablensky A, et al. Depression across cultures, in Culture and Depression. University of California Press 1985.
168. Marsella AJ. An interactional theory of psychopathology. In B Lubin, W Connor (Eds). Ecological Models in Clinical and Community Psychology. New York: John Wiley 1984.
169. Marsella AJ. Depressive experience and disorder across cultures. In H Triandis, J Draguns (Eds). Handbook of Crosscultural Psychology: Psychopathology (Vol 6). Boston: Allyn & Bacon, 1980.
170. Marsella AJ. The measurement of depressive experience and disorders across cultures. In AJ Marsella, R Hirschfeld, M Katz, The Measurement of Depression: Biological, Psychological, Behavioural, and Social Aspects. New York: Guilford Press 1987.

171. Maruta T, Osborne D, Swanson DW, Hailing JM. Chronic pain patients and spouses: Marital and sexual adjustment Mayo Clin Proc, 1981;56:307-10.
172. Maslow AH. Motivation & Personality. New York: Harper & Row 1970.
173. Mathews AM, Gelder MG, Johnston DW. Programmed Practice for Agoraphobia: Partners' Manual, London: Tavistock Publications 1981.
174. Matson JL, Andrasik M. Treatment Issues and Innovations in Mental Retardation (Ed). New York: Phenum Press 1983.
175. McGuire WJ. The nature of attitudes and attitude change. In G Lindzey, E Aronson (Eds). Handbook of Social Psychology. Vol. 3 (2nd Edition). Addison-Wesley: Reading Mass, 1969.
176. Mckellar P. Imagination and Thinking. London: Cohen and West 1957.
177. Mechanic D. Effects of Psychological distress on perceptions of physical health and use of medical and psychiatric facilities. Journal of Human Stress, 1978b;5:26-32.
178. Mechanic D. Medical Sociology (2nd ed). New York: Macmillan 1978a.
179. Mechanic D. The concept of illness behaviour. Journal of Chronic Diseases 1962;15:189.
180. Mehta M, Chawla HM. Behavioural intervention in asthma, a report of acase. Ind Jr Clinic Psych 1985;12(2):75-78.
181. Mehta M, Kumar D, Sethi SS. Family characteristics of children with Somatoform and Attention Deficit disorders. Abstracted in 13th international Association for Child and Adolescent Psychiatry and Allied Professions, San Francisco, USA 1994;17, SP-02-005.
182. Mehta M. Behaviour therapy for different type of phobias in Indian setting, DEI Research Journal of Educational and psychology, Special issue on Behaviour Therapy, 1986;3:1 57-62.
183. Mehta M. Identification of study styles of undergraduate medical students. Unpublished research report. KL Wig CMET, AIIMS, New Delhi 1995.
184. Mehta M. Student Learning Symposium on medical education, Ind. J. Pediatrics, 1994;61: 121-26.
185. Mehta M. Training Mothers of Mentally Retarded Children. Evaluation of Variables Determining Success. Indian Council of Medical Research, New Delhi 1987.
186. Meichenbaum D, Turk DC. The behavioural management of anxiety, anger and pain. In: PO Davidson (Ed). The behavioural management of anxiety, depression and pain. New York: Burner/Mazel 1976.
187. Meichenbaum D. Cognitive Behaviour Modification: An Integrative Approach. New York: Plenum Press 1977.
188. Meichenbaum DH. Self-instructional methods. In FH Kanfer, AP Goldstein. Helping people change: A textbook of methods. New York: Pergamon, 1975;357-91.
189. Melzack R, Torgerson WS. On the language of pain. Anesthesiology, 1971;34:50-59.
190. Melzack R, Wall PD. Pain mechanisms: A new theory. Science, 1965;150:971-79.
191. Melzack R. The McGill Pain Questionnaire. In: Melzack R (Ed): Pain measurement and assessment. New York: Raven Press 1983.
192. Michaels JW, Blommel JM, Brocato RM, Linkous RA, Rowe JS. Social facilitation and inhibition in a natural setting, Replications in Social Psychology, 1982;2:21-4.
193. Millon T, Green C, Meagher R. Handbook of Clinical Health Psychology. New York: Plenum Press 1982.
194. Millon T. Millon Clinical Multiaxial Inventory Manual, 3rd ed. Minneapolis, National Computer Systems 1983.
195. Milner B. Some effects of prefrontal lobectomy in man. Behaviour. New York: McGraw-Hill.
196. Minuchin S. Families and family therapy. Cambridge: Harvard University Press 1974.
197. Mischel W. On the future of personality measurement. American Psychologist, 1977;32: 246-54.
198. Monchy DC, Richardson R, Brown RA, Harden RN. Measuring attitudes of doctors: the doctor-patient rating. Med Educ 1988;22:231-39.
199. Moos RH (Ed). Coping with physical illness. New York: Plenum Press 1977.
    1 percent. Morton F. Describing conceptions of the world about us. Research report from the Institute of Education University of Gothenburg 1978.
200. Moos RH, Tsu VD. The crisis of physical illness: An overview. In: Moos RH (Ed): Coping with Physical Illness. New York. Plenum Medical 1977.

201. Nerenz DR, Leventhal H. Self-regulation theory in chronic illness. In: Burish T, Bradley L (Eds): Coping with Chronic Disease: Research and Applications. New York: Academic Press 1983.
202. Parkes CM. Bereavement and mental illness. Part IIA classification of bereavement reactions. Br J Med Psychol 1965;38:1.
203. Parsons T. Social structure and personality. London: Collier-Macmillan 1964.
204. Parsons T. The sick role and the role of the physician reconsidered. Milbank Memorial Fund Quarterly, 1975;53:257-58.
205. Pearlin LI, Schooler. The structure of coping. Journal of Health and Social Behaviour, 1978;19(1):2-21.
206. Pershad D. The Construction & Standardization of a Clinical Test of Memory. National Psychological Corporation, Agra 1977.
207. Philips C. Headache and personality. J Psychosomatic Research, 1976;20(6):535-42.
208. Piaget J. The Moral Judgment of the Child. London: Routledge and Kegan Paul 1932.
209. Pilowsky I. A general classification of abnormal illness behaviours. British Journal of Medical Psychology, 1978;51(2):131-37.
210. Platt S, Weyman A, Hirsch S, et al. The Social Behaviour Assessment Schedule (SBAS): Rationale, contents, scoring and reliability of a new interview schedule. Soc Psychiatry 1980;15:43-55.
211. Powell GF, Brasel JA, Blizzard RM. Emotional deprivation and growth retardation simulating idiopathic hypopituitarism. I. Clinical evaluation of the syndrome. New England Journal of Medicine, 1967;276:1271-78.
212. Ramsden P. Student learning and perception of the academic environment. Higher Educ; 1979;8:411-28.
213. Reisberg B, Ferris S, de Leon M, et al. The global deterioration scale (CDS): An instrument for the assessment of primary degenerative dementia (FDD). Am J Psychiatry; 1982;139:1136-39.
214. Reisberg B, Ferris S, de Leon M, et al. The global deterioration scale (CDS): An instrument for the assessment of primary degenerative dementia (PDD). Am J Psychiatry 1982;139:1136-39.
215. Reisberg B, Schneck M, Ferris S, et al. The brief cognitive rating scale (BCRS): Finding in primary degenerative dementia (PDD). Psychopharmacol Bull, 1983;19:47-50.
216. Reynolds W, Cormack D. Psychiatric and Mental Health Nursing, Theory and Practice Chapman and Hall, UK 1990.
217. Romano JM, Turner JA. Chronic pain and depression: Does the evidence support the relationship? Psychol. Bull, 1985;9718-34.
218. Rosen W, Mohs R, Davis K. A new rating scale for Alzheimer's disease. Am J Psychiatry, 1984;141:1356-64.
219. Rosensteil AK, Keefe FJ. The use of coping strategies in chronic low back pain patients: Relationships to patient characteristics and current adjustment. Pain, 1983;17:33-40.
220. Russell EW. A multiple scoring method for the assessment of complex memory functions. J Consult Clin Psychol 1975;43:800-09.
221. Salovey P, Mayer JD. Emotional intelligence. Imagination, cognition and personality 1990;9:185.
222. Sarason IG. Life Stress, self-preoccupation and social supports. In Sarason IG, Spielberger CD (Eds). Stress and anxiety. New York: Hemisphere Publishing 1980;73-94.
223. Schachter S, Singer J. Cognitive social and physiological determinants of emotional state. Psychological review. 1962;69:379-99.
224. Schellenberg JA. An invitation to social psychology. USA: Allyn and Bacon 1993.
225. Scott W. Measuring Mental Illness: Psychometric Assessment for Clinicians. American Psychiatric Press, Inc. 1989.
226. Seligman MEP. Helplessness: On depression, development and death. San Francisco: WH Freeman 1975.
227. Selye H. Stress in health and disease. Reading, MA: Butterworth 1976.
228. Selye H. The stress concept today. In IL Kutash, LB Schlesinger, et al (Eds). Handbook on stress and anxiety. San Francisco: Josey-Bass 1980;127-29.
229. Selye H. The stress of life. New York: McGRAw-Hill 1956.
230. Selzer ML. The Michigan Alcoholism Screening Test: the quest for a new diagnostic instrument. Am J Psychiatry 1971;127:1653-58.
231. Serban G. Social Stress and Functioning Inventory for Psychotic Disorders (SSFIPD): measurement and prediction of schizophrenics' community adjustment. Compr Psychiatry 1978;19:337-47.

232. Silverman D. Communication and medical practice: Social relations in the clinic. India: Sage Publication 1987.
233. Skevington SM. Psychological aspects of pain in rheumatoid arthritis: A review, Soc Sci Med, 1986;23:(6) 567-75.
234. Skinner BF. The behaviour of Organisms. New York: Appleton-Centure-Crofts 1938.
235. Skinner HA, Allen BA. Alcohol dependence syndrome: Measurement and validation. J Abnorm Psychol 1982;91:199.
236. Skinner HA, Horn JL. Alcohol Dependence Scale User's Guide. Toronto, Canada: Addiction Research Foundation 1984.
237. Skinner HA. The drug abuse screening test. Addict Behav 1982;7:363-71.
238. Solnit A. Change and the sense of time. In Anthony EJ, Chilands C (Eds): The child and his family: Children and Their Parents in a Changing World. New York: Wiley 1978.
239. Spitzer R, Williams J, Gibbon M, et al. Structured Clinical Interview for DSM-III-R-Patient Version. New York: Biometrics Research Department, New York State Psychiatric Institute 1988.
240. Spurgeon P, Roy D, Chapman T. Elements of Applied Psychology. Switzerland: Hardwood Academic Publishers 1994.
241. Stemberg RJ. Metaphors of Mind: Conceptions of the Nature of Intelligence. New York: Cambridge University Press 1984.
242. Sternberg RJ. Beyond IQ New York: Cambridge University Press 1985.
243. Stewart M, Roter D (Eds). Communicating with Medical Patients. Sage Publication 1989.
244. Thompson WD, Orvaschel H, Prusoff BA, et al. An evaluation of the family history method for ascertaining psychiatric disorders, Arch Gen Psychiatry 1982;39:53-58.
245. Thurstone LL. Primary Mental Abilities. Chicago: University of Chicago Press 1938.
246. Turk DC, Meichenbaum D, Genest M. Pain and behavioural medicine: A cognitive behavioural perspective. New York: Guilford Press 1983.
247. Turner JA, Chapman CR. Psychological interventions for chronic pain: A critical review. I. Relaxation training and biofeedback. Pain, 1981;12(1):1-21.
248. Turner JA, Chapman CR. Psychological interventions for chronic pain. A critical review-II. Operant conditioning, hypnosis, and cognitive-behaviour therapy. Pain, 1982;12(1):23-46.
249. Turner JA, Clancy S, Vitaliano PP. Relationships of stress, appraisal and coping, to chronic low-back pain. Behav Res Ther, 1987;25:281-88.
250. Vaughn C, Leff J. The measurement of expressed emotion in the families of psychiatric patients. British Journal of Social and Clinical Psychology 1976;15:157-65.
251. Verma K, IX Monte B, Adkoli BV, Nayar U, Kacker SK. Inquiry Driven Strategies for Innovation in Medical Education: Experiences in India. Indian J Pediatr 1993;60:739-49.
252. Wasir HS. Traditional Wisdom for Heart Care. New Delhi: Vikas Publishing House 1995.
253. Weakland J. O.K. - You have been a bad mother. In: Papp P (Ed): Family Therapy: Full Length Case Studies. New York: Gardner Press 1977.
254. Wechsler D. A standardized memory scale for clinical use. J Psychol 1945;19:87-95.
255. Wechsler D. The measurement of adult intelligence (3rd ed). Baltimore: Williams & Wilkins 1944.
256. Weissman M, Sholomskas M, John K. The assessment of social adjustment: an update. Arch Gen Psychiatry 1981;38:1250-58.
257. Wetzler S. Measuring Mental Illness: Psychometric Assessment for Clinicians (1982). Washington: American Psychiatric Press Inc 1989.
258. Wetzler S. Measuring Mental Illness: Psychometric Assessment for Clinicians. Washington: American Psychiatric Press, Inc. 1989.
259. Wooley SC, Blackwell B, Winget C. A learning theory model of chronic illness behaviour: Theory, treatment and research. Psychosomatic Medicine, 1978;40:379-401.
260. Wooley SC, Blackwell B, Winget C. A learning theory model of chronic illness A: Theory, treatment and research. Psychosomatic Medicine, 1978;40:379-401.
261. Wooley SC, Blackwell B. A Behavioural probe into social contingencies on a psychosomatic ward. Journal of Applied Behaviour Analysis, 1975;8:337-39.
262. World Health Organization. Doctor-patient interaction and communication. Geneva 1983.
263. Zung W. A self-rating depression scale. Arch Gen Psychiatry 1965;12:63-70.

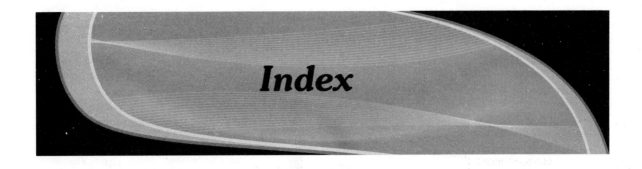

Index

A

Adolescence 116
   clinical applications 120
   ego and identity 119
   emotions 117
      adolescent love 117
      anger 117
      anxiety 117
      relationship with peers 118
      sexuality 117
   personality and social development 120
Adulthood 124
   stages in adult development 124
      age 30 transition 125
      early adult transition 124
      entering the adult world 125
      midlife transition 125
      setting down 125
Alcohol dependence scale 172
Assessment in behavioural sciences 161
   assessment interviews 163
   clinical observation 163
   goals 161
   personality tests 170
   psychological assessment 165
      attention and concentration 165
      memory assessment 165
      neuropsychological assessment 165
      perception 165
   psychological tests 163
      objectives 164
   questionnaires 171
   rating scales 170
   self-assessment 163
   semiprojective test 171
   sources 162
      physical evaluation 162
      psychosocial assessment 162
Attention 19
   attention deficit 23
   clinical applications 22
   factors facilitating attention 20
      external factors 20
      internal factors 20
   types 20
      automatic and conscious processing 21
      divided attention 21
      selective attention 20
      sustained attention 21
Attitudes 138
   assessment 143
      indirect methods 144
      observational rating scales 144
      rating scales 143
   developments 140
      family 140
      peers 140
   methods to change attitudes 142
   nature 138
   role of attitudes in nursing 139

B

Beck's cognitive model 196
Behaviour medicine 206
   applications 208
      chronic pain 208
      headache 208
   biopsychosocial contexts of problems 206
      aetiology 206
      compliance 207
      disease mechanism 206
      host-resistance 206
      intervention 207
      patient-decision making 206
   health promotion 209
      AIDS prevention 210
      diabetes 211
      exercise adherence 209
      management of stress 210
      medication adherence 210
      smoking cessation 209
   techniques 207
      self-monitoring 207
      stimulus control 207
Behaviour therapy 185
   applications 192
      behavioural training 193
      behavioural training for mentally subnormal children 192
   assessment 187
   characteristics 186

foundation 185
process 187
treatment methods 188
   aversion therapy 191
   biofeedback training 188
   contingency contracting 192
   exposure 189
   hypnosis 189
   operant conditioning 191
   procedure 190
   relaxation training 188
   social skills training 191
Behavioural sciences 1
   scope 3
      doctor-patient relationship 3
      health and illness behaviour 4
      hole of self-attention on symptom amplication 5
      human development 4
      illness-disability perception 5
      impact of social support 5
      importance of self-efficacy 5
      psychophysical relations 4
      social class and health behaviour 4
   subject content 2
Bereavement 134
   characteristics 137
   clinical applications 135
   stages 134

C

Cognitive behaviour therapy 196
   behavioural analysis 199
   clinical applications 203
   cognitive approaches 197
   cognitive learning therapies 198
   methods of assessment 199
   process 198
   self-monitoring 200
   strategies for treatment of depression 203
   techniques 200
      activity schedules 201
      distraction 201
      modelling 203
      problem solving 201
      rehearsal 202
      role-playing 202
      self-statements 201
      thought stopping 200
   theoretical basis 196
   treatment of anxiety 204
Coloured progressive matrices 174
Communication skills 212
   assessment 220
   components 213
      closing the interview 214
      empathy, and warmth 213
      greeting patients 213
      language 213
      listening 213
   specific situations 214
      breaking bad news 217
      information gathering 214
   strategies to communicate bad news 218
      allow patient time to integrate information 219
      never tell the patient a falsehood 219
      patient control over the quantity 219
      plan in mind before starting 218
      soften bad news with good news 219
Compliance 155
   assessment 159
   clinical application 159
      accommodation 160
      change in therapeutic regimen 160
      education 159
      enhancement of doctor-patient relationship 160
      modification of environmental and social factors 160
   factors related to compliance 158
      patient characteristics 158
      provider characteristics 159
   types 156
      contact with health provider 157
      lifestyle changes 157
      medication compliance 157
Coping with stress 93
   assessment of stress and coping 95
   clinical applications 95
      disease-related problem 97
      effect of stress on health 95
      sickness-related problems 97
   family coping 94
   stress-inoculation training 94
   vulnerability 97
Coronary heart disease 107
Counselling 177
   characteristics 181
      communication 181
      empathy 182
      warmth 181
   counselling in health care 183
   goals 179
   process 182
      change of utililsation 183
      closing phase 183
      counselling structure 183
      emphasis on strength 183
      necessary support 183
   respect 182
      client expectations 182
      genuineness 182

skills 179
   attending 180
   initiating 180
   passive listening 179
   perceiving 180
   responding 180
   summarising 180

D

Dartmouth pain questionnaire 235
Drug abuse screening test 172

E

Ellis based on rational emotive behaviour therapy 196
Emotion 77
   adrenal glands 79
   autonomic nervous system 78
      parasympathetic nervous system 79
      sympathetic nervous system 78
   clinical applicational 85
   cognitive factors 82
   emotional expression 84
      innate emotions expression 84
   general adaptation syndrome 80
   homeostatic balance 79
   intrapsychic aspects 81
   physiology 78
   role of learning in emotional arousal 83
   theoretical explanation 80
      Cannon-Bard theory of central neural processes 81
      James-Lange theory of bodily reactions 80
      Lasarus-Schachter theory 81
   types 83

F

Family 146
   affective involvement 149
   clinical application 153
   communication in families 150
   control styles 149
   family counselling 153
   family temperament 150
   family therapy 153
   pathology 150
   role of family in health and illness 147
   structure 146
   systems theory 151
      equifinality 151
      feedback 151
      homeostasis 151
      wholeness 151
   values and norms 149
Forgetting 28
   amnesia 30
      alcohol and drug abuse 30
      biological amnesias 30
      childhood amnesia 30
      defensive amnesia 31
      normal aging 31
      psychological amnesia 30
      senile dementia 30
      transient global amnesia 30
   clinical applications 33
      encoding 33
      retrieval 34
      storage 34
   clinical assessment 33
   interference 28
   methods to improve memory 31
      chunking 32
      making a story 32
      method of loci 31
      mnemonics 31
      pegword method 31
      remembering names and faces 32
      rhyming 32
   motivated forgetting 29

I

Illness behaviour 222
   abnormal illness behaviour 223
   causes of maladaptive illness behaviour 224
      disposition 224
      psychodynamic 225
      social learning 225
      sociocultural influences 224
   clinical applications 227
   management 226
   psychosocial adaptation to illness 225
   sick role 223
      absence pf responsibility 223
      being sick is undesirable 223
      seeking adequate help 223
Infancy and childhood 111
   cognitive development 112
      concrete operational stage 112
      preoperational stage 112
      sensory motor stage 112
      stage of formal operations 113
   psychosexual development 113
      anal stage 113
      latency period 114
      oral stage 113
      phallic stage 114
   psychosocial development 114
      autonomy vs shame, doubt 115
      generativity vs stagnation 115
      identity vs identity confusion 115
      industry vs inferiority 115
      initiative vs guilt 115
      integrity vs despair 116
      intimacy vs isolation 115
      trust vs mistrust 115

Intelligence 48
  clinical applications 56
  determinants of intelligence 53
    environment 54
    heredity 53
  emotional intelligence 51
  extremes of intelligence 54
    mental subnormality 54
  growth of intelligence 52
  intelligence quotient 51
  nature 48
    information processing
      theories 50
    multifactor theories 49
    primary mental abilities 49
    process oriented theories
      49
    two factor theory 49
  normal distribution of
    intelligence 56
  stability of intelligence 53

L

Learning 35
  avoid undue anxiety 43
  biological learning 41
    contraprepared 41
    prepared 41
    unprepared 41
  classical conditioning 36
    acquisition 36
    discrimination 36
    stimulus generalization 36
    stimulus substitution 36
  cognitive learning 39
    insight learning 40
    sign learning 40
  distribution of practice
    periods 43
  knowledge of results 43
  latent learning 41
  logical learning 43
  observational learning 40
  operant conditioning 37
    nature of reinforcers 37
    reinforcement 37
    schedule of reinforcement
      38

principles of learning 41
  contextual 42
  feedback 43
  individuality of learner 42
  role of motivation 42
  rational use of media 44
  social learning 40
Learning styles 44
  clinical applications 46
  role of teachers in facilitating
    learning 46
  student autonomy 45
  steps 45

M

McGill pain questionnaire (MPQ)
  235
Memory 24
  memory process 24
  memory systems 25
    episodic memory 27
    long-term memory 27
    rehearsal 27
    semantic memory 27
    sensory memory 26
    short-term memory 26
    working memory 26
  types 28
Memory questionnaires 167
Methods to deal with dying
  patients 133
Michigan alcoholism screening
  test 172
Middle adulthood 126
  physical changes 126
    intelligence and memory
      126
    parenthood and development 127
    personality 127
Motivation 67
  arousal and curiosity 72
  classification 70
    achievement motive 71
    aggression motive 71
    hunger motive 71
  clinical applications 73
  indications 67

models 67
  drive model 67
  homeostatic model 68
  humanistic model 69
  social cognitive model 70
motivational basis of addictive
  behaviour 74
  eating disorders 74
motives and conflict 72

O

Old age or the senescence 128
  clinical applications 130
  developmental tasks 128
  health changes 128
  personality changes 129
  psychological changes 128
    intelligence 128
    learning and memory 128
  social changes 130
  stressful life events 130

P

Perception 8
  clinical applications 16
    hallucinations 17
    pain perception 16
    perceptual function 16
    sensory defects 16
    sensory deprivation 17
  extrasensory perception 14
  perception as developmental
    process 13
  perceptual processes 8
    depth perception 9
    form perception 8
    movement perception 10
    visual pattern perception 9
  social perception 15
    attribution 15
Personality 100
  behaviour patterns and
    coronary heart
    disease 108
  clinical applications 109
  determinants 100
    environment 101
    heredity 101

personality related to illness 107
theories 102
   humanistic approach 106
   psychodynamic theories 102
   social learning theories 106
   trait and type theories 104
   type A and physiological reactivity 108
PGI memory scale 167
Psychological assessment of children 173
Psychology of pain 229
   coping with chronic pain 232
   gate control theory 230
   methods to assess pain profile 232
     behavioural analysis 235
     history of pain 233
     quantification of pain 233
     questionnaires 234
   pain in elderly 240
   physiological and psychosocial models of pain 230

psychological approaches to pain control 238
   biofeedback training 239
   cognitive-behavioural approach 239
   hypnosis 239
   operant therapy 238
   relaxation training 239
psychological evaluation 236
   depression 237
   life stress 237
   psychological dysfunction 237
   somatisation disorders 237

S

Sensation 7
Stress 88
   components 88
   executive stress 92
   family stress 91
   personality and stress 93
   stress-esteem 92
   test anxiety 92
   types 89
     daily hassles 90
     stressful life events 90

T

Thinking 58
   blocks in cognitive process 64
   clinical applications 65
   decision making 63
   different theories 62
     gestalt theory 62
     information processing theory 62
     learning theory 62
   functions 61
     problem solving 61
     reasoning 61
   judging 64
   neurological basis 60
   types 61
     convergent and divergent thinking 61
     purposive and fantasy thinking 61

W

Wechsler intelligence scale for children 174

Z

Zeigarnik effect 30